THE Men's Health

HARD-BODY

PLAN

THE ULTIMATE 12-WEEK PROGRAM
FOR BURNING FAT AND BUILDING MUSCLE

Featuring the <u>Hard-Body Diet</u> and the
Revolutionary New <u>Quick-Set Path to Power</u>

By Larry Keller and the Editors of Men's Health Books
Exercise Programs by Peter W. R. Lemon, Ph.D. • Food Programs by Thomas Incledon, M.S., R.D.

RODALE

Equipment courtesy of The Sports Shops at Nestor's, Whitehall, Pennsylvania; Pro-Formance Fitness Equipment, Allentown, Pennsylvania; and Willow Park Pools and Spas, Bethlehem, Pennsylvania

Library of Congress Cataloging-in-Publication Data

Keller, Larry.
    The men's health hard-body plan : the ultimate 12-week program for burning fat and building muscle : featuring the hard-body diet and the revolutionary new quick-set path to power / by Larry Keller and the editors of Men's Health Books ; exercise programs by Peter W. R. Lemon ; food programs by Thomas Incledon.
        p.   cm.
    Includes index.
    ISBN 1–57954–424–X hardcover
    ISBN 1–57954–229–8 paperback
    1. Men—Health and hygiene.   2. Physical fitness.   3. Weight training.
4. Nutrition.   I. Men's Health Books.   II. Title.
RA777.8 .K45   2000
613.7'0449—dc21   00–009333

Distributed to the book trade by St. Martin's Press

12 14 16 18 20 19 17 15 13   hardcover

      14 16 18 20 19 17 15   paperback

Visit us on the Web at www.menshealthbooks.com, or call us toll-free at (800) 848-4735.

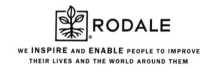

WE **INSPIRE** AND **ENABLE** PEOPLE TO IMPROVE
THEIR LIVES AND THE WORLD AROUND THEM

The Men's Health *Hard-Body Plan* Staff

MANAGING EDITOR: Ken Winston Caine

WRITERS: Rick Ansorge, Jeffrey Bouley, Ken Winston Caine, Susannah Hogendorn, Larry Keller, James McCommons, Eric Metcalf

ART DIRECTOR: Charles Beasley

COVER AND INTERIOR DESIGNER: Christopher Rhoads

PHOTO EDITOR: James A. Gallucci

PHOTOGRAPHERS: Mitch Mandel, Kurt Wilson (page 247)

STYLIST: Troy Schnyder

ASSISTANT RESEARCH MANAGER: Leah Flickinger

ASSISTANT MANAGER, EDITORIAL RESEARCH: Sandra Salera Lloyd

RESEARCH EDITOR: Deborah Pedron

LEAD RESEARCHERS: Deborah Pedron, Elizabeth B. Price

EDITORIAL RESEARCHERS: Molly Donaldson Brown, Anne Dixon, Karen Jacobs, Mary S. Mesaros, Joanne Policelli, Kirk Swanson, Rebecca Theodore

SENIOR COPY EDITOR: Susannah Hogendorn

EDITORIAL PRODUCTION MANAGER: Marilyn Hauptly

SENIOR LAYOUT DESIGNER: Donna G. Rossi

STUDIO MANAGER: Leslie M. Keefe

MANUFACTURING COORDINATORS: Brenda Miller, Jodi Schaffer, Patrick T. Smith

Rodale Active Living Books

VICE PRESIDENT AND PUBLISHER: Neil Wertheimer

EXECUTIVE EDITOR: Susan Clarey

EDITORIAL DIRECTOR: Michael Ward

MARKETING DIRECTOR: Janine Slaughter

PRODUCT MARKETING MANAGER: Kris Siessmayer

BOOK MANUFACTURING DIRECTOR: Helen Clogston

MANUFACTURING MANAGER: Eileen Bauder

RESEARCH MANAGER: Ann Gossy Yermish

COPY MANAGER: Lisa D. Andruscavage

PRODUCTION MANAGER: Robert V. Anderson Jr.

DIGITAL PROCESSING GROUP MANAGERS: Leslie M. Keefe, Thomas P. Aczel

OFFICE MANAGER: Jacqueline Dornblaser

OFFICE STAFF: Susan B. Dorschutz, Julie Kehs Minnix, Tara Schrantz, Catherine E. Strouse

CONTENTS

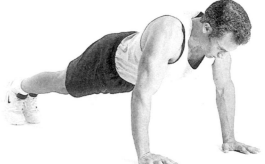

PART 4: THE HARD-BODY DIET

RESOURCES

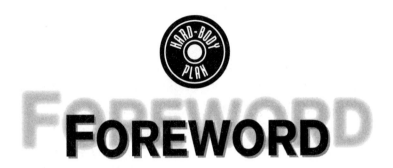

FOREWORD

I used to work for a fitness publishing company that was what you could call old school. I had a vague idea that we were doing things wrong there, but I could never quite figure out what we should have been doing instead.

Case in point: One day I came across one of my coworkers in the company gym. He was a good athlete but had never trained with weights before. Yet there he was, doing an array of arm exercises, set upon set of exercise after exercise. Finally, I asked him what he was doing.

"It's my arm day," he said.

Here was a guy who had been lifting weights for something like 3 weeks, and already he had an "arm day." And, presumably, a leg day, a chest day, maybe even a neck day.

It was like learning to drive in the fast lane of the Autobahn. Entering a toddler in the New York Marathon. Starting a life of crime by robbing Fort Knox. Oh, hell, fill in your own metaphor. My point is that it struck me as supremely wacky for a guy who had never lifted a weight to start off by doing advanced bodybuilding workouts.

But, then, that's the sort of advice that the muscle magazines were handing out in those days, and even smart guys were falling for it.

Take me, for example. I started pressing sand-filled, plastic-coated weights back in 1970, and it wasn't until 20 years later that I picked up body-building magazines and learned to do things wrong. Before that, I'd been doing things really, *really* wrong. It would be another few years before I would learn enough of the science to be able to confidently say that I knew how to do things right.

Had *The* Men's Health *Hard-Body Plan* existed all those years ago, I would have spared myself a lot of frustration, a smattering of injuries, and thousands of hours of time wasted on workouts that were poorly conceived and poorly executed. And I would have given my body the tools it needed to recover and grow more muscle.

First among those tools is the right food at the right times, and the Hard-Body Plan will show you how to eat for maximum muscle and minimum fat.

For anyone who is just starting out, this book is your entire learning curve. What people like me spent years and years learning, you'll have in a few hundred pages. You'll do productive workouts right from the beginning, make immediate progress, and get plenty of variety to keep your program from growing stale.

Or you can do things like I did and take more than 2 decades to sort things out. In that case, I'll see you on arm day.

—Lou Schuler, A.C.E.
Fitness Editor, *Men's Health* magazine

PART 1

THE NEW SCIENCE OF
STRENGTH TRAINING

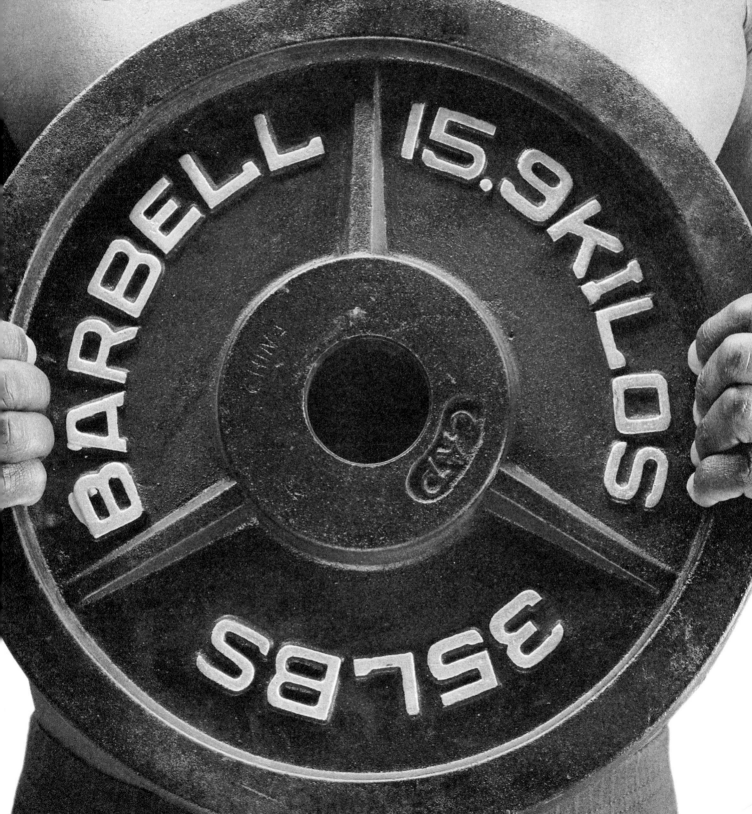

You WILL Get Stronger
THE ADVANCED SCIENCE OF STRENGTH

THE BODY OF SCIENTIFIC RESEARCH ABOUT BODYBUILDING—WHEN AND HOW TO LIFT WEIGHTS AND EAT SPECIFIC FOODS—HAS EXPLODED IN THE PAST 30 YEARS. THE HARD-BODY PLAN PROVIDES YOU WITH SOLID, CUTTING-EDGE SCIENCE.

Thirty years ago, Big Wally down at the seedy gym where the fighters worked out was the expert people turned to for advice on how to build muscle, burn off fat, and get a body into buff shape. Big Wally knew how much iron to pump and how often. Big Wally knew what to eat. Big Wally knew what strange supplements to take. People got results because some of what Big Wally taught was right . . . but some was dangerous.

Today, we know a lot more. Men and women in lab coats at top universities study this stuff. They conduct experiments and develop long-term research projects. Universities have whole departments devoted to different specialties within the field of muscle building and athletic performance. People get doctorates in muscle building. They call it exercise physiology.

This stuff is a science. And the Hard-Body Plan provides scientific precision from the surest science on the cutting edge.

We enlisted one of the top muscle docs in the world to draft the weight training program for *The Men's Health Hard-Body Plan:* Peter W. R. Lemon, Ph.D. He is a professor and head of research on exercise nutrition at the University of Western Ontario in Canada.

Dr. Lemon was in the vanguard of those studying exercise from a scientific perspective—he started in the late 1960s. He's not just a sci-guy. He's a musclehead, too. He lifts weights and has for more than 30 years.

Over those thirty-some years, he's heard and seen a mishmash of theories on how best to amass muscle and lop off love handles. But we're beyond speculative theories. Science now has definitive an-

MAGNIFICENT GROWTH OF MUSCLE RESEARCH

We all know now that muscle building is good for us. The general acceptance of this has been paralleled and perhaps propelled by the increase in the number of people studying all aspects of athletic performance, endurance, and health.

Peter Lemon, Ph.D., was an undergraduate student in the late 1960s and early 1970s, when the study of exercise, nutrition, and fitness was in its infancy. "When I took my first exercise physiology course, there were two textbooks in the field," he recalls. "There are probably 50 now—maybe more."

That's not the only harbinger of the tremendous growth in the scientific study of exercise and nutrition. Attendance at annual meetings of the American College of Sports Medicine has more than tripled in less than 2 decades.

In 1981, 1,650 people attended the conference. Not a bad turnout, right? Maybe, but at the organization's 1999 annual meeting, 5,400 attended.

That's as many people as you'll find some nights at a Montreal Expos baseball game.

Colleges and universities scramble to keep up with the interest in the study of athletic performance. Whereas once, physical education majors consisted almost solely of students planning to become elementary or high school teachers, nowadays, you may find students in these programs who are planning to become personal trainers, physical rehabilitation specialists, and preventive medicine practitioners.

swers. You're holding the solid science in your hands.

Science also knows what you should eat to maximize your weight training muscle gains and to trim your fat. We give you those answers too. And you may be surprised by some of them. "Nutrition is an area that has so much misinformation," says Dr. Lemon. "Everyone thinks it's simple. In reality, it's very complex."

That being the case, we had another expert, exercise physiology doctoral candidate Thomas Incledon, M.S., R.D., create the eating program for the Hard-Body Plan. Incledon is a registered dietitian, a certified strength and conditioning specialist, and the director of sports nutrition for Human Performance Specialists in Plantation, Florida. He has participated in numerous nutrition studies and written articles on diet and fitness.

So, what's the upshot of all this expertise? You're going to eat scientifically, and you may enjoy it more than you've ever enjoyed eating in your life. You're going to eat using the most efficient technology for fast muscle building. And you're going to experience results that go far beyond a better-built man in the mirror (but don't worry—that's the key part of the plan).

MUSCLING INTO THE LABORATORY

Along with new findings on how best to build muscle, science has also discovered myriad benefits from lifting weights. The more muscle you add, the higher your metabolism becomes, converting you into a more efficient weight-loss machine. Weight-bearing exercise slows bone loss, which may not seem important now but will be about the time you've lost your hair and your teeth. (Weight training, unfortunately, does not seem to slow loss of hair or teeth.)

Weight training and other forms of exercise also give you more energy and, of course, strength. Exercise even improves your mood. Skeptical? Well, researchers at Duke University Medical Center concluded that depressed patients who were placed on a 16-week program of exercise showed almost the same improvement as those who were given antidepressant medications or a combination of medications and exercise.

We're guessing that you want to lose flab and add muscle to look good or feel better. If it also helps you rant less at your wife or kids, that's gravy. So what we give you in the Hard-Body Plan is the latest, soundest thinking on building your body.

The Hard-Body Plan is your guide, your bible, to building bulk and shedding fat. It is packed with reliable information on how often and how much to lift, how often and how much to eat. Here's an overview. You'll find more in-depth information on these subjects as you dive into the program.

the maximum benefit from food's nutrients and give you the best shot possible at building muscle.

If you gorge yourself at the dinner table, your body simply can't absorb all the nutrients. You literally flush them down the drain.

Frequent meals, however, parcel out nutrients as needed and help your body maintain an anabolic or tissue-building state. Plus, eating several times a day raises your metabolism because your body has to burn calories to digest the food. This in turn helps you burn body fat. Your body will use those calories as fuel rather than storing them as fat.

We give you dozens of Hard-Body meals that are not only tasty and varied but also balanced, with a ratio of carbohydrates, protein, and fat that will best enable you to build muscle when you follow our weight training program. The formula is this: 15 percent protein, 20 to 25 percent fat, and the remaining 60 to 65 percent carbs.

GOOD EATS

Here's a feature of the Hard-Body Plan that we know you'll like. You get to eat often. In fact, we insist. Try six or seven times a day. Now, we're not talking six trips through Big Bertha's Bountiful Buffet every day. Because if you did that, the only thing bountiful would be the girth of your gut and the size of your butt.

But we are saying to eat often and eat less. By chowing down on six or seven easy-to-find or easy-to-fix designer meals and snacks throughout the day, you certainly won't be haunted by hunger as you follow this program. There are many good reasons for doing this, all supported by the latest research.

Smaller, more frequent meals spaced strategically throughout the day enable your body to get

KNOW YOUR NUTS

Nuts are a great way to get nutrients into your diet, but they can also deliver a quick jolt of fat if you eat too many of them. A serving of nuts is an ounce, and here's how that translates into individual nuts and calories:

Almonds: about 24 nuts, 164 calories

Cashews: about 18 medium nuts, 163 calories

Macadamias: about 11 nuts, 204 calories

Peanuts: about 68 small nuts, 165 calories

Pecans: about 15 halves, 195 calories

Walnuts (dried): about 14 halves, 185 calories

Maybe you were expecting a diet packed with protein. A lot of gym junkies believe that protein powers the path to bigger muscles fast. We know you've heard that. We know that high-protein diets have hit the heights of hype recently . . . again. And, in fact, protein *is* the crucial nutrient for repairing and building muscles. But you probably are getting plenty already.

The Hard-Body Plan is heavy on carbohydrates because carbs are more easily converted to energy by your body than protein is. Burning carbs for energy means that your body won't have to tap into protein as a source of fuel, so the protein will be available to repair muscle fibers and stimulate muscle growth—just what you want.

You needn't worry that this is a diet that only Kate Moss could love. It's hearty and healthy.

You might have, for example, a mushroom omelette with a slice of rye bread and some milk, coffee, and grapefruit in the morning; a tuna salad sandwich at lunch; and a chicken breast, baked potato (with butter!), veggies, and strawberries for dinner. Add in three or four hearty snacks—more like mini-meals—throughout the day. It's hardly a hardship diet, yet it's one that will help you lose weight when combined with your Hard-Body weight training program.

The other key component of the eating plan is timing. Research shows that consuming a mix of carbohydrates and protein before and immediately after your workout can be a boon to building muscle. That's because the combination of the two nutrients seems to lessen the harmful chemical reactions that result from the tiny tears in muscle fibers that occur when you lift weights. Result: You shorten the recovery period after exercise, have less soreness, and build bigger muscles faster.

What could be better than that?

In the Hard-Body Plan, you eat a snack containing a 4:1 ratio of carbs to protein within an hour of completing a workout. It's a no-sweat thing to do because you have so many options—anything from bagels to fruit or an energy bar.

We also realize that there are times when you're vacationing or on a business trip and you have to eat out a lot. That's a challenge to even the most diligent diet watcher, but we've made it easy for you. We show you how morning forays to Dunkin' Donuts and nocturnal visits to Taco Bell can be managed as part of the plan.

First, we provide you with lots of tips on how to keep your calories in check when traveling. (It's easy-to-remember stuff: Order salad dressings and potato toppings on the side, for example, so you can control how much to use to flavor your food. Or bank calories by eating a little less breakfast and lunch and fewer snacks if you know you're going out for dinner, so you can stay close to your calorie quota.)

Even better, we give you plenty of suggestions

HARD-BODY BAR GUIDE

Ever wonder how the expression *beer belly* came about? Check out how alcoholic beverages, including beer, stack up nutritionwise, and you'll understand.

Regular beer (12 ounces): 150 calories

Light beer (12 ounces): 78 to 131 calories

Gin, rum, vodka, or whiskey (1½ ounces, 80 proof): 100 calories

Red wine (3½ ounces): 75 calories

White wine (3½ ounces): 70 calories

for restaurant meals you can order that don't ooze fat with every bite. Better still, we aren't talking sprouts and alfalfa sandwiches with a dollop of cottage cheese on the side. No, with the Hard-Body Plan, you can eat lobster, steak, and fajitas—just not in the same meal. You will still eat well, and you'll eat smartly.

THE POOP ON PUMPING IRON

Eating wisely won't build muscles, of course, but food provides the fuel for your workouts and the nutrients for your recovery from them. And when it comes to weight training, the Hard-Body Plan offers a 12-week path to power whether you are a beginner, intermediate, or advanced weight lifter. How do we know? Because the workout program, like the

food program, is supported by scientific research and the real-life experiences of guys just like you.

The beauty of the Hard-Body Plan is that it is divided into weight training programs for beginner, intermediate, and advanced weight lifters. No matter what level you're at, you'll find an exercise regimen here to challenge you. In fact, there are more than 180 exercises altogether from which you may choose.

There are exercises with free weights. There are exercises with weight machines. There are even exercises with no weights, using everything from rubber tubing to milk jugs and your own body weight. And, of course, we offer fun cardio routines.

OFFICE MOVES

If you're chained to a desk all day and can't get free to go to the gym, here are a few exercises you can do at the office to keep loose and limber, courtesy of the American College of Sports Medicine:

• **Hands and fingers.** Make fists with your hands and hold them tight for about 2 seconds. Place your palms down, and spread and hold your fingers wide apart for 5 seconds. Don't extend your middle fingers when the boss lumbers by. Repeat the sequence five times.

• **Wrists.** Extend your arms in front of you and raise and lower your hands several times as if you're at a ball game doing the wave without leaving your seat. Then rotate your hands 10 times, alternating palms up and palms down. Repeat the sequence five times.

• **Shoulders.** Shrug your shoulders up toward your ears. In other words, mimic what you do when your boss asks you a question. Hold the position for about 2 seconds and then return to the starting position. Repeat the sequence five times. Don't do that, though, when the boss asks you a question, or you may find yourself looking for a new boss.

• **Lower back.** Still rooted to your chair, bend down between your legs toward the floor, reaching as far you can with your hands palms-flat. Hold briefly, then return slowly to the upright position. If a colleague asks what's up, tell him you thought you heard an air raid siren. Repeat the sequence five times, making sure that your chair is steady.

• **Hamstrings.** Join your hands together around your knees and pull your knees to your chest. Hold for about 5 seconds. Release your hands and return to the starting position. Repeat the sequence five times.

Here are the highlights. You'll find more in-depth discussions as you proceed through the program.

• **One-set lifting.** For beginners only, the Hard-Body Plan calls for doing a single set of each exercise.

• **Heavy weights.** Most of the time, you will be expected to perform no more than 10 repetitions of an exercise during a weight training set, regardless of whether you are doing one-set lifting or multiple sets. If you can do more repetitions, you will add additional weight so that you can do only 6 repetitions. As you get stronger and progress again to 10 repetitions, you will once again add enough weight that you can do only 6 repetitions.

• **Speed.** We have you move from one exercise to the next with the minimal amount of time needed for recovery before you lift again, and not a minute more. In fact, a minute is all you need between sets. Your workout will be more efficient and you'll finish faster so you can do other things.

• **Combo lifts.** For the more advanced lifter, we've included combo lifts (also known as super-sets). They entail moving directly from one exercise into another without rest. Result: a more intense workout and less time spent in the gym.

• **Forced reps.** Some of the exercise programs require you to lift to fatigue (muscle failure) and then try to power through one or two more repetitions. You need a training partner when you're ready for this.

• **Pyramids.** Occasionally, you will add weight and reduce the number of repetitions with each set to the point where you can manage but one repetition. As with forced reps, this taxes to the max the fibers that will grow your muscles.

As with the eating portion of the Hard-Body Plan, the weight training segment doesn't require you to endure a physical ordeal that rivals Navy SEALs training. That's not to say that it's easy. But it's doable. We've provided you with the latest science, the expertise. You have to provide the desire and discipline to stick with it. Do it. It's worth it. In a matter of weeks you'll see a powerful, Hard-Body Man staring back at you in the mirror. We think you'll like him.

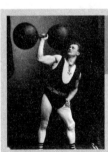

HARD-BODY FACT

Here's roughly how many calories a 175-pound man will burn during an hour of these activities:

Bicycling, 6 mph: 280	**Jumping rope: 750**	**Tennis, singles: 464**
Bicycling, 12 mph: 476	**Running in place: 754**	**Walking, 2 mph: 278**
Cross-country skiing: 812	**Running, 10 mph: 1,488**	**Walking, 3 mph: 371**
Jogging, 5½ mph: 858	**Swimming, 25 yards/min: 319**	**Walking, 4½ mph: 510**
Jogging, 7 mph: 1,067	**Swimming, 50 yards/min: 580**	

ANATOMY AND PHYSIOLOGY MADE EASY
ESSENTIAL LEARNINGS ABOUT MUSCLE GROWTH

THE INGREDIENTS OF MUSCLE BUILDING INCLUDE BLOOD, OXYGEN, HORMONES, CARBOHYDRATES, AND PROTEINS. MUSCLES CONSIST OF BUNDLES OF FAST-TWITCH AND SLOW-TWITCH FIBERS. EXERCISE FAST-TWITCH FIBERS TO BUILD STRENGTH AND MUSCLE SIZE. EXERCISE SLOW-TWITCH FIBERS FOR ENDURANCE.

Diana Ross once recorded a silly song in which she said she wanted a man with muscles. Well, Miss Motown, you're in luck. We've got hundreds of muscles. Of course, most of these aren't of the sexy, button-popping variety that Miss Ross panted about. We doubt, for example, that she became aroused thinking about involuntary muscles—such as those that enable us to digest our food and blink our eyes. Nor is she likely to have given much thought to cardiac muscles, the muscles that power the heart.

No, we and Diana Ross are interested in the development of voluntary or skeletal muscles. There are more than 600 of these muscles, which can be controlled by conscious thought. In other words, you can flex these muscles whenever you want.

Skeletal muscles are what you will be developing with the Hard-Body Plan. Pretend that you're a surgeon—or Hannibal Lecter—and you're stripping away the skin and looking at these muscles.

MUSCLES LAID BARE

First, notice the color. Those muscles that are composed primarily of fast-twitch fibers are paler than the slow-twitch, which are darker. Think of chicken breast versus chicken leg. We'll explain what this slow-twitch/fast-twitch stuff means a bit later.

See those stringy cords of tissue connected to your muscles? Those are tendons. They link muscles to bones . . . but not all muscles: Some muscles are attached to other muscles, and others—such as the 17 muscles you use to smile—are connected to your skin.

Now imagine that you are watching your exposed muscles at work. When you lift weights, you generate a stimulus within your central nervous system. Your muscle fibers then receive nerve impulses and the muscle contracts, or shortens. It is able to do this because it has a supply of glycogen, a form of stored carbohydrate, that it uses for energy. Your muscle fibers convert chemical energy into mechanical energy, causing the muscle to contract.

Your Hard-Body Plan capitalizes on this by including postworkout snacks to recharge your glycogen stores in half the time you otherwise would.

As you continue doing repetitions of an exercise, you see the muscle growing bigger before your very eyes. This is the pumped look that we all lust for in the gym—where your muscles seem inflated and your veins bulge as if you had a sack of serpents beneath your skin.

The pumped look occurs because the muscle has become engorged with blood that is rushing to it via capillaries. The blood carries with it the nutrients and oxygen needed for the growth and repair of muscle fibers. The pumped look you have after doing two or three sets of an exercise soon dissipates because the initial rush of blood empties out into your system.

You won't get that pumped look—or longer-lasting muscle growth—without pumping enough iron to tax the muscle fibers. No prob. We tax them in the Hard-Body Plan.

Muscles, like siblings in some families, always act in opposite ways. If you do a curl, your biceps contracts; but its opposite muscle, the triceps, relaxes. If you straighten your elbow, you'll extend or flex your triceps, but the biceps will relax.

Genetics overpowers desire when it comes to how much muscle you can pack on during a weight training program. We've all seen the guy who does minimal workouts and looks like he could compete on one of those gladiator shows, while another man trains harder and still looks like an accountant—albeit an accountant in good shape. If you're one of the latter, don't despair.

Yes, there are natural limits, but every body can build muscle. "Regardless of your body type, you can get bigger and stronger," says Peter Lemon, Ph.D., who drafted the exercise component of the Hard-Body Plan. "That applies to males and females and individuals of any age."

MIGHTY MORPHS

William Herbert Sheldon photographed 46,000 men and women to come up with his widely cited system for classifying body types. He identified 88 categories. To keep things simple, he grouped them into three main categories:

• **Endomorph.** Generally round and short in stature, guys in this group tend to have more fat cells than those in the other two groups.

• **Mesomorph.** These muscular men tend to add muscle easily and have wide shoulders, small waists, and low levels of body fat. Think of a running back in football or a competition bodybuilder as being this type.

• **Ectomorph.** These men are tall and lanky, like NBA players. They have a tougher time adding muscle bulk. One way for them to amass muscle faster while training is to consume 600 more calories—perhaps by eating four to six meals a day, says Thomas Incledon, M.S., R.D., the registered dietitian and certified strength and conditioning specialist who developed the Hard-Body Diet. (Smaller, more frequent meals are part of the Hard-Body Plan for everybody. And we tell you exactly

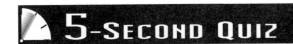

how to calculate whether you need more or fewer calories.)

Most of us have a combination of characteristics: We're part Endo, part Meso, and part Ecto but a bit more of one than the others, says Dr. Lemon. The dominating characteristics determine just how massive we will look, no matter how hard we work out.

FAST-TWITCH, SLOW-TWITCH, WE ALL TWITCH

The scientists who study strength are more likely to talk about the body's slow-twitch and fast-twitch muscle fibers than they are to talk about body types. The muscle fibers also are called Type I and Type II fibers, respectively. As many as three-quarters of us have a ratio of these fibers that falls between 60:40 and 40:60. Elite athletes, however, are typically outside these parameters. Some sprinters, for example, have been measured with 85 percent of their leg muscle fibers being fast-twitch.

"You should think of it as a continuum, with fast-twitch at one end being the very powerful, rapidly contracting muscle fibers that fatigue very quickly. At the other end are the muscle fibers that don't generate nearly as much force but have much more endurance. There probably are many types in between," says Dr. Lemon.

If you lift weights so heavy that you can only manage a few repetitions, you recruit the fast-twitch fibers. That's because they are brought into play when the slow-twitch fibers lack the force or power to finish the job. If you use lighter weights and perform a higher number of repetitions, you tap into the less powerful slow-twitch fibers.

Early in the Hard-Body Plan, you're going to do a lot of serious work recruiting those fast-twitch fibers. That's why the plan calls for you to perform single sets with heavy enough loads that you can only do six repetitions. Later, we're going to mix things up to keep the muscles alert and paying attention to the "grow, grow, grow" program.

If you typically lift nothing heavier than the TV remote in your daily routine, your muscles will break down old cells every 7 to 15 days. But if you lift weights or do other forms of resistance exercise, that process is accelerated since the exercise is causing microscopic tears in these fibers.

Given proper rest before the next workout, the muscle fibers repair themselves and come back bigger and stronger than before. That's why you need to gradually increase the load you lift in order to continue to see muscle growth.

Women usually don't bulk up the way men do when they lift weights, because they have fewer fast-twitch and slow-twitch fibers. They also have less testosterone. As you'd expect, then, men with high levels of testosterone see faster and bigger muscle gains than guys with less of the hormone.

As people age, they often exercise fewer of their fast-twitch fibers and develop a predominance of slow-twitch fibers. They probably could ward off much of this muscle fiber loss if they lifted weights during their forties and beyond. It's not known, however, whether fast-twitch fibers can be *regained* through weight training once they have been lost.

THE POWER OF THE PUMP

Researchers such as Dr. Lemon once thought that your potential for muscle development was pretty much predetermined by the number of fast-twitch and slow-twitch muscle fibers you were born with. That thinking has changed.

"There is more opportunity to manipulate muscle development than was once thought," says Dr. Lemon. We all have the potential to develop more of either type of fiber through specific exercises.

If, however, you have lots of endurance-enhancing slow-twitch fibers that are ideal for running a marathon, you probably won't be able to make yourself into a world-class sprinter by concentrating on weight training exercises that tax fast-twitch fibers. It won't happen, says Dr. Lemon, because you can't overcome the fact that the best sprinters got a head start genetically by having an unusually high number of fast-twitch muscle fibers. You could make yourself into a much more respectable sprinter, though.

Similarly, if you were born with a high percentage of fast-twitch fibers, you aren't likely to convert them all to slow-twitch via weight training or any other type of training. "But you could move along that continuum and become a decent endurance athlete," says Dr. Lemon.

THE FIBER QUESTION

Okay, back to the basics. Exercising a muscle causes tiny tears in the muscle fibers. As the muscle fibers heal, they come back bigger than before. That's how you accomplish muscle growth. But some scientists think that once a muscle fiber reaches a certain size, it splits, and that increases the number of fibers that you have

THE TWITCH SWITCH

Researchers now believe that you may be able to alter the ratio of fast-twitch and slow-twitch muscle fibers you were born with. This belief is due in part to the results of experiments on lab animals.

In certain studies, nerves from fast-twitch muscle fibers were surgically attached to slow-twitch fibers and vice versa. The result: The existing fibers took on the characteristics of the implants.

Other experiments have electrically stimulated slow-twitch muscle fibers as if they were fast-twitch fibers and vice versa. The researchers in these experiments found, for example, that if they hooked electrodes to a fast-twitch muscle such as the biceps and gave it low-intensity stimulation 12 hours a day, the muscle resembled a muscle with slow-twitch fibers.

What does this mean in the weight room? It's now thought that if you weight train a fast-twitch muscle as if it were a slow-twitch muscle (and vice versa), the muscle will change somewhat. So, if you exercise a slow-twitch muscle such as your quadriceps with heavy weight and low repetitions, it might gradually assume more fast-twitch characteristics.

available and makes room for even more muscle growth. This splitting process is known as hyperplasia.

We are all born with a different number of muscle fibers. A guy with, say, 25 percent more fibers than you has the potential to develop bigger muscles because he has more of these growth-inducing cells to recruit during his weight training. So if you could train some of your fibers to the point where they split, you in theory would increase your muscle-building potential.

Trouble is, it's not clear yet whether this really happens in humans. Studies on cats and rodents seem to show that they can increase their number of muscle fibers through weight training. You want a strong cat, buy it a miniature barbell set. You want a strong *you*, keep up with your lifting program and keep the faith. This fiber-splitting theory may actually pan out.

"It's a research question that is difficult to answer in humans because you have to remove and destroy the muscle, and you don't get many volunteers to do that," says Dr. Lemon. Here at *Men's Health*, we can think of a couple of editors we're willing to sacrifice for a controlled study, and you may know a few other people who should be enlisted.

THE MUSCLE IS THE MESSAGE

When you first start training with the Hard-Body Plan, you are likely to feel stronger before you see muscle growth. That's because your budding new body will undergo a neuromuscular response—another mouthful term.

Neuromuscular response means that as you start to pump iron, this new activity is telegraphed to your spinal cord and brain via nerves. The nerves tell the muscle being exercised that it must con-

tract, and the muscle follows these orders like a good soldier. Only then can the muscle relax. And only then will your muscle fibers respond to the stimulus of lifting weights.

"Your brain is telling your body what's going on," says Harvey Wallmann, a physical therapist and assistant professor and director of the department of physical therapy at the University of Nevada, Las Vegas. "Your body has to undergo that first."

Once it does, within just a couple of weight training sessions your nerves begin to communicate more efficiently with your muscle fibers, bringing more of them into play. This is half the formula for getting stronger.

The other half is creating more muscle mass, and this takes longer, typically a few weeks. That's because your body needs to synthesize the proteins that are used in muscle contractions. And that takes time.

So let's say that you've just started the Hard-Body Plan and you can do only six repetitions of an exercise with a particular weight. A couple of days later, you can do eight repetitions, and by the end of the week, you can do nine. Yet you look no different. Why? Your nervous system is already communicating better with your muscles—hence the increased number of repetitions—but you can't see the results of this increased strength because your body hasn't yet synthesized the proteins that are needed for those muscle contractions.

Within 3 weeks of starting your training program, you will likely feel significant strength gains.

It happens that quickly, says Dr. Lemon. You'll find that dragging loaded trash cans to the street has suddenly gotten easier. You'll find

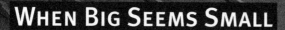

WHEN BIG SEEMS SMALL

It goes without saying that weight training benefits you both physically and mentally. But if you find yourself obsessed with pumping iron and never satisfied with your appearance, you may have the male equivalent of anorexia nervosa. It's called muscle dysmorphia.

Psychiatrists have found that a certain number of gym die-hards are never happy with how they look, no matter how much they bulk up. They may have the muscles of a superhero, but they wear loose-fitting clothing and work out alone at home in order to conceal their perceived puniness.

These men may give up jobs and relationships to spend more time in the gym. Some of them also experiment with esoteric diets and supplements and use steroids even after suffering side effects.

yourself sprinting up two flights of stairs where before one might have been your limit. You'll notice that you're stronger. But it may be a few more weeks before you actually see the changes in your body.

Of course, you need to train properly to get results. If you are lifting weights at 40 to 50 percent of your maximum capability, you will trigger the neuromuscular response but you may still look like Pee-Wee Herman "because you're not asking that muscle to do anything above and beyond what it could do on a normal basis," Wallmann says.

So you might try adding more weight to some of your exercise routines. The danger, of course, is in overdoing it. "In the early going, you'll probably be sore because sometimes it's a trial-and-error method," Wallmann says. "You don't know what you can do and can't do."

It's a balancing act. If you feel no soreness and see no muscle growth over a period of a few weeks, chances are that you need to add weight. But if you're feeling pain, not soreness, after workouts, you need to go lighter.

APPLYING THE SCIENCE
HOW THE HARD-BODY PLAN MAKES US STRONGER FASTER

THE HARD-BODY PLAN INCORPORATES THE LATEST THINKING IN WEIGHT TRAINING. IT FEATURES COMBO LIFTS, FORCED REPETITIONS, PYRAMIDS, AND OTHER TECHNIQUES TO MAXIMIZE MUSCLE GROWTH.

By now you have a general picture of the Hard-Body Plan and how and why muscles grow. This chapter explains in detail key features of the program, which, as followed, will transform you into a Hard-Body Man in just 12 weeks.

ONE-SET LIFTING

Conventional thinking in weight training has long held that you need to perform at least three sets of an exercise in order to really develop muscles. But modern science has concluded that, at least as far as short-term training programs are concerned, this notion is as outdated as the fallacy that overweight people shouldn't start lifting weights until they've slimmed down, for fear that they'll bulk up further.

Indeed, two researchers at Adelphi University in Garden City, New York, reviewed 35 studies comparing multiple-set lifting with single-set lifting. Thirty-three of the 35 studies found no significant difference in the level of strength increase among people performing the two types of exercise. Their conclusion: Most of the evidence suggests that for training programs of 4 to 25 weeks, there is no significant increase in strength or muscle growth as a result of training with single versus multiple sets.

We use that science in the Hard-Body Plan. We

direct men at the beginner level to do one-set lifting. This provides three benefits:

- You can complete a workout in less time.
- You do less work.
- You reduce your risk of injury.

If it's so great, then why are we recommending one-set lifting only for novice weight trainers? Because your muscles are going to cry out for variety as you move into more advanced lifting.

One-set lifting is challenging enough to stimulate muscle growth in beginners, says Peter Lemon, Ph.D., designer of the Hard-Body Plan. Eventually, though, muscles adapt to the workout you're putting them through, and you need to find additional ways to overload them.

To overload them, we're going to add more sets as you advance. That's what Dr. Lemon prescribes for intermediate and advanced lifters.

STRONGER FASTER

Probably the most common excuse that men give for not working out is that they're too busy.

But many of these same men spend a lot of time in the gym when they don't have to. "You can cut down dramatically on the time it takes to do the exercises," says Dr. Lemon.

The Hard-Body Plan helps you manage your workout time more efficiently so that you can get to work, play with the kids, make love to your wife, and still stay in shape.

The key, says Dr. Lemon, is to avoid dawdling between exercises. Remember, you're in a gym, not a museum. So move it. Your muscles need recovery time, but not much. "I'm expecting people to move from one exercise to the next with very little rest," says Dr. Lemon. What's very little? "About a minute of rest is ideal."

That's not the only way that the Hard-Body Plan saves you time in the gym. We include a number of combo lifts, also called supersets. A combo lift combines into one exercise two free-weight exercises

THE GOLD STANDARD

What McDonald's is to fast food and Wal-Mart is to retailers, Gold's is to gyms: ubiquitous. And profitable.

The first Gold's Gym was opened by Joe Gold in 1965 near Muscle Beach in Venice, California. The health clubs continued to grow like a gym rat's muscles. Gold sold the chain in 1979. The new owners began franchising the gyms in 1980, so now there are hundreds of Gold's owners.

Today there are more than 500 Gold's Gyms around the world. The original in Venice is still there. But there are also Gold's in such disparate cities as Cairo, Moscow, London, Seoul, and Mexico City. Gold's claims to have more than 2 million members.

Sports and entertainment celebrities who have been Gold's members include Muhammad Ali, Billy Crystal, Rebecca De Mornay, Janet Jackson, Michael Jordan, Michelle Pfeiffer, Keanu Reeves, Arnold Schwarzenegger, and Brooke Shields.

And the Gold's Gym trademark is on everything from nutritional drinks and supplements to home exercise equipment, personal care products, and clothing.

Who knew that physical fitness could be such a gold mine?

that work either the same muscle group or different groups at the same time. It's sort of a "buy one, get one free" approach to weight lifting.

So, for example, if you're at the advanced stage in weight training, we'll have you do dumbbell curls and then, without setting the dumbbells down, execute some dumbbell raises.

Combo lifts combine two exercises and skip the rest between them. It's "go, go, go." This keeps your gym time down. And it increases your training intensity. That's a good thing.

Some guys even do tri-sets or giant sets, three or four exercises in a row without resting. Maybe you can handle that challenge. But heed this warning: Only attempt this if you are at an advanced level of weight training. Otherwise you increase the risk of injury, says Dr. Lemon.

The beauty of combo lifts is that you can devise your own. "You're limited only by your own creativity," says Dr. Lemon.

Two-Day Delay

While the Hard-Body Plan stresses little rest between exercises, it does require you to rest 48 hours between workouts of the same muscle groups. There is no point in, say, training your chest and upper arms and then hitting the same muscle groups again the very next day.

If you train the same muscles every day, "you get little improvement and, in some cases, a drop-off in strength," says Dr. Lemon. That's a bad thing.

It happens because your muscles haven't had time to adapt to the stimulation of the previous day's workout. When you work a muscle group intensely, the muscle fibers tear. You grow muscle—and grow stronger—as the muscles repair themselves. You have to give them time to do that.

You can, however, work out up to 6 days a week if you wish. Just time it so that you don't train the same muscle groups on consecutive days. One

day you can do, say, arms and shoulders, and the next day legs and butt. This is called a split routine.

Besides allowing your muscle fibers to recover, there is another reason not to overdo the lifting: You'll avoid burnout. "If you train really hard every day, you're not going to do as well, and you're going to give up because it's hard work," says Dr. Lemon.

THE VALUE OF VARIETY

You wouldn't want to eat the same thing for dinner every night, right? Or listen to the same song over and over? Well, working out is the same way. Men want variety. "It gets very boring if you have the same eight exercises, session after session," says Dr. Lemon.

The Hard-Body Plan gives you a vast assortment of exercises—try 182 exercises for the beginner, intermediate, and advanced groups combined. From week to week, we shake it up. You will find plenty here to keep things interesting. That variety isn't limited to the *number* of exercises. It's also a factor in how you do them. If you want to do free weights, there're dozens of lifts here. Weight machines? Ditto. And if you find yourself unable to lift weights (maybe you're on vacation), we've included lots of exercises using no weights. All three methods are designed to firm your body and build up muscles. And we've added the essential warmup and cooldown exercises to help you avoid injury.

This eclectic mix of exercises keeps life interesting and builds muscle faster. Isn't that what you want from a weight training program? Here's how it works.

As explained in detail in the chapter Essential Learnings about Muscle Growth beginning on page 9, muscles consist largely of fast-twitch and slow-twitch fibers. The fast-twitch grow fastest by far. But if you limit yourself to exercises that tax only

BEFORE THERE WAS ARNOLD

Think Arnold Schwarzenegger was the first bodybuilder to parlay his muscles into a successful film career? Think again.

The late Steve Reeves was Mr. America in 1947 and Mr. Universe in 1950. He then went on to star in 18 movies between 1954 and 1968. Most were action flicks set in the time of ancient Greece or Rome, such as *Hercules* and *The Last Days of Pompeii*.

After Reeves injured his shoulder in a chariot spill during one film, he married a Polish countess and retired to a ranch near San Diego to raise horses. Unable to work out with heavy weights because of the accident, he took up power walking and wrote a book on the subject.

Reeves was still handsome and muscular right up to his death at age 74 in 2000. And he's not forgotten. In 1995—45 years after his last bodybuilding title, 27 years after his last movie—the Steve Reeves International Society was created. The fan club claims more than 1,000 members.

the fast-twitch fibers, you are denying yourself the chance to develop the muscle to its full potential, says Dr. Lemon.

The more muscle fibers you recruit, the bigger your muscles grow and the more symmetrical they will look. "Both of these things will make you look better," says Dr. Lemon.

It's only by doing a number of *different* movements that you recruit the maximum number of muscle fibers and enable the muscle to grow to its full potential.

Plus, slow-twitch fibers boost your endurance, which comes in pretty handy whether you're playing sports, making love, or hiking in the country. Hence the need for variety in your weight training routine to hit all the parts of a muscle group.

A wide-ranging program with lots of variety is vital. In How to Determine the Right Amount of Weight on page 21, you'll learn about how and why you may hit a plateau, a point where you just don't seem to be making gains any longer. The Hard-Body Plan teaches you to mix up your exercises in a way that will bust a plateau faster than you can spell Schwarzenegger. Some examples:

• **10-6 routines.** Most of the time, you will work toward doing 10 repetitions in a weight training set. Once you can do 10, you will add weight so that you can do only 6 repetitions. When your strength increases and you can do 10 reps again, add more weight and perform 6 reps once again.

"It's designed to force you to keep the intensity as high as you can," says Dr. Lemon. "There is no question that the intensity of the workout is what is critical to the muscle adaptation that occurs." As you become stronger—and you will—you must increase either the weight that you're lifting or the number of repetitions. In most cases, Dr. Lemon favors increasing the load. But not always.

• **Lighter loads, more reps.** Once a week or so, reduce the amount of the load you're lifting and perform more repetitions—say, 15 to 20. This will challenge some of the slow-twitch muscle fibers that aren't being recruited when you do 6 to 10 repetitions. You'll feel a different sort of muscle fatigue with the higher number of repetitions, and you'll keep your workout interesting.

• **Pyramids.** In weight training, you can perform pyramids or reverse pyramids. Neither originated with the Egyptians, and Dr. Lemon is partial to the former. With pyramids, you add weight and reduce repetitions after each set of an exercise.

So, for example, you might start off with a set of 10 repetitions, then add weight and do 6 repetitions, then add weight again and perform 3 repetitions, then add weight again and maybe do only 1 repetition. This process tends to hit a very high number of your muscle fibers, Dr. Lemon says.

• **Combo lifts.** As we said above, combo lifts are an intense muscle workout because you do two exercises as one, with no resting in between.

• **Forced reps.** As we mentioned earlier, this entails lifting weight to fatigue (also called going to muscle failure), then squeezing out another repetition or two. "As some of the muscle fibers become fatigued, you can recruit other ones," says Dr. Lemon. "Usually it's a muscle fiber that normally doesn't get recruited."

You need a training partner to do forced reps, to help you lift the weight on those last ones. Or do it on weight machines. Don't try this if you are a beginner or exercising alone with free weights. You could very well be pinned under the weight if you can't complete a repetition.

PICK A PARTNER

You don't need a training partner to follow the Hard-Body Plan, but Dr. Lemon recommends one. Here's why:

• **Safety.** Whether you're powering up a forced rep or your palms are slippery, there are times when you may drop your load or come close to it when you are lifting free weights. A partner can spot for you so that you don't lose a load, or he can help extricate you if you do. And if a partner's there, you'll both laugh about it. If the partner's not there, you might cry. We know these things.

• **Motivation.** "Probably most important is the social aspect of having a partner," says Dr. Lemon. A partner makes training more enjoyable. And a partner motivates you. If you're inventing excuses to avoid the gym, your partner can shame you into going. And once you are working out, you can challenge each other to see who can lift more weight, perform more repetitions, and the like.

You can even go one step further in your use of a partner if you hire a professional trainer who is qualified to give you real-time professional advice about your workouts: whether you should be going lighter or heavier, how many repetitions are too many or too few, and so on. If you do hire a pro, some evidence suggests that you might have more productive workouts. William Kraemer, Ph.D., conducted a study at Pennsylvania State University in which weight lifters were divided into two groups for a 12-week program. One was under the supervision of a personal trainer—a certified strength and conditioning specialist (C.S.C.S.). Those in the other group went solo. By the end, the

5-SECOND QUIZ

How many men in America say that they pump iron with barbells at least 100 days a year?

Answer: Nearly 6.8 million, according to the Sporting Goods Manufacturers Association.

supervised lifters had made significantly better progress with maximum single bench press and squat weights than the unsupervised group.

THE POSITIVE THING ABOUT THE NEGATIVE

To get the maximum benefit from the Hard-Body Plan, go slow on the negative. What does that mean? The *negative phase* in weight lifting refers to the lowering of weight. So when you do the bench press, the negative phase is when you lower the bar. This is also called the eccentric phase. When you lift the bar, you are in the concentric phase.

Try lowering the weight at *half the speed* with which you raise it, Dr. Lemon suggests. This creates resistance to the downward force of gravity and superstimulates muscle growth, he says.

In the bench press, some guys bounce the weight off their chest in the negative phase to gain momentum for the subsequent upward lift. Don't do this. To get the full benefit, you must control the weight and the muscles involved as you lower it.

While the negative phase is a terrific muscle builder, it shouldn't be attempted with superheavy weights until you've progressed to the advanced level in the Hard-Body Plan. Dr. Lemon defines *superheavy* as a weight that you can't lift more than six times with proper form.

MUSCLES BIG AND SMALL

To add still more variety to your Hard-Body Plan workouts, from time to time you can change the order in which you exercise various muscle groups, says Dr. Lemon. But try to start your sessions with large muscle groups, then move to smaller muscle groups. If you do it the other way around, you may be too fatigued to do the larger muscles justice.

So if you are exercising your legs, first do the thighs, which have huge quadriceps and hamstring muscles. Then do the much smaller calf muscles.

Similarly, if you are training your arms, start with the biceps and triceps, then move on to your forearms and wrists.

There you have it. All you need to do in order to build a better body is get with the program. What are you waiting for?

LOAD BEARING

HOW TO DETERMINE THE RIGHT AMOUNT OF WEIGHT

USE LIGHT WEIGHTS WHEN STARTING A WEIGHT TRAINING REGIMEN, AND MASTER THE FORM AND TECHNIQUE OF EACH EXERCISE. THEN INCREASE THE AMOUNT OF THE LOAD TO AN AMOUNT THAT YOU CAN DO FOR ONLY 6 TO 10 REPETITIONS. WHEN 10 GETS EASY—AND IT WILL—IT'S TIME TO UP THE WEIGHT.

The lowdown on loads is simple. Never lift more than you can handle.

But how do you know what you can handle? That's simple too. You start easy and work your way up.

What are the rules of thumb? That's a bit more complicated. They vary depending on your fitness level and where you are in your individual weight lifting program.

BEGINNER'S BASICS

Take it easy. Really. That's the right way to start. "A lot of beginners will try to lift as much weight as they can, and they frequently use dif-

ferent muscles than the exercise is designed for," cautions Peter Lemon, Ph.D., the architect of the Hard-Body Plan.

Let's say that you're training your biceps by doing barbell curls, and you begin with a heavy weight. A lot of guys do this. And they develop this rocking motion that helps them swing the bar up toward their chest. Wrong. Barbell curls are not about rocking. "Rocking brings in large muscles in the back and legs, which you really aren't trying to train with that exercise," says Dr. Lemon.

Doing the exercise incorrectly won't even help you inadvertently develop those back and leg muscles. "You're not training them intensely because the weight you have is relatively light for those large muscles," Dr. Lemon explains.

To avoid this common mistake, use light weights for the first two or three weight training sessions and concentrate on mastering the proper form and technique for the exercises, says Dr. Lemon. Once you've done that, select a weight you can lift between 6 and 10 times. Dr. Lemon says:

"If you pick a weight and you do 3 repetitions and you're fatigued, then you drop down in weight. If you pick a weight that you can do 12 or 15 times, then you increase the weight."

Once you can do several sets of 10 repetitions, you can add more weight. The new load should be such that you can do about 6 to 10 repetitions again, Dr. Lemon says.

If you can do 10 repetitions, you are lifting about 72 percent of your 1-rep maximum—the greatest amount of weight you can lift one time. Six reps amounts to roughly 85 percent of your 1-rep max. It's at these higher percentages that you are especially taxing the high-twitch muscle fibers that grow so fast. And that's the idea. If you do 15 to 20 repetitions of an exercise, you're performing at 50 to 60 percent of your 1-rep max. Now you're hitting more of the slow-twitch muscle fibers that promote endurance but grow less quickly.

It's especially important for novices to use proper technique in their weight training programs. They can become easily discouraged if, because of poor form, they don't see results in a few weeks. If you work out in a gym, ask the trainer to keep an eye on you and let you know when your form is wrong. If you're working out at home, just keep at it. And read the instructions for each exercise again every few days so that you'll keep proper form in mind.

As a general rule, you should add about 10 percent to the load when increasing the amount of weight you are going to lift in any given exercise, says Patrick Mediate, a certified strength and conditioning specialist and eastern regional coordinator for the National Strength and Conditioning Association.

If you can get to the 6-week mark, you probably won't have to convince yourself to keep going with your program. Once you see results, it's easier to get yourself motivated to go to the gym.

ONCE IS NOT ENOUGH

Here's something you should not incorporate into your weight training program, especially if you're a beginner: one-repetition lifts.

Some men deliberately do an exercise—say, the bench press—with so much weight on the bar that one repetition is all they can manage. Unless you're training for the Olympics or one of those strongman events, don't bother.

"I don't see much advantage to doing that," says Peter Lemon, Ph.D., architect of the Hard-Body Plan. "If you're going to do damage to a muscle or to the heart or the brain stem, it's going to happen, more likely, with these massive, all-out efforts.

"You can get the same training benefits with lighter weight and more repetitions. Even if you're interested in how much you've improved, if you do a five- or six-repetition-maximum test, that's much safer and can still show progress. If you can do 200 pounds six times today and you can do 250 pounds six times a month later, you can still chart your progress that way."

SHIP-SHAPE SHOWMAN

We told you that one-repetition lifts with huge amounts of weight in order to develop massive power are not a good idea for most men. John Wooten may be an exception.

The Boston man makes it his business to stage stunts demonstrating his strength. He has pulled a Boeing 747 jet and a 280-ton train. More recently, Wooten—who is in his early fifties and proclaims himself the world's strongest man—pulled a 16,000-ton cruise ship 70 feet with a rope from a dock while the ship was in the water.

The 6-foot, 290-pound Wooten is a cancer survivor, has only one lung, and suffers from asthma. He says that he began lifting weights at age 12 and still eats spinach at least once a week.

MAINTENANCE MAN

Odds are that you aren't following a weight training program to get bowling ball biceps and bulging veins that look like ropes. But you probably do want to reach a level where you look and feel better. Once you do, should you then keep lifting the same load in each exercise to maintain the status quo? No.

"You should try to change your workout anyway," says Mediate. This is crucial because if you don't adjust the amount of weight you're lifting, your muscles eventually stop adapting to the stimulus you place on them.

To avoid this, go a little heavier with the weights for a few weeks, doing fewer repetitions. Or try lighter weights and more reps for a while. Change the order in which you do your exercises. Or perform some new exercises that work the same muscle groups.

PLATEAU BUSTING

How do you know whether you've reached a plateau? If you're lifting the same amount of weight as last month for the same number of repetitions and you just can't seem to add any, that's a plateau. Maybe a month ago you were doing 10 repetitions of 140-pound bench presses, and today you're stuck on that number.

Plateaus happen—guaranteed—if you don't alter your workout, says Thomas Baechle, Ed.D., chairman of the exercise science department at Creighton University in Omaha, Nebraska. "After a period of time, the body will adapt. The same stimulus that initially created the strength gains will not be strong enough to continue the changes. As the muscles get stronger, fewer fibers are needed to do the same load. If you don't increase the load, then those fibers that initially had to be called in to lift the barbell will become lazy. They just will not get involved to the same extent."

So all those muscle fibers that teamed up to help you make those tough lifts are now kicking back and snoozing and falling out of shape. You've got to wake them up.

Adds Dr. Lemon: "The theory is that by creating some shock to the system, the muscles are stimulated to make further gains." How do you do this? Take it from Rick Huegli, former head strength and conditioning coach at the University of Washington in Seattle:

"An appropriate workout is going to have variation to it, so that it's not the same every week. Otherwise, you're going to plateau and get stale and it will be status quo for you."

Just to be sure that you keep up the changes, Huegli advises you to do some paperwork.

THE BENCH-PRESS BAROMETER

Most of us have heard the old adage: If you can bench-press your body weight, you're a pretty strong guy.

But is it true? Sort of.

A better indication of overall strength is to be able to lift your body weight in exercises such as dips, pushups, pullups, and squats, says trainer Patrick Mediate. The bench press is more indicative of shoulder strength than of overall body power, he says.

"If you can go down in a full single-leg squat with your right leg and then your left leg, you're pretty strong," says Mediate.

"It's helpful to have a menu of exercises broken down into body parts, muscle groups, and objectives in the front of your workout log. Then you've got something to refer to and work from," he says. In other words, think it through and chart out some viable variations.

If you are working out at home, you can hang a blackboard (or whiteboard) in your gym and chart some routines and variations on it as a reminder.

To increase the intensity of your workouts—and put those siesta-taking muscle fibers back to work—use the same techniques we described earlier for maintaining what muscle you have built. Change the order in which you do exercises, and lift less weight but do more repetitions or sets. Or you can try doing your repetitions more slowly. The Hard-Body Plan routines offer ample opportunity to vary your lifts.

Some men may even find that they can increase the load on some exercises—the very exercises on which they have reached an impasse. Dr. Lemon explains:

"Even though you can't do 10 repetitions, increase the weight anyway. Often, you'll find someone who's doing 6 to 8 repetitions with a certain weight. They increase the weight and they can still do 7 or 8 repetitions. It's just kind of a psychological plateau. We probably only use a fraction of our potential strength."

Plateaus also come from overtraining, Dr. Baechle says. You could be doing too many sets too soon, and your body has not had time to adapt.

Getting sufficient rest between workout sessions is crucial for continued muscle growth. "Rest is just as important as the training stimulus itself," says Dr. Baechle. The Hard-Body Plan honors this principle, so you can train hard and muscle up fast. In our programs, no muscle groups are exercised on consecutive days.

ARE WE READY?
WHEN–AND WHEN NOT–
TO LIFT

YOU'VE EATEN A SMALL MEAL RECENTLY; YOU'RE WEARING COMFORTABLE, LOOSE-FITTING CLOTHING; AND YOU'RE PSYCHING UP TO GIVE IT YOUR BEST. YOU'RE READY TO LIFT. MINOR COLDS AND SORENESS ARE NO EXCUSE. TOUGH THEM OUT.

The gym membership card is in your sports bag. Or you've built the perfect home gym. You're motivated. You've got the Hard-Body Plan theory down pat, and you're ready to morph into a man of muscle. Now the questions are: When should you work out to get the best results? When should you not? What else do you need to do to ensure that you're ready?

To answer the last question, not much. If you're middle-aged and you or members of your family have certain medical conditions, you should consult your doctor before beginning the Hard-Body Plan or any other workout regimen. To give you a clearer idea of what we mean, the American College of Sports Medicine says that you should get your physician's permission if you answer yes to more than one of the following questions:

• Are you over the age of 45?
• Has your father or a brother suffered a heart attack before age 55, or has your mother or a sister had a heart attack before age 65?
• Do you smoke?
• Has your blood pressure been measured at greater than 140 over 90, or do you take high blood pressure medication?
• Is your total cholesterol greater than 240?
• Are you physically inactive—that is, do you get less than 30 minutes of exercise on 3 or fewer days per week?
• Are you more than 20 pounds overweight?

Did you answer yes to two or more of those questions? Most likely your doc wants you to exercise, but ask to make sure.

MEALS MATTER

Even if you don't eat before you lift weights, you will add muscle. But it's a good idea to eat first. If you train on an empty stomach in the morning, for example, you will have lost a significant amount of carbohydrates from fasting overnight. This can cause low blood glucose that could make you feel so light-headed that you'll think you have brains made of shaving cream. Eating carbohydrate-rich food beforehand will give you more energy, and it's a key part of the Hard-Body eating plan.

Eating is also important after a workout, to replace carbohydrates that you use up during your session. And there is some evidence that protein may help in the muscle repair and building process after a workout session. As you'll see in part 3 of this book, the Hard-Body Plan recommends that you eat within 15 to 60 minutes after a workout. So eat.

You will eat more efficiently, too, if you have several snacks or small meals throughout the day rather than three big meals. This way, you're never too full to train. The Hard-Body Plan features six or seven meals a day. You won't go hungry here. But you won't fatten up, either. We feed you right, according to the latest sensible science in sports nutrition.

TIMING ISN'T EVERYTHING

Some guys ponder what time of day to lift with the gravity of an undertaker surveying an accident victim. This is something that you should devote as much thought to as, oh, what color of T-shirt to wear to the gym. May we suggest salmon pink with dark mauve trim and matching shoes?

There have in fact been at least a couple of studies suggesting that nighttime is the right time

to pump iron. The thinking is that your ratio of anabolic to catabolic hormones is most conducive to building muscle in the evening. *Anabolic* hormones build up muscle fibers, *catabolic* hormones break 'em down. And there, in one little biological nutshell, is the whole theory of muscle making: Build 'em up, tear 'em down, build 'em up, and on and on.

"The time of day plays a role, but it may not be the determining factor," says Peter Lemon, Ph.D., architect of the Hard-Body Plan. More important than *when* you do it is *whether* you do it, he says.

Regardless of what time of day you train, *train,* and you will get bigger and stronger. It's more important to exercise when it's convenient, so that you'll find it easy to stick with it.

What about working out twice a day? This is something that hard-core bodybuilders sometimes do, working one or two muscle groups per session and alternating muscle groups each session. There's nothing at all wrong with it, but most guys don't have the time or inclination for such a rigorous regimen, says Dr. Lemon.

SORENESS AND SICKNESS

Your muscles are sore from your last workout. You have a cold and your head feels like a block of concrete. Good reasons to skip a workout, right? Maybe, maybe not.

Soreness and weight lifting go together like Elizabeth Taylor and marriage, especially when you are just starting a weight training program. Men tend to lift too much weight at first rather than gradually increasing the load. So they get sore. Lower the intensity and work through it, advises Harvey Wallmann, a physical therapy professor at the University of Nevada, Las Vegas. "Sore muscles are weak and damaged, and continuing to train at a high intensity can lead to further damage and injury," he says.

"In the early going, you may be somewhat sore because sometimes it's a trial-and-error method," says Wallmann. "You don't know what you can do and can't do."

The key is to recognize the difference between soreness and pain. "Soreness isn't bad," says Wallmann. "Pain is bad. Pain is telling your body, 'Don't do this anymore.'" With soreness, however, you should probably work through it, using lighter weights until it passes. In fact, doing light repetitions may actually help you feel better because it can clear the lactic acid that can build up in your muscles and cause soreness.

Before you begin a workout, loosen up a sore muscle with moist heat. Afterward, apply ice wrapped in a towel to the same area for no more than 20 minutes.

That's solid advice from Patrick Mediate, eastern regional coordinator for the National Strength and Conditioning Association.

If you continue to have soreness, don't be macho, man. You can develop tendinitis or even have tendons pull away from bones with some weight lifting injuries. In case you're wondering, the parts of the body most often injured during weight training are the fingers. That's followed by the back and the shoulders.

To minimize soreness in the first place, stretch before, after, and even in between exercises. There is some evidence that muscle repair is hampered somewhat if you don't stretch. There's a right and a wrong way to stretch, too. We tell you how to do it right in Warming Up and Cooling Down on page 41.

If you have a cold, you can probably continue to exercise without making the symptoms worse. In one study, researchers inoculated 50 volunteers with a cold-causing virus and then separated them into two groups. One group exercised, one was sedentary.

The differences in how long each group's cold symptoms lasted weren't statistically significant, researchers concluded. So they offer the following advice.

WHEN TO LIGHTEN UP

Muscle pain—especially if you don't notice it until a couple of days after a workout—is just one symptom of overuse syndrome, which is where you lift too much weight too fast. There's an easy solution: Lighten the load.

You may also need to lighten your load if you often feel restless or if you have trouble sleeping, an elevated heart rate when resting, a lack of appetite, and general fatigue and irritability, says Patrick Mediate, eastern regional coordinator for the National Strength and Conditioning Association.

Some men who can't sleep because of their overly strenuous workouts think that their insomnia is caused by not training hard enough, so they push themselves even harder, says Mediate. "It's a vicious cycle and they get hurt even worse."

Go ahead and exercise while you have a cold, as long as your symptoms are "above the neck" ones, such as a runny nose, sneezing, or a sore throat. But start at a lower intensity than normal.

If the symptoms lessen in the first few minutes, you can increase the intensity accordingly.

If you have "below the neck" symptoms, however, such as fever, vomiting, diarrhea, or a productive cough, lay off the workouts. Let the illness run its course before you resume your workouts.

COP AN ATTITUDE

Even if you're feeling physically fine, you won't be ready to lift weights unless you're mentally ready. If you're not, you will find all sorts of ways to rationalize blowing a workout.

"Maintaining your motivation level is a huge factor," says Dr. Lemon. "There's got to be some reason why you're doing this, either for your health, to look better on the beach, or whatever. Keep reaching back for that; it will help motivate you."

The key is to get through the first 6 weeks without quitting.

"You kind of get hooked after a while. If you can somehow keep people going for about 6 weeks, they usually have enough internal motivation to continue," he says.

The flip side, however, is as ugly as Mike Ditka in a tutu. "When people miss one workout, they find that the next one is easier to miss," says Dr. Lemon. "Then pretty soon they've missed five in a row. You have to avoid that kind of downward spiral."

As we point out elsewhere, Dr. Lemon is a firm believer in having a partner or a group of people to work out with. The group spirit and social obligation keep you motivated and on track with your training program.

STYLE POINTERS

One good thing about weight training is that you don't have to tap into your 401(k) plan to outfit yourself for the gym. You can be as minimalist as you want.

Loose-fitting shorts and a T-shirt are a good start. They should be lightweight and absorb perspiration. But snug-fitting shorts also have an upside. "Generally the spandex stuff is good because

---

HOME SWEET HOME

According to one survey, roughly 18 million Americans exercise at home at least twice a week. Here are some reasons they give for having a home gym as opposed to going to a gym.

- **Convenience.** No need to drive to a club to exercise.
- **Control.** No scheduling, no waiting to use equipment, and no sharing of lockers or showers.
- **Cost.** A home gym can cost upward of $5,000 to equip, but health club memberships can exceed that after a few years.
- **Cocooning.** Some people want to spend more time at home with their families.

it keeps the heat in and prevents some injuries," says Mediate.

Wear hard-toed shoes with slip-resistant soles. A cross-trainer is much better than a running shoe, which is designed to run forward only, Mediate says. Running shoes can produce ankle and knee injuries.

Some guys like to wear gloves when they lift weights. Gloves are of limited value, serving mostly to help your grip when you're hoisting particularly heavy loads.

Most guys shouldn't bother wearing a weight belt. "Initially, if they get used to crutches like that, they won't get the full benefit of lifting," says Mediate. That's because weight belts can actually inhibit the strengthening of your lower-back muscles and abdominal muscles. They're sometimes helpful after a back injury, though, offering support and stability so you can get back to lifting sooner. And they can help if you are lifting a very heavy weight for a low number of reps. A caution, though: If you *need* the belt to lift that heavy weight, chances are that the weight is simply too heavy and you should go lighter.

Now you have the right gym gear. If for some reason you still want to put off lifting, there's one more safety check that can kill some time. You could wander around the gym inspecting the equipment. Check the undersides to see whether you can find any warning labels, and read those. Look for frayed cables, stripped bolts, and missing collars. See that Exercycle over there? Give it a test. Let's make sure that it's working right. Let's see if it can handle, say, 5 or 10 minutes of serious pedaling. You're on your way, Hard-Body Man.

THE FULL-BODY MUSCLE PLAN
PUTTING IT ALL TOGETHER

THE HARD-BODY PLAN PROVIDES A SMORGASBORD OF EXERCISES TO GIVE YOU A FULL-BODY WORKOUT REGARDLESS OF YOUR LEVEL OF EXPERIENCE. FOLLOW THE PLAN AND YOU _WILL_ ADD MUSCLE.

Right here at your fingertips you have your Hard-Body Plan. But what now? How do you use it for optimal results? We're glad you asked.

First thing first: Decide whether you're a beginner-, intermediate-, or advanced-level weight trainer. This is important because the number and types of exercises vary with each. You don't want to be a novice and start out trying the intermediate or advanced program. Chances are that you'll find it too hard and quit. So build up to it gradually.

Similarly, if you've been weight training for some time now, you probably don't need to start with the beginner program. It's designed so that you can see some quick, early improvements to your physique that you can fine-tune later. But if you've already been pumping iron for a while, these initial exercises may be old hat. If you do start with the beginner program and it's too easy, move right on up to the next level so that you don't

get bored and quit, says Peter Lemon, Ph.D., architect of the Hard-Body Plan.

BEGINNER

By far the most powerful aspect of the Hard-Body Plan for beginners is one-set lifting. As we explain elsewhere, performing one set of an exercise if you're a novice is enough to develop more muscle. And it's a quick routine, which is convenient when you're just beginning to work lifting into your life and schedule.

You work each muscle group two or three times a week, starting with a load for each exercise that is heavy enough that you can lift it only six times.

When you get to 7 repetitions, that's okay. When you get to 8 repetitions, that's okay. But when you are strong enough to perform 10 repetitions, it's time to pile on the weight. Add enough weight that you once again can do only 6 repetitions.

Why? In order to progress as you become stronger, you have to keep increasing the number of repetitions you are doing or increase the amount of weight you are lifting. The first course of action will add to your endurance. But if it's bigger muscles you want—and the sooner the better—then you must increase the load. "Keep the intensity as high as you can," says Dr. Lemon.

INTERMEDIATE

As you would expect, the weight training sessions become more difficult when you move to the intermediate level. Instead of performing a single set of each exercise, you now do three sets (including your warmup) of 6 to 10 repetitions of each exercise.

We also introduce some new concepts into your workout routines. We recommend experimenting with one or two partial repetitions at the end of each set when you are too fatigued to complete a full repetition. Called lifting to muscle failure, this technique is especially effective at recruiting and stressing large numbers of the muscle fibers, which in turn stimulates dramatic growth. "I really believe that stressing the muscle beyond where most people do is beneficial," says Dr. Lemon. You need a partner to help with this, however, especially if you are doing this with free weights.

Another way intermediate lifters face increasing challenge is with combo lifts, also known as supersets. A superset entails doing two different exercises in succession without a rest. Supersets increase the

intensity of a workout, provide variety, and cut down on your time in the gym. Dr. Lemon says:

"There's no question that the intensity of the workout is what's critical to the muscle adaptation that occurs."

Sure, you can do a moderate workout long enough that you expend the same energy as in a shorter, more intense workout, but why? You'll see more dramatic results with the quicker but harder training session.

Another muscle-building variation for intermediate lifters is just that: variation. We regularly instruct you to shake up your routine and lift a lighter than normal load for 15 to 20 repetitions instead of your usual 6 to 10 repetitions. Another variation: Increase the load on successive sets and reduce the number of repetitions. These are called pyramids and are yet another way to intensify and shake up your workout.

ADVANCED

The advanced level of the Hard-Body Plan incorporates many of the concepts you learned at the intermediate level, such as lifting to failure. But advanced lifters do more advanced and challenging exercises, and they use more weight.

You'll expect and appreciate a tougher workout if and when you move to the advanced level. And at this point you'll be pretty comfortable in the gym and you'll enjoy the extra time there. But advancement to the advanced level isn't absolutely required.

Most guys don't advance to the advanced phase, nor do they need to, says Dr. Lemon.

You want tough? Try these: French curls and lying triceps extensions for your arms, behind-the-neck presses for your shoulders, barbell overhead pulls for your chest, good mornings for your back, and squats for your thighs. And those are just some of the more difficult exercises you will do as an advanced lifter. Once you master them, you'll appreciate the variety and the challenge they provide.

As you get stronger, you'll want to not only lift greater loads but also try an increasing number of exercises. No problem. We keep piling them on. You'll find more exercises in the intermediate phase than in the beginner portion of the Hard-Body Plan, and more exercises in the advanced segment than in either of the other two.

COMMON DENOMINATORS

There are some things that the beginner, intermediate, and advanced routines have in common. One is that each of these routines provides a full-body workout. No muscle group is neglected.

This is important for several reasons. If you develop one muscle group and neglect another, you leave yourself vulnerable to injury. Train your hamstrings and neglect your quadriceps and you will be more prone to muscle pulls in your upper legs, not to mention the possibility of chronic lower-back pain. Develop your chest and ignore your back—and a lot of guys do—and you may find yourself slouching meekly into middle age with rotten posture. If we catch you doing that, we'll confiscate your copy of this book.

In the Hard-Body Plan, you will change exercises each week for each muscle group at each level, rotating your way through three different weekly programs, so that you repeat many exercises only every fourth week.

You're going to like what this accomplishes. You'll really work the muscles and hit most or all of the growth-inducing muscle fibers as you cycle through the various weekly programs. As a result, your muscles will look bigger, better, and more symmetrical.

You'll see great results because, like the rest of life, your workout will always be changing. If your workout didn't change, your muscles would adapt to the same exercises done over and over and quit growing. "You have to keep tricking the muscle because it will respond by adapting to the new stimulus," says Dr. Lemon. "Then it stops responding

GOING THROUGH A PHASE

When should you be ready to move from the beginner to the intermediate phase of the Hard-Body Plan, or from the intermediate to the advanced stage? There's no hard-and-fast rule. Men develop muscles and strength at various speeds, depending on their genetic makeup and how hard they work out, says Peter Lemon, Ph.D.

But somebody who is training pretty seriously will probably be ready to move from the beginner to the intermediate phase after 12 weeks of following the Hard-Body Plan, says Dr. Lemon, who drafted the program.

"A lot of people never get out of the intermediate category," he says. "Advanced is pretty serious. It's not your average person. Certainly, doing the intermediate is excellent if you keep doing that."

Even a man who is content to remain at the beginner level of the Hard-Body Plan will see improvement. Although he won't continue to build muscle, he will maintain the gains he's made. "You're still going to be much better off than you were," says Dr. Lemon.

if the stimulus stays the same. You have to keep changing that to confuse the muscle so it will keep responding.

"This is why I recommend that you not only do heavy weights for a few reps but that you also sometimes do lighter weights many times," says Dr. Lemon. "You recruit the different types of fibers and therefore get adaptations in all the fibers you have, not just one type. You'll not only get a bigger overall muscle, you'll also cause an adaptation so that you have changes in endurance as well as strength."

Working all the muscle groups promotes muscle growth—called hypertrophy by the guys with *Ph.D.* after their names—for another reason. A full-body workout prompts a greater hormonal response. Some researchers think that if you train only a couple of small muscle groups, growth-promoting hormones will be released in amounts too small to matter. "Some of the hormones are intimately involved in the growth process," says Dr. Lemon. You want these hormones released.

If that's not reason enough to do a whole-body workout, here's yet another. It wasn't long ago that skeptics—most likely guys with licorice stick arms and toothpick legs—claimed that lifting weights made a guy muscle-bound: that is, that lifting would give you big, stiff, inflexible limbs and abs. Working all the muscle groups not only prevents this from happening, it makes you *more* flexible as well as bigger and stronger.

There's one other thing that all the phases of the Hard-Body Plan have in common: rest.

It's tempting to do curls 3 days in a row in our zeal for bigger arms, or to bench-press 5 days a week to develop a powerful chest and shoulders. But it doesn't work.

IN THE MOOD

You know that weight training will help you look better and feel physically better. But there's also evidence to suggest that lifting weights may lift your mood. And we're not talking Olympic-size loads, either.

Researchers divided 84 volunteers into three groups. One of the three groups lifted weights. They did 12 to 20 repetitions of the bench press, leg press, torso-arm pulldown, and overhead press exercises with a recovery period of 45 to 75 seconds between sets and exercises.

Three hours later, the participants in this group had less anxiety, depression, and anger than did the other two groups, researchers concluded. And the improved mental state of the volunteers was *not* dependent on whether they had weight lifting experience.

The truth is, those methods will hurt, not help, in our quest for a hard body. That's because lifting weights causes microscopic tears in those muscle fibers that must be repaired for muscle growth to occur. The repairs occur one way: with rest.

The Hard-Body Plan addresses this need for muscle fibers to recover from a workout by requiring you to wait at least 48 hours before exercising a specific muscle group a second time. In other words, if you work your biceps, triceps, and chest on Monday, it will be at least Wednesday before you do so again.

Where else can you get a day off for every day you work?

THE MIRROR MAN
HOW TO GAUGE
YOUR SUCCESS

SOMETIMES YOU KNOW YOUR WEIGHT TRAINING PROGRAM IS WORKING SIMPLY BECAUSE YOU CAN SEE BULKIER BICEPS OR PUMPED-UP PECS WHEN YOU LOOK IN THE MIRROR. BUT THE MOST RELIABLE WAY TO ASSESS YOUR SUCCESS IS TO KEEP A TRAINING LOG OR DIARY.

A key to measuring your progress with the Hard-Body Plan is to be clear about what you want to accomplish, says Rick Huegli, former head strength and conditioning coach at the University of Washington in Seattle. Establish your goals and objectives, then plan your workout regimen and look for results accordingly.

"If your objective isn't very clear, then you might just put in your time and get stale with it," Huegli says.

Let's say that your goal is to become stronger. You'll know that you're succeeding if you are doing more sets and repetitions or lifting heavier weights than when you began your program. If you're less sore than you used to be and your body recovers

faster from a workout, this too is a sign that you are gaining strength. Initially, you may have been simply hurting after a workout. Now, like the song says, you hurt so good.

"The formula can be simple: Are you accomplishing more work than you had accomplished before?" Huegli says.

On the other hand, once you've reached a certain level in your weight training, you may be content not to add more weight or additional repetitions or sets to your routines. By sticking with the status quo, you can maintain what strength and muscle development you've gained, and this too can be considered a success if that is the goal you have set.

Regardless of your goals, you should be able to see more firmness or tone after just a couple of weeks of pumping iron.

"You don't feel as flabby," says Harvey Wall-mann, assistant professor and director of the department of physical therapy at the University of Nevada, Las Vegas.

And then, what you're really looking for—increased muscle mass—usually is apparent in 4 to 6 weeks, Wallmann adds.

You'll lose flab, but don't count on the scales to tell you that. You'll *see* it. You very well may not lose weight as you become more fit. That's because muscle mass weighs more than fat. But adding muscle also enables you to burn more fat. Notice: It *enables* you to burn fat but doesn't guarantee it. To increase fat burning, you need to combine aerobic exercise—things like walking, running, and stairclimbing—with your weight training regimen. We tell you fun ways to do that in the chapter called Cardio Routines beginning on page 236.

Don't get discouraged if the mirror doesn't seem to reflect the body you want to see as quickly as you think you should see it. It's happening just the same. And we can prove it. Here's Huegli's method.

The best way to gauge your gains—and losses—is to keep a 6-month or 1-year workout log. Here you'll record data detailing what you've done during your workouts.

You will be more likely to maintain a log if you look at it not as a chore but as something fun, says Thomas Baechle, Ed.D., chairman of the exercise science department at Creighton University in Omaha, Nebraska.

"You've got to rest between sets anyway," Dr. Baechle points out. "So, if you just get in the habit of filling in the log during rest periods, it's really not work."

A log can help in these ways:

● **It motivates you to stick to your training program.** "I think, for the average person, it represents a commitment to his training. It really is fun to look back after a few months or a year to see where you were and where you are now," Dr. Baechle says.

● **It documents your progress.** Maybe you're less concerned about strength but want a buff bod and muscles that are a marvel. By using your log to periodically record your body weight and the measurements of your chest, biceps, and the like, you can document your transformation into the Incredible Hunk.

● **It provides comparative data.** Even if your muscles aren't bursting through your shirts, you'll know whether you're getting stronger by comparing data you enter in your log. If you were doing three sets of 10 repetitions of an exercise 3 months ago, and now you're performing 15 repetitions, you have empirical evidence of your increased strength.

● **It helps you modify your program.** Your training regimen should have variety. Maybe you think you're diligently mixing up the exercises you do, but a review of the log may show that your regimen has grown as predictable as summer reruns. If so, consider adding new exercises, changing the number of sets and repetitions you do, or performing the exercises in a different order.

And that's yet another advantage of keeping a workout log. If you significantly modify your exercise routine, the log will give you a baseline from

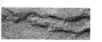

the prior training method that you can compare with the newer way of training.

Plus, if you keep a workout log, you needn't rely on your memory to determine whether you are resting enough between workouts and exercising each muscle group enough to get a balanced workout.

A workout log can be whatever you make it. Huegli suggests a bound notebook, 8½ by 11 inches or even smaller—say, the size of a paperback novel. It should be neither so big that you won't carry it to the gym nor so small that it's hard to cram information on a page. How many columns you include depends on how much data you wish to record. At the very least, you should have a column reflecting the date, plus additional columns for the types of exercises done that day and the number of sets, reps, and weight—called the load—as well as for comments.

You might also want to have a column showing your warmup and cooldown routines, Huegli adds.

Also consider writing down how long you rest between sets, the order of the exercises, and perhaps what you eat before you lift. But keep the log relatively simple or you may avoid using it, advises Patrick Mediate, eastern regional coordinator for the National Strength and Conditioning Association.

You can compose your own log or you can search bookstores and the Internet. But we've made it easy for you by preparing a Hard-Body Plan Workout Log that you can photocopy and attach to a clipboard.

How often you write in the log depends on your patience—or lack thereof—for the paperwork involved. You can record data every time you work out or perhaps for a week or two every month or so. Dr. Baechle strongly favors the first option.

"The process really keeps you focused," he says. Regardless of how often you write in your log, write often enough and with enough detail to make valid comparisons.

Even if you don't keep a workout log and see no immediate changes in your body, there will be other signs that your weight training plan is working.

You'll begin to have more energy and you'll be more alert. You'll just generally feel better. Here are some signs of progress:

• With your newfound stamina, you have the energy to be a 60-minute man during sex.

• You're no longer whipped after mowing the yard. Now you find yourself wishing that you had an acre of land.

• You're so strong after shoveling your sidewalk that you do your neighbor's too—and you don't even like him.

• After a long day at work, you manage to remain awake through a sappy network movie of the week.

• When you climb a couple of flights of stairs, you no longer gasp like you're scaling Mount Everest. In fact, you're hardly winded.

• You sleep better. Even your wife and dog's snoring doesn't interrupt your slumber.

• You have a feeling of well-being. You may not swagger or strut, but you feel better about yourself. You're becoming a Hard-Body Man and you like the way it feels. "There's an emotional payoff to physical fitness," says Huegli.

"It's a confidence builder," adds Mediate. "Men become more aggressive in their jobs. Their social lives will improve."

HARD-BODY PLAN WORKOUT LOG

DATE

EXERCISE	SETS	REPS	WEIGHT	NOTES

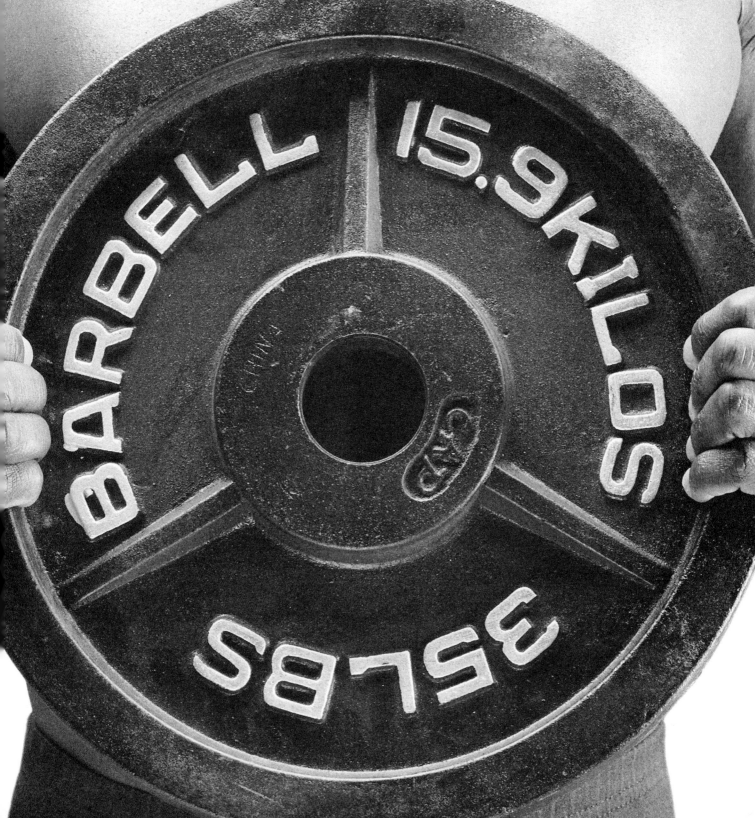

PART 2
FULL-BODY
MUSCLE PLANS

What's Right and What's Wrong
Warming Up
and Cooling Down

Start with a little aerobic exercise. Follow it with some stretching and then some lifting with light weights. Do this daily before you start tossing the big weights around.

Here's fitness fanatic Jack LaLanne talking to *Outside* magazine a few years ago on the subject of warming up before working out.

"Warming up is the biggest bunch of horseshit I've ever heard in my life. Fifteen minutes to warm up! Does a lion warm up when he's hungry? 'Uh-oh, here comes an antelope. Better warm up.' No! He just goes out and eats the sucker."

We like Jack LaLanne. We appreciate his colorful straightforwardness. But we think he needs to watch lions a little longer.

"That lion takes a snooze, and what do you see when he wakes up? He stretches," says Rick Huegli, former head strength and conditioning coach at the University of Washington. "The better you warm up, the better you're going to perform."

Most workout wonks agree with Huegli and say that you need to do some warming up before you pump iron.

Here's why. When you warm up, you pump blood into your muscles and elevate their temperature. This in turn makes them less susceptible to painful pulls and tears. "Common sense indicates that if the muscle is warmed up, the body is better prepared to more effectively recruit the muscle for exercise, and there might be less chance of damaging the muscle," says Thomas Baechle, Ed.D., chairman of the exercise science department at Creighton University in Omaha, Nebraska.

The Stretching Truth

We're going to mention this first because a lot of guys were taught wrong. You may have been told to always stretch before a workout. Don't. That is, don't stretch first thing. Don't stretch a muscle that isn't already warmed up, says Peter Lemon, Ph.D., designer of the Hard-Body exercise plan.

We do want you to stretch. But we want you to warm up the muscles first with some light aerobics. Then, your stretches should be specific to the muscles you'll be working, and they should also be relatively brief. Brief doesn't mean careless, though: You can cause injuries to the very muscles you're trying to protect if you stretch too vigorously, too roughly, or too far. "I've seen individuals who have actually pulled muscles when they were stretching," says Dr. Lemon.

We don't want you pulling muscles, but a few minutes of stretching before and after pumping iron—along with a program that trains muscle groups equally—clearly promotes flexibility and prevents you from suffering what critics once carped would inevitably happen to those who lift weights: becoming muscle-bound.

Static stretching is safest. That means that you gently, slowly stretch a muscle through its full range of motion—the entire movement through which a body part rotates around a joint, for instance. Stretch to the point at which you feel resistance or tightness; hold; and then ease off. Do not stretch to the point of pain.

Do each stretch once or twice, and hold the maximum position 10 seconds, Dr. Lemon advises. In subsequent stretching sessions, you can gradually stretch farther, increasing your flexibility.

The easiest way to hurt yourself is to bounce while stretching. Bouncing causes a reflex contraction that can cause a muscle pull or tear. "You can stretch the muscle longer if you do it slowly because you don't kick in this reflex," says Dr. Lemon.

AEROBICS

The best way to give your body an overall, general warmup before lifting is to do aerobic exercise. That doesn't mean jumping around to loud music as if there's cayenne pepper in your jock, unless you particularly like cayenne pepper and loud music. Treadmills and stationary bicycles give you a less frenetic aerobic workout. You can try other aerobics machines, too. Or do some light jogging and walking, and swing your arms a bit. How long do you need to do this aerobic stuff? Here's what Dr. Lemon advises:

Whatever aerobic activity you choose, do it until you break into a sweat. For most guys, that's about 5 to 7 minutes.

Fast-paced exercise is good for your heart and lungs. If you extend it a bit—to say, 20 minutes—it counts not only as a warmup but also as part of the aerobic exercise that the Hard-Body Plan calls for to help you maximize the benefits of your weight training program.

STRETCHED TO THE LIMIT

We told you that stretching too far can lead to injury. Here's another reason not to overdo it: It may weaken your workout.

When 30 subjects in a joint Louisiana State and Brigham Young University study stretched vigorously for 20 minutes before a workout, they lost strength during weight training.

And in another study done in Finland, 20 men who stretched for an hour before exercise had 85 percent slower reaction times.

LIGHT LIFTING

Here are two cool ways to warm up the muscles you'll stress during your workout.

• **Use weights.** Do the very exercise you're going to perform first, but with half the weight, Dr. Baechle says. Let's say that you're planning to do several repetitions of the bench press at 120 pounds. Start off by doing a few reps at 60 pounds. This allows you to stretch the muscles in a very specific way, and it warms you up quickly. This warmup is acutally built into the Hard-Body workouts in the next chapter.

• **Use your body.** You also can put your own body weight to use as a warmup tool. Maybe you intend to start your workout with 10 bench-press repetitions. Don't want to fuss with moving plates on and off the bar? Hit the floor. Do 30 pushups for a warmup, then bench-press with the full load.

Even if you're the sort of guy who's so busy that you have to schedule sex with your wife, you can take a few extra minutes to warm up before working out. Because that's all you need—a few extra minutes. And you already know how to schedule things.

The best warmup takes 10 minutes: Do some aerobic exercise, stretch, and lift light weights working the specific muscle group that you're going to exercise. Do the warmup routine in that order.

A warmup before lifting weights is especially critical if you're planning to lift a heavy load and do few repetitions. "The higher the weight and the fewer the number of repetitions, the more chance you have for injury if you're not warmed up," Dr. Lemon warns.

COOLDOWN

Like warming up before lifting, cooling down afterward is overlooked by a lot of men. Here's why it's important. Either during or immediately following weight training, there is a huge increase in bloodflow to the muscles. That's what gives you that pumped feeling and appearance.

The trouble is that now there is less blood and oxygen returning to the heart since so much of it is in the muscle. When you abruptly stop lifting or doing other exercise, the blood simply pools in the muscle. Your heart needs some of the oxygen that's bound to the hemoglobin in your blood. If it doesn't get that oxygen, you could have a heart attack. You could even die, and let's face it, dying blows the whole workout.

It's a pretty dire scenario but one that's easy to avoid. When you finish a weight training workout, do some light aerobic exercise or a few reps with light weights—or even walk around a bit, advises Dr. Lemon. This will squeeze blood back into your blood vessels and toward your heart. For most men, a mere 5 minutes of this cooldown activity will do the job.

UPPER BODY

FOUR-WAY NECK TWIST AND TILT

Stand with your back straight and your legs shoulder-width apart. Your neck should be straight and your shoulders relaxed.

[A] Slowly turn your head to the right as far as it will comfortably go. Hold for 10 seconds. Then repeat, turning your head to the left. Return to the starting position.

[B] Without bending your upper body, tuck your chin into your chest until you feel a mild pull in the back of your neck. Hold for 10 seconds.

[C] Slowly tilt your head back until you are looking straight up, but not so far back that your head rests on your shoulders. Hold for 10 seconds, then relax.

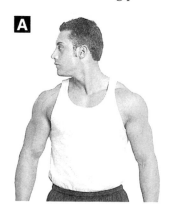
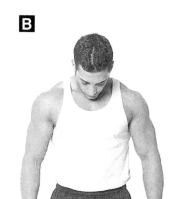
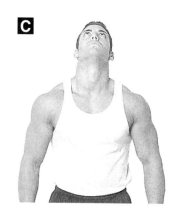

OVERHEAD SHOULDER STRETCH

[A] Stand erect with your shoulders back, chest out, and feet about shoulder-width apart. Raise your right arm overhead, bend your elbow, and rest your right hand behind your neck, just between your shoulder blades. Keep your left hand at your side.

[B] Use your left hand to gently push on your right elbow, edging it toward the center of your body and farther down behind your neck. Switch arms and repeat.

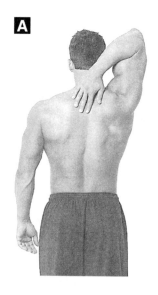
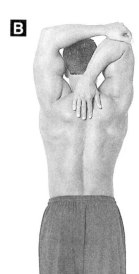

CHEST STRETCH

Place your hands on both sides of a doorway at shoulder height. Keep your chest and head up and your knees slightly bent.

Move your upper body forward until you feel a comfortable stretch. Hold the position for 10 seconds, but do not hold your breath. Do once.

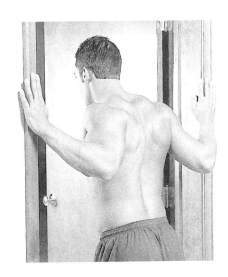

LOWER BODY

SPINAL TWIST

Sit on the floor with both legs extended.

[A] Bend your right leg over your left leg, keeping your right foot flat on the floor outside your left knee. Place your left elbow on the outside of your right knee, and extend your right arm behind you with your palm flat on the floor for support.

[B] Twist your upper body to the right by slowly looking over your right shoulder. Apply pressure with your left elbow on the outside of your right knee as you twist. Keep your upper body straight. Hold, then switch sides and repeat.

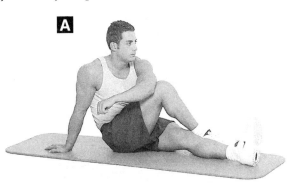

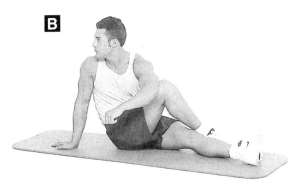

LYING LEG PULL

[A] Lie on your back with your forearms under your thighs. Pull your knees as close to your chest as they will comfortably go. This stretches your lower back.

[B] Keeping your knees close to your chest, extend your legs over your head. This extends the stretch to include your hamstrings and butt muscles. Hold for 10 seconds, then return to the starting position.

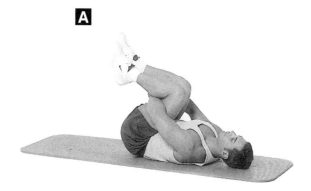

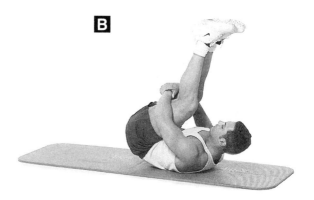

BUTTERFLY STRETCH

To do a butterfly stretch, sit on the floor with your legs bent frog-style, the soles of your feet pressed together. Gently press your knees toward the floor with your elbows or hands. Hold.

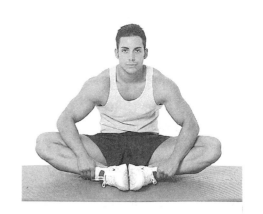

HAMSTRING STRETCH

Sit on the edge of a bed or bench with your right leg extended on the bench and your left foot on the floor. Rest your right hand on your right knee, then slowly slide your fingers to your toes, reaching as far as is comfortable. Hold. Switch legs and repeat. (This position takes stress off your lower back, unlike similar exercises in which you sit on the floor.)

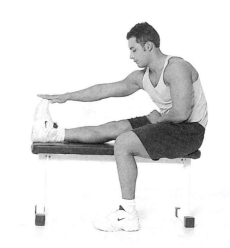

THIGH PULL

Stand touching a chair or wall for support. Bend your right knee and grab your right foot with your left hand, pulling your foot up so that your heel presses against your butt. Hold. Switch legs and repeat.

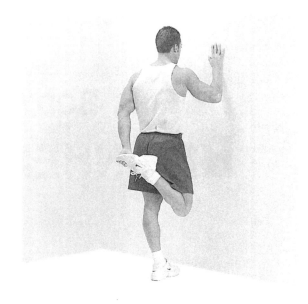

CALF STRETCH

Stand slightly away from a wall and lean on it with your forearms, your head resting on your hands. Place your right foot in front of you, leg bent, your left leg straight behind you.

Slowly move your hips forward until you feel a stretch in the calf of your left leg. Keep your left heel flat and your toes pointed straight ahead. Hold an easy stretch for 10 seconds. Switch legs and repeat.

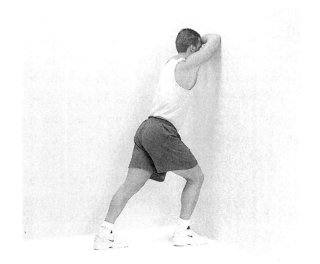

FULL-BODY MUSCLE PLAN
BEGINNER WORKOUT

Expect quick muscle growth from this powerful, one-set lifting program for beginners.

In the beginner and intermediate programs, you do a different variation of the full-body workout each week for 3 weeks. We call these Workout 1, Workout 2, and Workout 3. Then you start the cycle over again with Workout 1. By rotating through three different weekly workouts, you go 3 full weeks before repeating most exercises. That's part of the program's unique design to encourage the most rapid, efficient muscle growth.

How does the rotation work?

Week 1, you do Workout 1. Week 2, you do Workout 2. Week 3, you do Workout 3. Week 4, you do Workout 1. Week 5, you do Workout 2. Week 6, you do Workout 3 . . . and so on, simply cycling through the three workouts every 3 weeks until you have worked through all 12 weeks of the program. Then, you may move on to the Intermediate Workout (see page 52).

INSTRUCTIONS

This program is designed as a 3-days-a-week workout. It can be adapted to a 2-days-a-week workout. We'll tell you how to do that after we explain the basics of the program.

1. Do some aerobics and stretching, then do a warmup set (6 to 10 repetitions) of each exercise using light weights.

2. After the warmup, find a starting load that is hard to lift 6 times. This may take some experimenting on your first day. Once you find this load, you'll use it until it becomes too easy. Complete one set of 6 repetitions for each exercise. Perform the positive phase (also known as the concentric or lifting phase) of each exercise as quickly as possible while maintaining proper form. Perform the negative (or eccentric or lowering) phase much more slowly, to a count of four.

3. Increase the number of repetitions to 10 for each exercise as you build strength and can do so while maintaining proper form.

4. When you can do 10 repetitions of an exercise, increase the weight on your next session and drop back to doing 6 repetitions. Again, over time, work your way up to 10. Each time you reach 10, you can increase the weight.

5. Allow at least 48 hours between training sessions to ensure sufficient recovery.

6. Follow the weekly variations in the exercises, as this more fully trains the entire muscle area and more quickly builds muscle.

To convert this to a 2-days-a-week program, add exercises 1 to 3 from Day 3 to the Day 1 routine; then add all of the Day 5 exercises to the remaining Day 3 exercises (exercises 4 to 7).

WORKOUT 1

DAY 1: ARMS AND SHOULDERS

1. OVERHEAD PRESS WITH BARBELL (PAGE 98)

2. UPRIGHT ROW (PAGE 100)

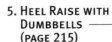

3. SIDE DELTOID RAISE (PAGE 96)

4. LYING TRICEPS EXTENSION (PAGE 73)

5. BARBELL CURL (PAGE 69)

6. FOREARM CURL (PAGE 74)

7. REVERSE FOREARM CURL (PAGE 75)

DAY 2: REST AND RECOVERY

DAY 3: BUTT, THIGHS, AND LEGS

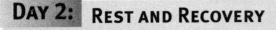

1. LATERAL LUNGE WITH BARBELL (PAGE 180)

2. HACK SQUAT (PAGE 195)

3. LEG CURL WITH ANKLE WEIGHTS (PAGE 199)

4. LEG EXTENSION WITH ANKLE WEIGHTS (PAGE 198)

5. HEEL RAISE WITH DUMBBELLS (PAGE 215)

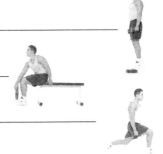

6. ANKLE FLEXION WITH WEIGHT PLATE (PAGE 216)

7. STATIONARY LUNGE WITH DUMBBELLS (PAGE 181)

DAY 4: REST AND RECOVERY

DAY 5: CHEST, ABS, AND BACK

1. BENCH PRESS (PAGE 118)

2. DUMBBELL FLY (PAGE 117)

3. WIDE-GRIP ROW (PAGE 158)

4. DUMBBELL SWING (PAGE 161)

5. DUMBBELL TRUNK TWIST (PAGE 140)

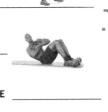

6. OBLIQUE TRUNK ROTATION WITH WEIGHT PLATE (PAGE 138)

7. LEG RAISE WITH ANKLE WEIGHTS (PAGE 139)

DAY 6: REST AND RECOVERY

DAY 7: REST AND RECOVERY

WORKOUT 2

DAY 1: ARMS AND SHOULDERS

1. DUMBBELL MILITARY PRESS (PAGE 99)

2. DUMBBELL RAISE (PAGE 100)

3. FRONT DELTOID RAISE (PAGE 96)

4. LYING CROSS-SHOULDER TRICEPS EXTENSION (PAGE 72)

5. REVERSE-GRIP BARBELL CURL (PAGE 69)

6. WRIST ROLLER (PAGE 75)

DAY 2: REST AND RECOVERY

DAY 3: BUTT, THIGHS, AND LEGS

1. HACK SQUAT (PAGE 195)

2. LEG EXTENSION WITH ANKLE WEIGHTS (PAGE 198)

3. FRONT SQUAT (PAGE 197)

4. SEATED HEEL RAISE WITH BARBELL (PAGE 215)

5. ANKLE FLEXION WITH WEIGHT PLATE (PAGE 216)

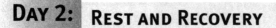

6. DUCK SQUAT WITH DUMBBELL (PAGE 179)

7. BENCH LATERAL STEPUP WITH DUMBBELLS (PAGE 196)

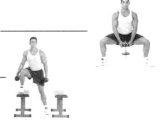

DAY 4: REST AND RECOVERY

DAY 5: CHEST, ABS, AND BACK

1. INCLINE BENCH PRESS (PAGE 119)

2. DUMBBELL FLY (PAGE 117)

3. ONE-ARM DUMBBELL ROW (PAGE 160)

4. T-BAR ROW WITH BARBELL (PAGE 159)

5. DUMBBELL SIDE BEND (PAGE 140)

6. CURL-UP WITH WEIGHT PLATE (PAGE 138)

DAY 6: REST AND RECOVERY

DAY 7: REST AND RECOVERY

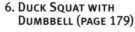

WORKOUT 3

DAY 1: ARMS AND SHOULDERS

1. BEHIND-THE-NECK PRESS WITH BARBELL (PAGE 97)

2. SHRUG (PAGE 99)

3. SIDE DELTOID RAISE (PAGE 96)

4. FRENCH CURL (PAGE 73)

5. PREACHER CURL (PAGE 71)

6. FOREARM CURL (PAGE 74)

7. REVERSE FOREARM CURL (PAGE 75)

DAY 2: REST AND RECOVERY

DAY 3: BUTT, THIGHS, AND LEGS

1. HACK SQUAT (PAGE 195)

2. LEG CURL WITH ANKLE WEIGHTS (PAGE 199)

3. LEG EXTENSION WITH ANKLE WEIGHTS (PAGE 198)

4. SEATED HEEL RAISE WITH BARBELL (PAGE 215)

5. ANKLE FLEXION WITH WEIGHT PLATE (PAGE 216)

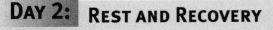

6. STATIONARY LUNGE WITH DUMBBELLS (PAGE 181)

7. STANDING KICKBACK WITH ANKLE WEIGHTS (PAGE 179)

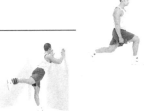

DAY 4: REST AND RECOVERY

DAY 5: CHEST, ABS, AND BACK

1. DECLINE BENCH PRESS (PAGE 120)

2. DUMBBELL FLY (PAGE 117)

3. GOOD MORNING (PAGE 159)

4. ONE-ARM DUMBBELL ROW (PAGE 160)

5. DUMBBELL TRUNK TWIST (PAGE 140)

6. OBLIQUE TRUNK ROTATION WITH WEIGHT PLATE (PAGE 138)

7. DUMBBELL SIDE BEND (PAGE 140)

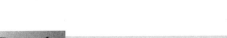

DAY 6: REST AND RECOVERY

DAY 7: REST AND RECOVERY

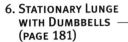

FULL-BODY MUSCLE PLAN
INTERMEDIATE WORKOUT

How we move to multiple sets to supercharge muscle growth, and we definitely train 3 days a week. Still, we cycle through three different week-long programs and, for the most part, only repeat the same exercises once every third week.

INSTRUCTIONS

1. Train three times a week. Allow sufficient recovery by waiting at least 48 hours between sessions when training the same part of the body.

2. Always start with some aerobics and stretching, then do a warmup set by performing one set of 6 to 10 repetitions with a light to moderate load. This minimizes the chances of a muscle strain or pull during the subsequent training period.

3. Including your warmup set, your standard intermediate routine is three sets of 6 to 10 repetitions for each exercise listed. The starting load after the warmup set should be one that is hard to lift 6 times. As your strength increases, increase reps per set until you can do 10 reps while maintaining proper form. Then, for your next session, increase the load and drop back to 6 reps.

Perform the positive phase (also known as the concentric or lifting phase) of each exercise as quickly as possible while maintaining proper form,

and perform the negative (or eccentric or lowering) phase much more slowly (to a count of four).

4. Vary your routines. You may train more frequently if you wish—for instance, 4 or 5 days per week—but to do so you must rotate through different body areas in order to allow each area 48 hours of recovery time. This type of rotation is called a split routine. Another variation is to do combo lifts, also called supersets, two exercises in succession (one rep of each) without a rest. You can do almost any two exercises this way. Combo lifts increase the intensity of a workout, create some variety, and can shorten your workout session.

Yet another variation, called pyramids, is to use a lighter load than usual and do 15 to 20 repetitions in the first set, then increase the load on successive sets and reduce the number of repetitions. So, for example, in set 1, you might do 10 repetitions with 200 pounds; in set 2, you might do 7 repetitions with 250 pounds; and in set 3, you might do 4 repetitions with 300 pounds.

5. As you gain training experience, you might try experimenting with 1 or 2 partial repetitions at the end of each set, at the point where you can no longer complete a full repetition. This is called going to muscle failure, and it may enhance muscle development. *Note:* When you are going to muscle failure, you need the assistance of a partner for safety. Don't take risks.

WORKOUT 1

DAY 1: ARMS AND SHOULDERS

1. OVERHEAD PRESS WITH BARBELL (PAGE 98)

2. UPRIGHT ROW (PAGE 100)

3. SIDE DELTOID RAISE (PAGE 96)

4. DUMBBELL KICKBACK (PAGE 72)

5. PREACHER CURL (PAGE 71)

6. FOREARM CURL (PAGE 74)

7. REVERSE FOREARM CURL (PAGE 75)

DAY 2: REST AND RECOVERY

DAY 3: BUTT, THIGHS, AND LEGS

1. HACK SQUAT (PAGE 195)

2. LEG CURL WITH ANKLE WEIGHTS (PAGE 199)

3. LEG EXTENSION WITH ANKLE WEIGHTS (PAGE 198)

4. HEEL RAISE WITH DUMBBELLS (PAGE 215)

5. ANKLE FLEXION WITH WEIGHT PLATE (PAGE 216)

6. STATIONARY LUNGE WITH DUMBBELLS (PAGE 181)

7. LATERAL LUNGE WITH BARBELL (PAGE 180)

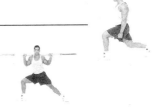

DAY 4: REST AND RECOVERY

DAY 5: CHEST, ABS, AND BACK

1. INCLINE BENCH PRESS (PAGE 119)

2. DUMBBELL FLY (PAGE 117)

3. ONE-ARM DUMBBELL ROW (PAGE 160)

4. T-BAR ROW WITH BARBELL (PAGE 159)

5. DUMBBELL TRUNK TWIST (PAGE 140)

6. OBLIQUE TRUNK ROTATION WITH WEIGHT PLATE (PAGE 138)

7. DUMBBELL SIDE BEND (PAGE 140)

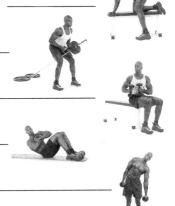

DAY 6: REST AND RECOVERY

DAY 7: REST AND RECOVERY

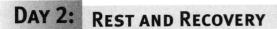

WORKOUT 2

DAY 1: ARMS AND SHOULDERS

1. DUMBBELL MILITARY _____
   PRESS (PAGE 99)

2. DUMBBELL RAISE _____
   (PAGE 100)

3. FRONT DELTOID _____
   RAISE (PAGE 96)

4. LYING CROSS-
   SHOULDER TRICEPS ———
   EXTENSION (PAGE 72)

5. REVERSE-GRIP
   BARBELL CURL ———————
   (PAGE 69)

6. WRIST ROLLER _____
   (PAGE 75)

DAY 2: REST AND RECOVERY

DAY 3: BUTT, THIGHS, AND LEGS

1. BENCH LATERAL
   STEPUP WITH ——————————
   DUMBBELLS
   (PAGE 196)

2. HACK SQUAT _____
   (PAGE 195)

3. LEG EXTENSION
   WITH ANKLE ——————
   WEIGHTS (PAGE 198)

4. FRONT SQUAT _____
   (PAGE 197)

5. SEATED HEEL RAISE
   WITH BARBELL ——————————
   (PAGE 215)

6. ANKLE FLEXION WITH
   WEIGHT PLATE ———————
   (PAGE 216)

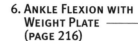

7. DUCK SQUAT
   WITH DUMBBELL ———
   (PAGE 179)

DAY 4: REST AND RECOVERY

DAY 5: CHEST, ABS, AND BACK

1. INCLINE BENCH PRESS_____
   (PAGE 119)

2. DUMBBELL FLY _____
   (PAGE 117)

3. ONE-ARM DUMBBELL _____
   ROW (PAGE 160)

4. T-BAR ROW
   WITH BARBELL ———
   (PAGE 159)

5. DUMBBELL SIDE
   BEND (PAGE 140) ——————

6. CURL-UP WITH
   WEIGHT PLATE ———
   (PAGE 138)

DAY 6: REST AND RECOVERY

DAY 7: REST AND RECOVERY

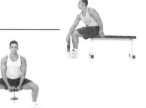
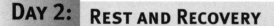

WORKOUT 3

DAY 1: ARMS AND SHOULDERS

1. **BEHIND-THE-NECK PRESS WITH BARBELL** (PAGE 97)

2. **SHRUG** (PAGE 99)

3. **SIDE DELTOID RAISE** (PAGE 96)

4. **FRENCH CURL** (PAGE 73)

5. **PREACHER CURL** (PAGE 71)

6. **FOREARM CURL** (PAGE 74)

7. **REVERSE FOREARM CURL** (PAGE 75)

DAY 2: REST AND RECOVERY

DAY 3: BUTT, THIGHS, AND LEGS

1. **HACK SQUAT** (PAGE 195)

2. **LEG CURL WITH ANKLE WEIGHTS** (PAGE 199)

3. **LEG EXTENSION WITH ANKLE WEIGHTS** (PAGE 198)

4. **SEATED HEEL RAISE WITH BARBELL** (PAGE 215)

5. **ANKLE FLEXION WITH WEIGHT PLATE** (PAGE 216)

6. **STATIONARY LUNGE WITH DUMBBELLS** (PAGE 181)

7. **STANDING KICKBACK WITH ANKLE WEIGHTS** (PAGE 179)

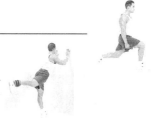

DAY 4: REST AND RECOVERY

DAY 5: CHEST, ABS, AND BACK

1. **DECLINE BENCH PRESS** (PAGE 120)

2. **DUMBBELL FLY** (PAGE 117)

3. **GOOD MORNING** (PAGE 159)

4. **ONE-ARM DUMBBELL ROW** (PAGE 160)

5. **DUMBBELL TRUNK TWIST** (PAGE 140)

6. **OBLIQUE TRUNK ROTATION WITH WEIGHT PLATE** (PAGE 138)

7. **DUMBBELL SIDE BEND** (PAGE 140)

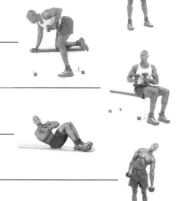

DAY 6: REST AND RECOVERY

DAY 7: REST AND RECOVERY

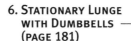
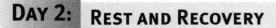

FULL-BODY MUSCLE PLAN
ADVANCED WORKOUT

This is for extremely serious, committed musclemen. We're adding tough moves, new exercises, tri-sets and giant sets, and more. Ready for the challenge?

At the advanced level, you do a 2-day split routine. You train legs, butt, thighs, chest, triceps, and abs on Day 1, and train back, shoulders, biceps, and forearms on Day 2. Then you rest 2 days and start again. You'll rest again on Day 7.

As in the beginner and intermediate levels, you rotate between the weeklong workouts. There are only two advanced workouts to rotate between, though. Do one one week and the other the next. Keep rotating forever and ever if you want to make monster muscle.

INSTRUCTIONS

1. Train 4 days a week. Allow sufficient recovery by waiting at least 48 hours between sessions when training the same part of the body.

2. Your standard advanced routine is to complete three sets of 6 to 10 repetitions for each exercise listed. After your aerobics and stretching, the first set is a warmup using lighter weights. The starting load for the second and third sets should be one that is difficult to lift 6 times. As your strength increases, increase the repetitions per set until you can do 10 reps, and then for your next session increase the load and drop back to 6 reps.

Perform the positive phase (also known as the concentric or lifting phase) of each exercise as quickly as possible while maintaining proper form, and perform the negative (or eccentric or lowering) phase much more slowly (to a count of four).

3. Do 1 or 2 partial repetitions at the end of each set when you reach the point where you can no longer complete a full repetition. This is called going to muscle failure, and it may enhance muscle development. *Note:* You always need the assistance of a partner for safety purposes when doing partial repetitions.

4. Vary your workouts as at the intermediate level, and add tri-sets and giant sets. Tri-sets are like combo lifts except that you add an exercise so you are doing three in succession without rest. With giant sets, you do four exercises in succession without rest between them.

WORKOUT 1

DAY 1: LEGS, BUTT, THIGHS, CHEST, TRICEPS, AND ABS

1. SQUAT (PAGE 195)

2. HACK SQUAT (PAGE 195)

3. LEG CURL WITH ANKLE WEIGHTS (PAGE 199)

4. LEG EXTENSION WITH ANKLE WEIGHTS (PAGE 198)

5. HEEL RAISE WITH DUMBBELLS (PAGE 215)

6. ANKLE FLEXION WITH WEIGHT PLATE (PAGE 216)

7. STATIONARY LUNGE WITH DUMBBELLS (PAGE 181)

8. INCLINE BENCH PRESS (PAGE 119)

9. DUMBBELL FLY (PAGE 117)

10. FRENCH CURL (PAGE 73)

11. ROWING CRUNCH WITH ANKLE WEIGHTS (PAGE 139)

12. OBLIQUE TRUNK ROTATION WITH WEIGHT PLATE (PAGE 138)

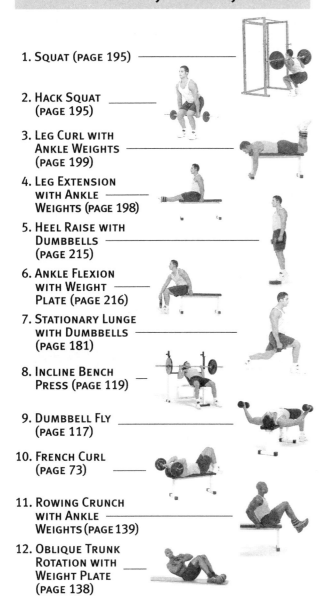

DAY 2: BACK, SHOULDERS, BICEPS, AND FOREARMS

1. UPRIGHT ROW (PAGE 100)

2. SIDE DELTOID RAISE (PAGE 96)

3. SHRUG (PAGE 99)

4. FRONT DELTOID RAISE (PAGE 96)

5. BEHIND-THE-NECK PRESS WITH BARBELL (PAGE 97)

6. T-BAR ROW WITH BARBELL (PAGE 159)

7. DUMBBELL SWING (PAGE 161)

8. WIDE-GRIP ROW (PAGE 158)

9. ONE-ARM DUMBBELL ROW (PAGE 160)

10. PREACHER CURL (PAGE 71)

11. REVERSE-GRIP BARBELL CURL (PAGE 69)

12. FOREARM CURL (PAGE 74)

13. REVERSE FOREARM CURL (PAGE 75)

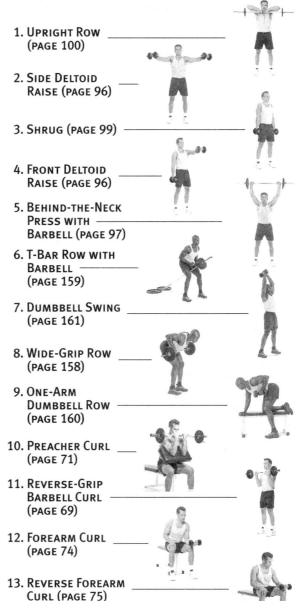

DAY 3:   REST AND RECOVERY

DAY 4:   REST AND RECOVERY

DAY 5:   LEGS, BUTT, THIGHS, CHEST, TRICEPS, AND ABS

1. FRONT SQUAT _____ (PAGE 197)

2. GOOD MORNING ____ (PAGE 159)

3. DUCK SQUAT WITH DUMBBELL _____ (PAGE 179)

4. LEG CURL WITH ANKLE WEIGHTS _____ (PAGE 199)

5. DUMBBELL POWER LUNGE (PAGE 197) _____

6. SEATED HEEL RAISE WITH BARBELL _____ (PAGE 215)

7. ANKLE FLEXION WITH WEIGHT _____ PLATE (PAGE 216)

8. LATERAL LUNGE WITH BARBELL _____ (PAGE 180)

9. DECLINE BENCH PRESS (PAGE 120) _____

10. DUMBBELL FLY _____ (PAGE 117)

11. DUMBBELL KICKBACK _____ (PAGE 72)

12. LEG RAISE WITH ANKLE WEIGHTS _____ (PAGE 139)

13. OBLIQUE TRUNK ROTATION WITH _____ WEIGHT PLATE (PAGE 138)

DAY 6:   BACK, SHOULDERS, BICEPS, AND FOREARMS

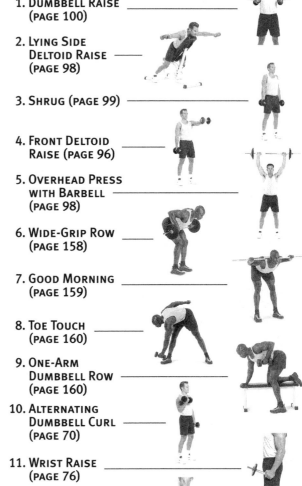

1. DUMBBELL RAISE _____ (PAGE 100)

2. LYING SIDE DELTOID RAISE _____ (PAGE 98)

3. SHRUG (PAGE 99) _____

4. FRONT DELTOID RAISE (PAGE 96) _____

5. OVERHEAD PRESS WITH BARBELL _____ (PAGE 98)

6. WIDE-GRIP ROW _____ (PAGE 158)

7. GOOD MORNING _____ (PAGE 159)

8. TOE TOUCH _____ (PAGE 160)

9. ONE-ARM DUMBBELL ROW _____ (PAGE 160)

10. ALTERNATING DUMBBELL CURL _____ (PAGE 70)

11. WRIST RAISE _____ (PAGE 76)

12. REVERSE WRIST _____ RAISE (PAGE 76)

DAY 7:   REST AND RECOVERY

WORKOUT 2

DAY 1: LEGS, BUTT, THIGHS, CHEST, TRICEPS, AND ABS

1. SQUAT (PAGE 195)

2. HACK SQUAT (PAGE 195)

3. LEG CURL WITH ANKLE WEIGHTS (PAGE 199)

4. LEG EXTENSION WITH ANKLE WEIGHTS (PAGE 198)

5. HEEL RAISE WITH DUMBBELLS (PAGE 215)

6. ANKLE FLEXION WITH WEIGHT PLATE (PAGE 216)

7. STATIONARY LUNGE WITH DUMBBELLS (PAGE 181)

8. INCLINE BENCH PRESS (PAGE 119)

9. DUMBBELL FLY (PAGE 117)

10. LYING CROSS-SHOULDER TRICEPS EXTENSION (PAGE 72)

11. PARALLEL DIP WITH WEIGHT PLATE (PAGE 74)

12. DUMBBELL TRUNK TWIST (PAGE 140)

13. DUMBBELL SIDE BEND (PAGE 140)

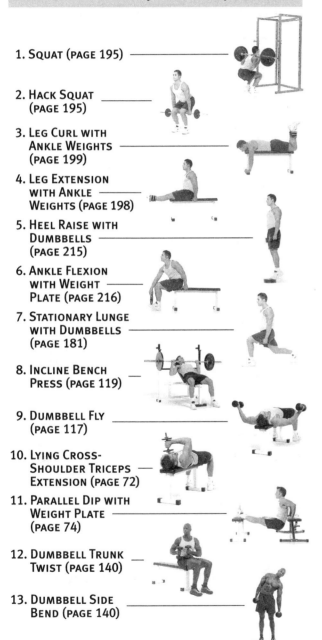

DAY 2: BACK, SHOULDERS, BICEPS, AND FOREARMS

1. UPRIGHT ROW (PAGE 100)

2. SIDE DELTOID RAISE (PAGE 96)

3. SHRUG (PAGE 99)

4. FRONT DELTOID RAISE (PAGE 96)

5. BEHIND-THE-NECK PRESS WITH BARBELL (PAGE 97)

6. T-BAR ROW WITH BARBELL (PAGE 159)

7. DUMBBELL SWING (PAGE 161)

8. WIDE-GRIP ROW (PAGE 158)

9. ONE-ARM DUMBBELL ROW (PAGE 160)

10. PREACHER CURL (PAGE 71)

11. REVERSE-GRIP BARBELL CURL (PAGE 69)

12. FOREARM CURL (PAGE 74)

13. REVERSE FOREARM CURL (PAGE 75)

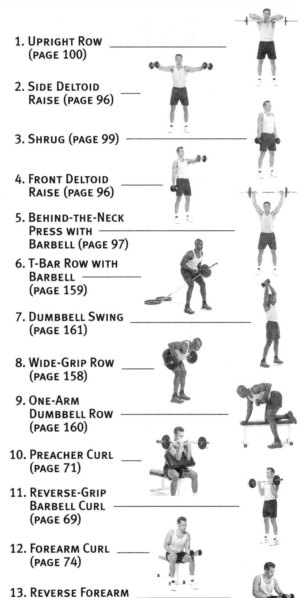

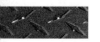

DAY 3: REST AND RECOVERY

DAY 4: REST AND RECOVERY

DAY 5: LEGS, BUTT, THIGHS, CHEST, TRICEPS, AND ABS

1. **FRONT SQUAT** (PAGE 197) _____
2. **GOOD MORNING** ____ (PAGE 159)
3. **DUCK SQUAT WITH DUMBBELL** _____ (PAGE 179)
4. **LEG CURL WITH ANKLE WEIGHTS** ____ (PAGE 199)
5. **DUMBBELL POWER LUNGE** (PAGE 197) _____
6. **SEATED HEEL RAISE WITH BARBELL** ____ (PAGE 215)
7. **ANKLE FLEXION WITH WEIGHT PLATE** (PAGE 216) _____
8. **LATERAL LUNGE WITH BARBELL** ____ (PAGE 180)
9. **DECLINE BENCH PRESS** (PAGE 120) _____
10. **DUMBBELL FLY** ____ (PAGE 117)
11. **DUMBBELL KICKBACK** _____ (PAGE 72)
12. **LEG RAISE WITH ANKLE WEIGHTS** ____ (PAGE 139)
13. **DUMBBELL TRUNK TWIST** (PAGE 140) _____

DAY 6: BACK, SHOULDERS, BICEPS, AND FOREARMS

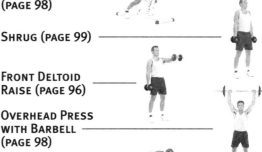
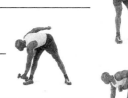
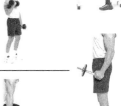

1. **DUMBBELL RAISE** _____ (PAGE 100)
2. **LYING SIDE DELTOID RAISE** ____ (PAGE 98)
3. **SHRUG** (PAGE 99) _____
4. **FRONT DELTOID RAISE** (PAGE 96) _____
5. **OVERHEAD PRESS WITH BARBELL** ____ (PAGE 98)
6. **WIDE-GRIP ROW** (PAGE 158) _____
7. **GOOD MORNING** _____ (PAGE 159)
8. **TOE TOUCH** ____ (PAGE 160)
9. **ONE-ARM DUMBBELL ROW** _____ (PAGE 160)
10. **ALTERNATING DUMBBELL CURL** ____ (PAGE 70)
11. **WRIST RAISE** _____ (PAGE 76)
12. **REVERSE WRIST RAISE** ____ (PAGE 76)

DAY 7: REST AND RECOVERY

MOLDING IT TO YOUR LIFE, GOALS, NEEDS
PERSONALIZING THE PLAN

ADJUST THE HARD-BODY PLAN TO MEET YOUR SPECIFIC NEEDS. ADD NEW EXERCISES, DO EXERCISES LONGER OR WITH HEAVIER OR LIGHTER WEIGHTS. BUT DO STAY WITHIN THE CONFINES OF THE PLAN. IT PROVIDES A BALANCED, TOTAL-BODY WORKOUT.

You're a maverick, right? The kind of guy who wears a coat and tie to work on casual Fridays. The sort who braids his ear hair rather than trimming it. A man who—when he's really feeling rowdy—eats dessert before the main course. You wild man, you. So chances are that if you stick with the Hard-Body Plan, you'll want to modify it at some point. Tweak it. Fine-tune it to suit your evolving needs. We've got two words to say to that: No problem.

Here are some reasons why you might want to personalize the Hard-Body Plan and some ways to do so.

VARIETY

You'll find more exercises in each phase of the Hard-Body Plan—beginner, intermediate, and ad-vanced—than you'll ever do over the course of a week of working out. But if you want still more va-riety, you can mix and match from exercises listed in all three levels of lifting. And, if you don't feel like exercising with machines, you can do the equivalent no- or free-weight exercises, or vice versa.

"Some of the advanced exercises are more dif-ficult and could be a problem for a beginner," says Peter Lemon, Ph.D.

"Going the other way will not be a problem," Dr. Lemon says. "You will have mastered those ex-ercises along the way."

We can't emphasize this enough: Changing your weight training routine is not only good, it's also necessary to keep your muscles growing. Oth-erwise you will hit a plateau and stop making progress. And you may get bored and quit and revert back to your former body—the one that caused people to mistake you for John Goodman.

SPORTS

You may do more sitting at your job than a cross-country trucker, but you still play a sport or two on weekends. Good idea. And if you want to improve your performance on the court or the field, you might be thinking that it's wise to tailor your workouts to the muscle groups that most come into play during these sports.

We've made it easier for you to do so in the chapter called Functional Fitness beginning on page 253. It tells you which muscle groups are most taxed by each of the activities listed and which exercises will bolster those muscles.

Let's say that you play a fast-paced game of full-court basketball once a week. You might want to do a few more squats for leg and hip thrust, and leg curls to avoid blowing out a hamstring, as well as some aerobic training to increase your stamina. Bowling strikes your fancy? Consider emphasizing exercises that give you arm and shoulder power, such as alternating dumbbell curls and the dumbbell military press. You're stuck with being a lineman when you play touch football? Do extra squats with heavy weights so that you can flatten your obnoxious brother-in-law on the other side of the ball.

Maybe you play a sport that requires a lot of endurance as opposed to brute strength. You could increase the number of weight training sessions in which you lift lighter loads and perform, say, 20 to 25 repetitions.

But if endurance is the major component of your activity, don't overdo heavy lifting. Otherwise you will build some unnecessary muscle that could be counterproductive because you have to carry the extra weight, says Dr. Lemon.

Instead, you might supplement your weight training with exercises that incorporate your weekend sport. If you go cycling on weekends, spend additional time pedaling up hills in the evenings or in the gym on a recumbent bike. And make more time than you otherwise might for cardio exercises: treadmills, stairclimbers, and the like in the gym, or walking up stairs or running in the park. These heart-pounding exercises increase your stamina.

Training for a particular sport provides you with lots of room to improvise a unique workout that can supplement your Hard-Body Plan. For instance, Dr. Lemon has softball players swing a medicine ball like a bat, releasing it when they go through the strike zone. This more closely dupli-

GYMS AND GERMS

Go ahead and personalize the Hard-Body Plan, but don't get too personal with germs around the gym. Here are the 10 best ways to contract a disease at the gym, according to Georgia Tech University's *Sports Medicine & Performance Newsletter.*

1. Go to the gym when it's most crowded.
2. Wear shoes and socks that retain moisture.
3. Rub your eyes with your hands.
4. Don't place a towel between your body and a workout bench.
5. Wear the same athletic shoes every day.
6. Share towels and water bottles.
7. Don't use shower slippers.
8. Never wash your hands at the gym.
9. Only partially dry off after a workout.
10. When you towel off, start at the bottom and work up.

cates hitting a ball than weight training exercises do. And, he says, it prestretches muscles in a way that generates more force.

Dr. Lemon also has pitchers throw weighted softballs to help them develop more velocity when they hurl regulation balls. If you try this, however, don't use a superheavy ball. "If you get too heavy, it changes the mechanics of the movement," he says.

Here's another exercise you can devise to give yourself an edge if you play in a softball league. Practice swinging a bat that has a weighted rope attached to it. The rope gets fastened to a pulley 10 feet behind you, with weights attached to the rope below the pulley. You can also try this with a golf club to strengthen your golf swing.

JOB

You may also want to refine the Hard-Body Plan if you work at a job that has specific physical challenges. The more your exercises can simulate the movements you do on the job, the more useful and relevant the plan will be for you, says Dr. Lemon.

● **Firefighter.** To better enable you to carry hoses and tools up stairs and ladders, you might be wise to do some extra squats and leg curls to strengthen your quadriceps and hamstrings. You could also include an extra set of barbell curls, parallel dips, and bench presses to provide you with the upper-body strength to carry or drag a body and swing an ax.

Whether you're training for a sport or a job, always look for exercises that closely mirror the activity that you will be doing. Since firefighters sometimes chop holes in roofs with axes, consider driving a stake into the ground with a sledgehammer that is at least 25 percent heavier than your regular ax, suggests Dr. Lemon. You can move

on to heavier sledgehammers as your strength increases, but make sure that the movement remains the same. If the weight is so heavy that the mechanics of the movement change, your gains will not transfer to the desired activity. So, don't use a tool that weighs too much, or you will risk altering the movement you want to mimic.

● **Letter carrier.** You could add an additional set of shrugs for strong shoulders that enable you to lug a heavy pouch full of magazines and letters if you don't have a motorized route. And maybe practice running short sprints to develop the explosive, quick acceleration you need to escape demented dogs.

● **Office worker.** Whether you're an executive or a data entry clerk, you don't need much strength or stamina to master your desk job. But all that sitting can aggravate lower-back pain. Consider doing more crunches and leg raises to strengthen your abs. Weak abdominal muscles often are the cause of lower-back pain.

● **Meat cutter.** All that carving and cutting, slicing and dicing is done more easily if you have strong forearms and wrists. Do extra forearm curls and wrist rollers.

● **Lawyer.** Yeah, we know that hoisting all those legal briefs hardly requires you to be a Hard-Body Man. But if you try cases before juries, it doesn't hurt to present a powerful image. A well-developed chest and shoulders can do the job. Spend a little more time on the bench press and the dumbbell military press.

CAVEATS

While modifying the Hard-Body Plan is well and good, you still need to stay within the framework of the program, or you risk failing to get the results you seek. Let's say, for example, that your job or the sport you play requires a good deal more upper-body than lower-body strength. Should you train only your upper body? No.

"Maintain a balance," says Dr. Lemon.

You may also be tempted to personalize the Hard-Body Plan by skipping leg exercises, particularly if you aren't seeing quick or impressive gains. "It's true for many people that the legs don't respond as well as the arms and chest," says Dr. Lemon.

Maybe you're thinking, "As long as I maintain an upper-body balance—chest and back, biceps and triceps—what difference does it make?"

"From the standpoint of overall health, the lower body represents a large percentage of the total muscle mass," says Dr. Lemon. "Anything you do, you've got to support your weight with your lower body."

This has important implications for men as they age. As we grow older, we lose muscle mass, and, with it, our metabolic rate drops. That in turn causes us to get fatter if our dietary intake remains similar. But by continuing to work *all* of our muscle groups, we can burn fat calories more efficiently.

And that's not all. Training the lower body gives us balance. As we age, this can make the difference between stumbling slightly when we stub a toe or tumbling to the ground and perhaps breaking some bones. And speaking of bones, weight training will keep them strong and less likely to become brittle and breakable as we grow older.

"That may not seem very important for a 25-year-old, but 25-year-olds are going to be 75-year-olds at some point," says Dr. Lemon. "If you establish a habit early on and maintain it, there is no question that you'll be better off."

So, sure, go ahead and fine-tune the Hard-Body Plan if you want. But not too much. And not to the point where you exclude any muscle groups.

QUICK-SET PATH TO
POWERFUL ARMS

THE BICEPS ARE THE ARMS' BIG ATTENTION-GETTERS, BUT DON'T SKIMP ON DEVELOPING YOUR OTHER ARM MUSCLES. WORKING THE SUPPORTING PLAYERS WILL GIVE YOU A MORE SYMMETRICAL APPEARANCE AND HELP YOU AVOID INJURY DUE TO A MUSCLE IMBALANCE.

Watch guys in the weight room and it's easy to see what body part most of us work hardest: the arms. We want biceps like a longshoreman's, forearms like a blacksmith's.

"From a vanity standpoint, they're the muscles guys concentrate on the most," says John Abdo, a trainer of personal trainers in Santa Barbara, California.

Muscular arms are useful as well as aesthetically pleasing—for moving furniture, for helping your honey wrest that stubborn lid off the salsa jar, and for making some oaf think twice about picking a fight with you.

Powerful arms also help you to better perform some exercises aimed at developing other parts of your body. Seated rows, for example, develop your lats and upper back, but it helps to have strong arms to pull the pulley handle toward you.

Work your arm muscles last during an upper-body workout. Otherwise, they may fail you when you need them to perform heavy-lifting exercises for your chest and back muscles.

Here are some facts about each of the arms' muscle groups—stuff that's good to know as you watch them grow.

UPPER ARMS

The gaudiest arm muscles are the biceps. If somebody asked you to make a muscle, it's the biceps muscles, of course, that you would flex. Think of them as Karl Malone and your other arm muscles as the subtler but equally important John Stockton. Very different, but a team.

The biceps actually is two muscles. In fact, its name means "two heads." The *biceps brachii* provides the "head" of the muscle, while the larger *brachialis* supports it underneath. Both are part of the elbow flexor muscle group that helps you bend your arm and bring your hand to your shoulder.

If you are just starting with a weight training program, it's better to begin with too little rather than too much weight. Too much weight leads to poor technique and greater risk of pulling a muscle.

Beginning weight lifters sometimes focus too much attention and effort on their biceps and try to force growth too quickly. Better to start out a little light and go up in weight later. It's easier and safer.

Bodacious biceps are great, but don't work them at the exclusion of your triceps. The triceps muscles run along the back sides of your upper arms and have three "heads."

On each arm, the triceps is the biceps' counterpart. It's part of the elbow extensor group that enables you to straighten out your arm and extend your hand away from your body. When you flex your biceps, the triceps relaxes. If you contract your triceps, your biceps goes limp.

Ignoring your triceps while you pump up the biceps increases your chance of injury, especially if you play sports. It's a common mistake men make.

By developing your biceps and triceps muscles in a balanced way, you'll maintain healthy shoulder and elbow joints.

"The triceps is a very impressive muscle," Abdo says. "It adds balance and symmetry not just to the arms but to how they tie into the shoulder." Unlike the biceps, a well-developed triceps muscle doesn't have to be flexed to stand out, Abdo adds. "A lot of times you can show a good definition just from a standing position, without having to bend the elbow at all."

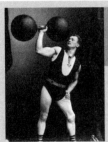

The record for the most pushups in 24 hours is 46,001, according to the *Guinness Book of Records*. The record number done in 1 year: more than 1.5 million. The most one-armed pushups: 8,794 in 5 hours.

LOWER ARMS

Unless you worship Popeye, chances are that you spend no more time considering your forearms than you do pondering what the salty sailor saw in Olive Oyl. Yet your forearms consist of three main muscle groups—brachioradialis, flexors, and extensors—that permit you to bend your wrists and squeeze and extend your fingers.

This in turn lets you have a firm handshake, make a fist, and grip a golf club or a bat.

Strong forearms also help you lift weights that work other muscles. "To some extent, grip strength has to be there in order to go up in weight," says Joe Ogilvie, a fitness instructor at Canyon Ranch in Lenox, Massachusetts, and Chelsea Piers Sports Center in New York City. "If your forearms fatigue too early, you're not going to be able to strengthen your biceps."

For some men, forearms develop easily. That's because almost every upper-body exercise requires a gripping action, so forearms and wrists benefit almost by accident. But these are isometric contractions. Abdo says:

It's best to include specific forearm and wrist exercises that include movement. Doing so will not only improve the appearance of your forearms but also help prevent elbow injuries such as "tennis elbow" that actually are forearm injuries.

Unless you participate in arm wrestling, rock climbing, golf, or another sport requiring a powerful grip, save forearm exercises for last, Ogilvie and Abdo advise. Since the forearm has small muscle groups, it fatigues easily.

BICEPS ► FREE WEIGHTS

HAMMER CURL

This exercise also works other elbow flexor muscles on the front of your arms.

[**A**] Stand straight with your feet shoulder-width apart and your knees slightly bent. Hold a dumbbell in each hand, with your arms fully extended at your sides and your palms facing in.

[**B**] Slowly curl the dumbbells until the ends touch your shoulders. Don't rotate your wrists while curling; do keep your upper arms and elbows stationary. Hold for a second, then lower the dumbbells slowly with a controlled motion to the starting position.

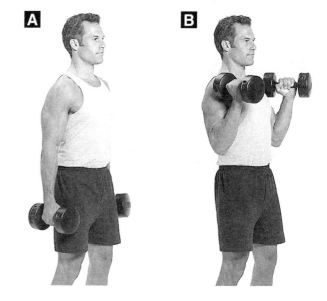

CONCENTRATION CURL

This exercise also works other elbow flexors.

[**A**] Sit in a chair or at the end of a weight bench with your feet a little more than shoulder-width apart. Hold a dumbbell in your left hand, your palm facing up and your arm fully extended. Rest your left elbow on your left inner thigh. With your right hand on your right thigh, bend forward slightly, keeping your back straight.

[**B**] Slowly curl the dumbbell up toward your shoulder, keeping your upper arm perpendicular to the floor. Hold for a second, then lower the dumbbell slowly with a controlled motion to the starting position.

Finish the set, then switch arms.

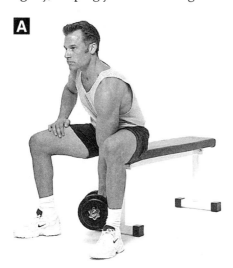

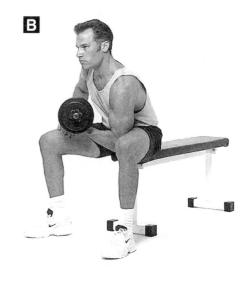

BARBELL CURL

This move strengthens other elbow flexors too.

[**A**] Stand straight with your knees slightly bent. Hold a barbell underhand (palms up), with your hands about shoulder-width apart. Your arms should be extended, and the barbell should be at your thighs.

[**B**] Keeping your elbows close to your body, use your biceps to curl the bar slowly up toward your chin. Keep your wrists straight throughout the curl, and don't sway your back or rock your body for momentum. Hold for a second, then lower the barbell slowly with a controlled motion to the starting position.

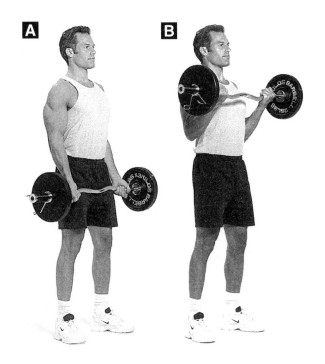

REVERSE-GRIP BARBELL CURL

Another great exercise for the elbow flexor muscle group on the front of your arms.

[**A**] Stand with your feet shoulder-width apart and your knees slightly bent. Hold a barbell in an overhand grip, with your hands spaced shoulder-width apart. Your arms should be fully extended, with the bar resting against your upper thighs. Keep your elbows close to your sides.

[**B**] Slowly curl the bar toward your chin. Hold for a second at the top of the lift, then lower the bar slowly with a controlled motion to the starting position.

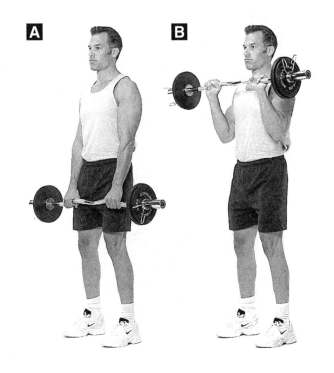

ALTERNATING DUMBBELL CURL

This is another exercise that works your elbow flexors.

Stand straight with your feet shoulder-width apart and your knees slightly bent. Hold a dumbbell in each hand with your arms down at your sides and your palms facing in.

[**A**] Slowly curl the left dumbbell up toward your collarbone. As you do the curl, rotate your arm so that your palm faces up. Hold for a second at the top of the lift, then lower the weight slowly with a controlled motion to the starting position.

[**B**] Repeat with your right arm.

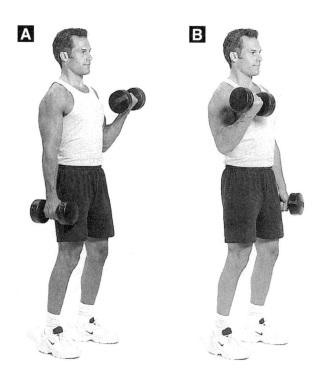

INCLINE DUMBBELL CURL

This gives your biceps a good workout.

[**A**] Holding a dumbbell in each hand, sit on an incline bench, keeping your head and upper body in full contact with the bench. Your feet should be flat on the floor. Let your arms hang down, fully extended and perpendicular to the floor, with your palms facing your body.

[**B**] Slowly curl the dumbbells up to your shoulders, keeping your upper arms stationary and your elbows pointed down. Your palms should turn up during the lift until they face your shoulders. Hold for a second, then slowly lower your arms with a controlled motion to the starting position.

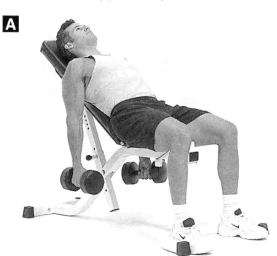

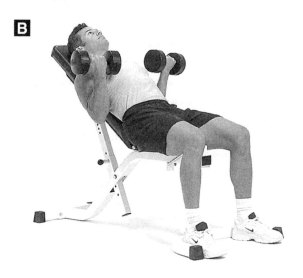

PREACHER CURL

This move works your elbow flexors, on the front of your arms.

[A] Sit on a bench with your arms hanging over a platform. Your elbows should be low on the platform, with your armpits almost touching the pad. Hold a curling bar with your palms facing up and your hands spaced closer together than shoulder width.

[B] Slowly curl the bar toward your chin, keeping your upper arms in contact with the pad. Hold for a second, then lower slowly with a controlled motion to the starting position.

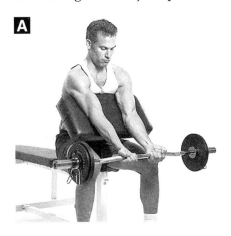

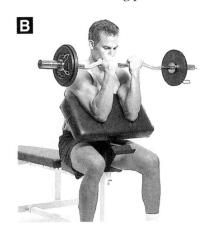

TRICEPS ► FREE WEIGHTS

SEATED OVERHEAD TRICEPS EXTENSION

This exercise works the elbow extensor muscles on the back of your arms. If your weight plates are removable, make sure the collars are tight.

[A] Sit on a bench with your feet firmly on the ground. Hold a dumbbell overhead, palms up. Keep your upper torso erect, facing forward, with a slight, natural forward lean in your lower back.

[B] Keeping your upper body in place and your upper arms close to your head, slowly lower the dumbbell behind you in a semicircular motion until your forearms are as close to your biceps as possible. You may lean slightly forward to help offset the weight, but don't sway or arch your back. Your elbows should face forward. Hold for a second, then raise the weight to the starting position.

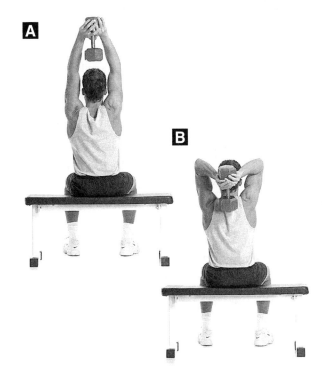

DUMBBELL KICKBACK

This exercise works your elbow extensors.

[**A**] Holding a dumbbell in your left hand, support yourself on an exercise bench with your right knee and your right hand. Keep your left foot on the ground, with your back straight and parallel to the floor. Your left arm should be bent 90 degrees.

[**B**] Slowly straighten your left arm and extend the weight behind your body, keeping your upper arm parallel to the floor. You should feel your left arm's triceps muscle fully contract. Then slowly bend your left arm again, bringing the weight back to the starting position.

Finish the set, then switch arms.

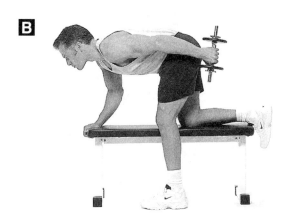

LYING CROSS-SHOULDER TRICEPS EXTENSION

This exercise works your elbow extensors. Note: *Overhead lifts can be dangerous. If your weight plates are removable, make sure the collars are tight. Beginners should use light weights and a spotter. Definitely use a spotter with heavier weights.*

[**A**] Lie on a bench with your head near one end, keeping your knees bent and your feet flat on the floor. Hold a dumbbell in your right hand, with your right arm extended straight up from your body and your palm facing your feet.

[**B**] Keeping your upper arm and your elbow stationary, slowly lower the dumbbell across your upper chest until the end touches your left shoulder. Then slowly extend your arm back to the starting position.

Finish the set, then switch arms.

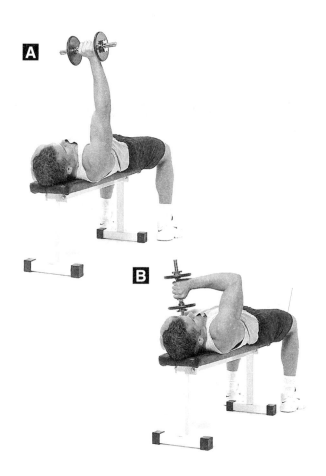

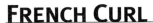

FRENCH CURL

This move works your elbow extensors. Caution: *To avoid facial injury, beginners should use light weights. A spotter is always a good idea.*

[A] Lie on your back on a weight bench with your knees bent and your feet resting on the bench. Hold a curling bar over your chest, with your palms facing up and away from you and your arms fully extended. Grip the bar with your hands spaced 4 to 6 inches apart.

[B] Keeping your upper arms stationary, slowly bend your elbows, lowering the weight toward the top of your head. Then slowly return the bar to the starting position.

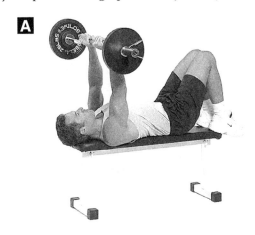

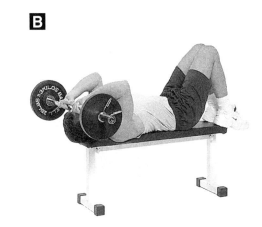

LYING TRICEPS EXTENSION

This move works the elbow extensors. Note: *Use less weight than you would for a French curl, and make sure the weight collars are tight.*

[A] Lie on your back on a bench with your head slightly over the end of the bench and your feet flat on the floor. Hold a dumbbell with both your thumbs around the bar and the weight resting on your palms. Extend your arms at about a 180-degree angle but not locked, the weight over the top of your head. Keep the bar vertical.

[B] Keeping your upper arms stationary, slowly bend your elbows, lowering the weight until it is behind your head. Hold for a second, then slowly return to the starting position.

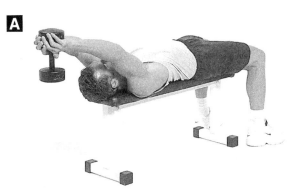

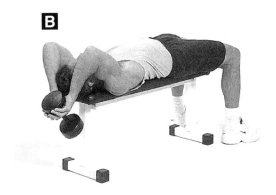

PARALLEL DIP WITH WEIGHT PLATE

This exercise strengthens the elbow extensor muscles on the back of your arms. Note: *If you have wrist problems, don't do this exercise.*

Place two exercise benches or two heavy chairs side by side, 3 to 4 feet apart.

[**A**] Sit on one bench and place a weight plate in your lap. Hold on to the edge of the bench with your arms shoulder-width apart and plant your heels firmly on the facing bench, about 6 inches in from the edge, suspending your butt slightly in front of your hands.

[**B**] Slowly bend your arms and lower your body toward the floor. Go as low as you can without touching the floor. Then slowly extend your arms, raising yourself back to the starting position.

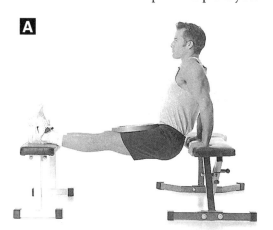

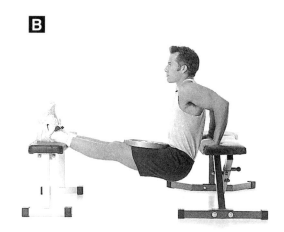

FOREARMS ► FREE WEIGHTS

FOREARM CURL

This exercise works the wrist flexor muscles on the front of your forearms. It also can be done with both hands and a barbell.

[**A**] Sit at the end of a bench with your legs slightly farther than hip-width apart. Hold a dumbbell in your left hand, palm up, and rest your right hand on your right thigh. Your left wrist should be slightly over your left knee so that you can bend your wrist through its full range of motion. The top of your left forearm should rest against your thigh. Your upper body should be upright, but you may lean slightly into your left leg for comfort.

[**B**] Slowly curl the dumbbell in a semicircular motion up toward your body as far as you can without letting your arm rise up off your thigh. At the top of the curl, hold for a second, then lower to the starting position.

Finish the set, then switch hands.

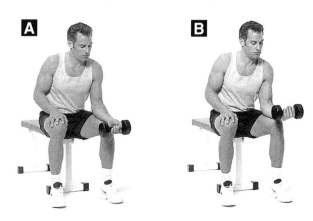

REVERSE FOREARM CURL

This exercise works your wrist extensors, on the back of your forearms. Note: *Use a lighter weight for this than you would for a normal forearm curl.*

[**A**] Sit at the end of a bench with your legs slightly farther than hip-width apart. Hold a dumbbell in your left hand, palm down, and rest your right hand on your right thigh. Your left wrist should be slightly over your left knee so that you can bend your wrist through its full range of motion. The meaty bottom part of your left forearm should rest against your thigh, and your upper body should be fairly upright, but you may lean slightly into your left leg for comfort.

[**B**] Slowly curl the dumbbell in a semicircular motion up toward your body as far as you can without letting your arm rise up off your thigh. At the top of the curl, hold for a second, then lower to the starting position.

Finish the set, then switch hands.

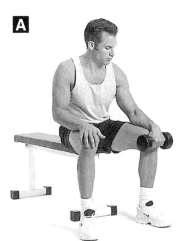

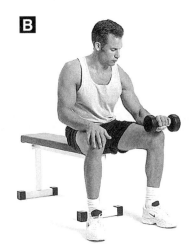

WRIST ROLLER

This move builds strength in your wrist flexors and extensors.

[**A**] Stand upright with your feet about shoulder-width apart. Hold the wrist roller in both hands (palms down) with your arms extended in front of you. The weight should be dangling in front of you.

[**B**] Slowly roll the weight up with your wrists, using long, exaggerated up-and-down movements with your wrists to work their full range of motion. Keep the rest of your body stationary; don't sway your body or drop your arms. When the weight reaches the top, slowly lower it using the same motion.

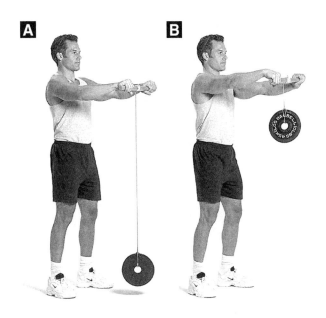

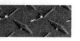

WRIST RAISE

This lift is also known as radial deviation; it works the muscles and tendons around your forearm's radius bone.

[**A**] Stand with your left arm at your side, grasping a hammer or a dumbbell with a weight on one end only. The weighted end should be in front of your hand.

[**B**] Slowly raise and lower the weight through a comfortable range of motion. Don't move your elbow or shoulder—all movement should occur at the wrist.

Finish the set, then switch arms.

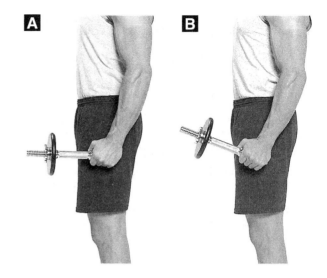

REVERSE WRIST RAISE

Also known as ulnar deviation, this exercise works the muscles and tendons around the ulna, the forearm bone next to the radius.

[**A**] Stand with your right arm at your side, holding the same weight you used for the wrist raise—but now the weighted end should be behind your hand.

[**B**] Slowly raise and lower the weight, using only your wrist. Again, don't move your elbow or shoulder.

Finish the set, then switch arms.

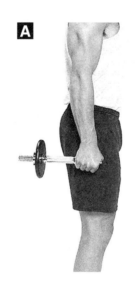
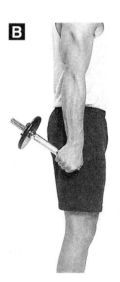

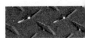

BICEPS ► MACHINES

CABLE CURL

This exercise also works other elbow flexor muscles on the front of your arms.

[**A**] Stand facing a low pulley with a bar handle on the cable. Place your feet shoulder-width apart about 1½ feet from the pulley post. Keep your knees bent and your back straight. Hold the bar underhand with both hands, your arms fully extended. Your shoulders should lean back slightly.

[**B**] Keeping your upper arms tight against your body and perpendicular to the ground, slowly curl the bar toward your chest. Pause for a second at the top, then slowly lower the bar to the starting position.

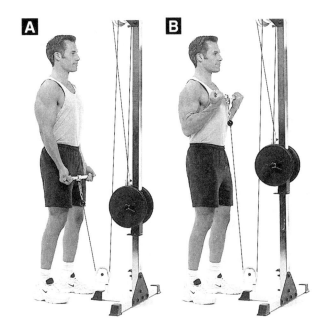

REVERSE-GRIP CABLE CURL

This exercise works other elbow flexors too.

[**A**] Stand facing a low pulley with a bar handle on the cable. Place your feet shoulder-width apart about 1½ feet from the pulley post. Keep your knees bent and your back straight. Hold the bar overhand with your hands about shoulder-width apart, your arms fully extended, and the bar resting against your upper thighs. Keep your elbows close to your sides.

[**B**] Slowly curl the bar toward your collarbone. Pause for a second at the top, then slowly lower the bar to the starting position.

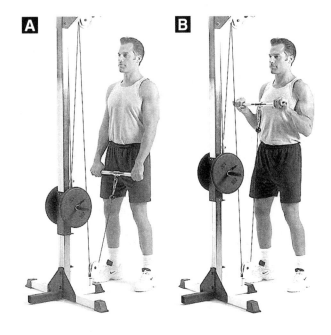

LYING CABLE CURL

This move also works other elbow flexors.

Position a weight bench so that one end is close to a multistation weight machine with a D-handle overhead pulley cable.

[A] Lie on your back on the bench, with your knees bent. Place your right hand under the small of your back for support, and hold the bar under-

hand with your left hand, your left arm fully extended. This is the starting position.

[B] Slowly curl the handle toward your shoulder. Pause for a second at the top of the movement, then slowly return to the starting position.

Finish the set, then switch arms.

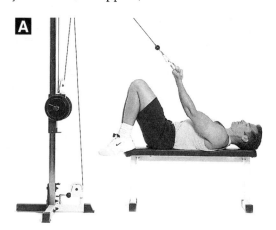

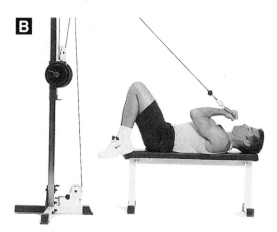

CONCENTRATION CABLE CURL

This exercise strengthens your elbow flexors.

Position a weight bench so that one end is close to a multistation weight machine with a D-handle low pulley cable.

[A] Sit on the bench with your feet a little more than shoulder-width apart. Hold the handle in your left hand, your palm facing up and your arm fully extended. Rest your left elbow on your left

inner thigh. With your right hand on your right thigh, bend forward slightly, keeping your back straight.

[B] Slowly curl the handle up toward your shoulder, keeping your upper arm perpendicular to the floor. Hold for a second, then slowly lower the handle to the starting position.

Finish the set, then switch arms.

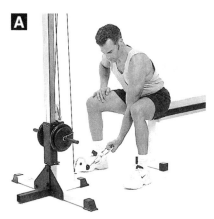

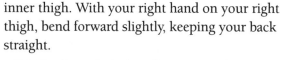

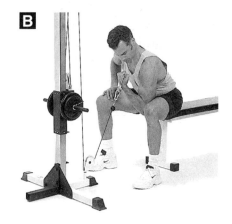

TRICEPS ► MACHINES

CABLE PUSHDOWN

This exercise also works other elbow extensor muscles on the back of your arms.

[**A**] Stand facing an overhead pulley with a bar handle on the cable, your legs shoulder-width apart and knees slightly bent. Hold the bar with both hands in a narrow, palms-down grip. Your forearms should be parallel to the floor. Keep your elbows and upper arms close to your body.

[**B**] Slowly and smoothly straighten your arms, pressing the bar down as far as you can without locking your elbows. Keep your wrists locked and straight. Hold for a second at the fully straightened position, then slowly allow the bar to rise to the starting position.

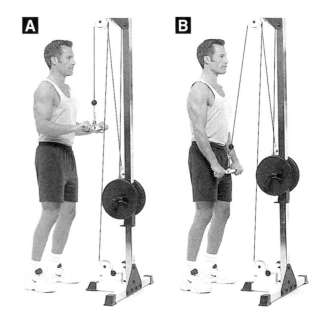

CABLE PULLDOWN

This move works other elbow extensors too.

[**A**] Stand sideways in front of an overhead pulley with a D handle on the cable. Your right shoulder should be closest to the equipment, your legs shoulder-width apart, and your knees slightly bent. Grip the handle with your left hand, your palm facing your body. Keep your upper arm vertical, with your elbow bent at about 45 degrees.

Take a step back so that the cable can move in a straight path across the front of your body, and bend forward slightly at the hips. Keep your back straight.

[**B**] Very slowly pull the handle down across your body until your arm is fully extended. Hold for a second, then slowly return to the starting position.

Finish the set, then turn around and switch arms.

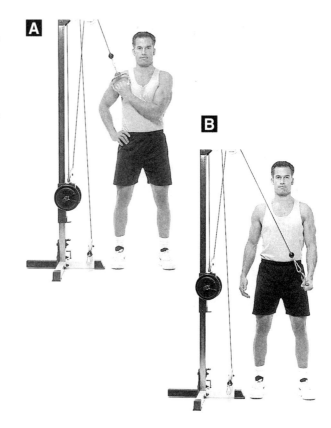

CABLE PUSH

This exercise also works other elbow extensors.

Position a weight bench close to a multistation weight machine, perpendicular to the front of the machine. While standing, grab the rope handle on the overhead pulley cable with both hands.

[**A**] Holding the handle, kneel at the bench and bend your elbows 90 degrees so that your fore-

arms are perpendicular to the floor. This is the starting position.

[**B**] Slowly push the handle downward until your forearms are fully extended. Hold for a second, then slowly return to the starting position.

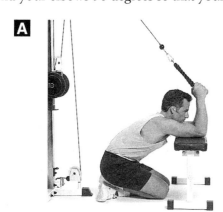 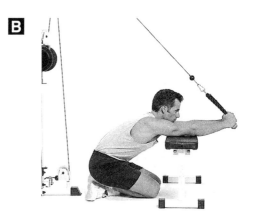

FRENCH CABLE CURL

This exercise works other elbow extensors too.

Position a weight bench so that one end is about a foot from a multistation weight machine with a bar-handle low pulley cable. While standing, grab the bar.

[**A**] Lie on your back on the bench with your head pointed toward the machine, your knees bent, and your feet resting on the bench. Grip the

bar with your palms facing up and away from you, your hands about 4 to 6 inches apart. Your elbows should be bent 90 degrees, with the bar just over the top of your head and your upper arms perpendicular to the floor.

[**B**] Slowly unbend your elbows until your arms extend directly out from your shoulders. Hold for a second, then slowly return to the starting position.

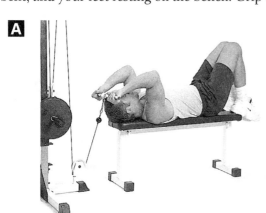 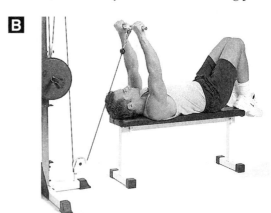

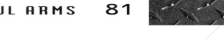

LYING CROSS-SHOULDER TRICEPS CABLE EXTENSION

This exercise works your elbow extensors.

Position one end of a weight bench near a D-handle low pulley cable. (For your right-arm sets, the bench should be slightly to the left of the machine.) While standing, grab the D handle overhand with your right hand.

[**A**] Lie on your back on the bench with your head pointed toward the machine, your knees bent, and your feet flat on the floor. Keeping your upper arm perpendicular to the floor, bend your elbow until one end of the handle touches your left shoulder.

[**B**] Keeping your upper arm and elbow stationary, slowly extend your arm until it points straight up from your body, your palm pointing toward your feet. Pause, then slowly lower.

Finish the set, then switch arms.

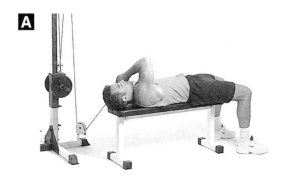

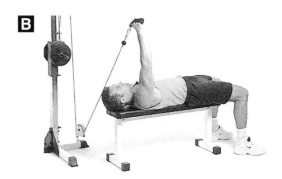

FOREARMS ► MACHINES

FOREARM CABLE CURL

This lift works your wrist flexors, muscles on the front of your forearms.

Position a weight bench so that one end is about a foot from a bar-handle low pulley cable.

[**A**] Sit at the end of the bench with your legs slightly wider than shoulder-width apart. Hold the bar palms-up with your hands about shoulder-width apart. Your wrists should be slightly over your knees so you can bend them through their full range of motion, and the tops of your forearms should rest on your thighs. Your upper body should be upright, but you may lean slightly into your legs for comfort.

[**B**] Curl the bar in a semicircular motion up toward your body as far as you can without letting your forearms rise up off your thighs. At the top of the curl, hold for a second, then lower.

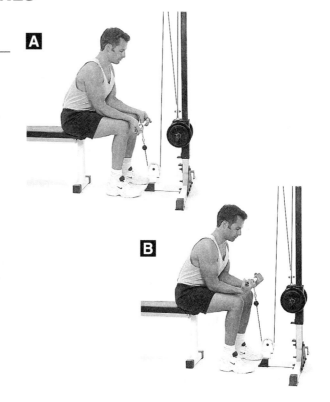

REVERSE FOREARM CABLE CURL

This exercise works your wrist extensors, muscles on the back of your forearms. Use less weight for this than you would for a normal forearm curl.

Position a weight bench so that one end is about a foot from a multistation weight machine with a bar-handle low pulley cable.

[**A**] Sit at the end of the bench with your legs slightly wider than shoulder-width apart. Hold the bar palms-down with your hands about shoulder-width apart. Your wrists should be slightly over

your knees so you can bend them through their full range of motion, and the meaty bottom parts of your forearms should rest against your thighs. Your upper body should be fairly upright, but you may lean slightly into your legs for comfort.

[**B**] Curl the bar in a semicircular motion up toward your body as far as you can without letting your forearms rise up off your thighs. At the top of the curl, hold for a second, then lower to the starting position.

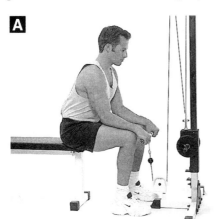

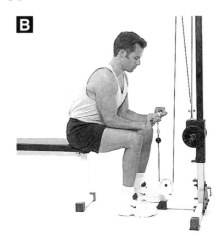

BICEPS ► NO WEIGHTS

BICEPS CURL WITH TUBING

This exercise works the elbow flexor, muscles on the front of your arms.

[**A**] Spread your feet shoulder-width apart and hook exercise tubing under each foot, grasping the handles with your arms fully extended.

[**B**] With your arms at your sides and your palms facing your body, slowly curl your right arm up, keeping your right elbow against your side. As your right hand passes your thigh, turn your wrist so that your palm faces up. Continue the curl until your hand reaches shoulder height. Slowly lower your arm to the starting position.

Finish the set, then switch arms.

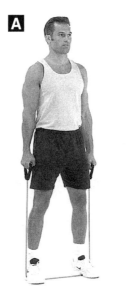

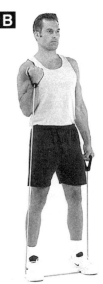

INCLINE CURL WITH TUBING

This exercise strengthens your elbow flexors.

Run a length of exercise tubing underneath the long bar that connects the feet of an incline bench.

[**A**] Sit on the bench and grasp the tubing's handles. (If necessary, run the tubing under the bottom of the seat, and take up any slack by wrapping the tubing around your hands.) Keep your head and upper body in full contact with the bench and your feet flat on the floor. Let your arms hang down, fully extended and perpendicular to the floor, with your palms facing your body.

[**B**] Slowly curl the tubing up to your shoulders, keeping your upper arms stationary and your elbows pointed down. Your palms should turn up during the curl until they face your shoulders. Hold for a second at the top, then slowly lower your arms to the starting position.

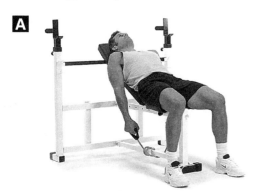

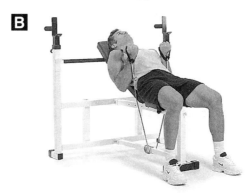

TRICEPS ► NO WEIGHTS

DESK DIP

This move strengthens your elbow extensors, on the back of your arms.

[**A**] Stand with your back to a sturdy desk and brace your palms on the edge, just outside the width of your hips. Keep your body rigid and slide your feet forward until your butt just clears the edge of the desk. Support your weight on your heels. This is the starting position.

[**B**] Slowly bend your elbows and lower your butt toward the floor, until your elbows are bent at a 90-degree angle. Push yourself back up to the starting position.

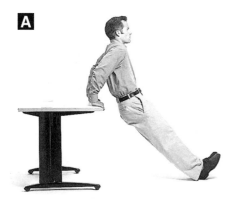

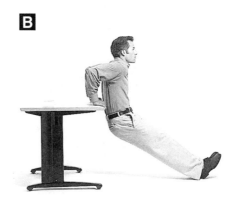

TRICEPS PRESS WITH TUBING

This exercise builds your elbow extensors.

Grasp one handle of exercise tubing with your right hand. Put that hand behind your neck and let the tubing fall down the center of your back, along your spine.

[**A**] Reach behind with your left hand and grasp the tubing at a spot that feels comfortable, probably near the small of your back. Hold the tubing tightly there so that it can't slip.

[**B**] Slowly raise your right hand above your head, keeping your elbow close to your head. Don't lock your elbow in the open position, but when it's almost fully extended, stop and slowly return to the starting position.

Finish the set, then switch arms.

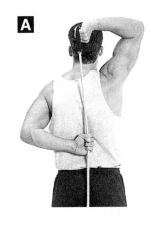

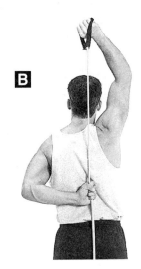

FRENCH CURL WITH TUBING

This move builds your elbow extensors.

Run a length of exercise tubing underneath the long bar that connects the feet of a weight bench.

[**A**] Lie on the bench with your feet touching the floor, and grasp the tubing's handles over your head, with your elbows bent and your palms facing away from you. (If necessary, run the tubing under the bottom of the bench itself, and take up any slack by wrapping the tubing around your hands.) Your hands should be about 4 to 6 inches apart.

[**B**] Keeping your upper arms stationary, slowly uncurl your arms over your chest until they are fully extended. Hold for a second, then slowly return to the starting position.

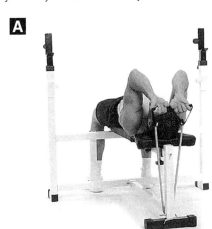

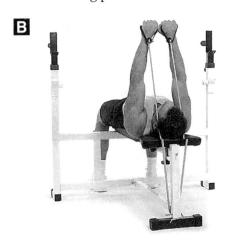

FOREARMS ► NO WEIGHTS

FOREARM CURL WITH TUBING

This move builds your wrist flexors, on the front of your forearms.

Sit at the end of a bench with your legs slightly farther than hip-width apart. Secure a length of exercise tubing under both feet.

[**A**] Hold the handles with your hands palms-up and your wrists slightly over your knees so you can bend your wrists through their full range of motion. The tops of your forearms should rest against your thighs, and your upper body should be fairly upright, but you may lean slightly into your legs for comfort.

[**B**] Slowly curl the tubing handles in a semicircular motion up toward your body as far as you can without letting your arms rise up off your thighs. At the top of the curl, hold for a second, then lower the handles to the starting position.

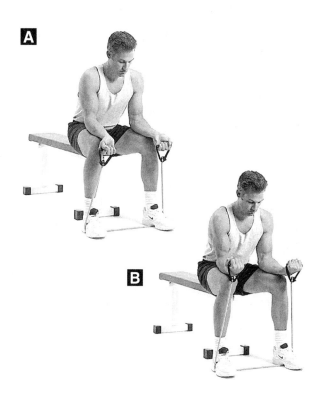

REVERSE FOREARM CURL WITH TUBING

This exercise builds your wrist extensors.

Sit at the end of a bench with your legs slightly farther than hip-width apart. Secure a length of exercise tubing under both feet.

[**A**] Hold the handles with your hands palms-down and your wrists slightly over your knees so you can bend your wrists through their full range of motion. The meaty bottom parts of your forearms should rest against your thighs, and your upper body should be fairly upright, but you may lean slightly into your legs for comfort.

[**B**] Slowly curl the tubing handles in a semicircular motion up toward your body as far as you can without letting your arms rise up off your thighs. At the top of the curl, pause, then lower.

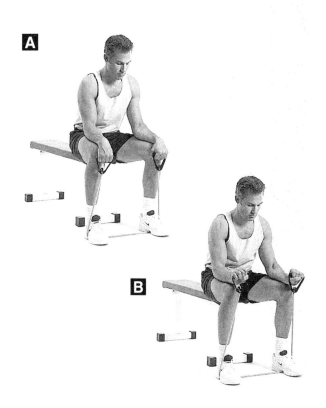

WRIST ROLLER WITH TUBING

This exercise works both the wrist flexors and wrist extensors.

Attach one end of a length of exercise tubing to the middle of a wrist roller bar, and secure the other end of the tubing under one foot. Stand upright, your feet about shoulder-width apart, and extend your arms in front of you, holding the wrist roller with both hands palms-down.

Slowly roll the bar in one direction using long, exaggerated up-and-down movements to work your wrists' full range of motion. Keep the rest of your body stationary; don't sway your body or drop your arms. When you can't roll the tubing any tighter, reverse the direction of the winding movement.

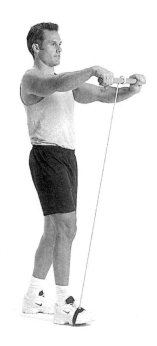

POWERFUL ARMS
BEGINNER WORKOUT

We recommend that you train with the balanced, full-body plan on page 48. If you need to concentrate specifically on arm work, though, this program will produce quick gains. Choose one exercise routine to follow: free weights, machines, or no weights.

INSTRUCTIONS

1. Do the complete exercise routine 2 or 3 days a week. Wait at least 48 hours between sessions. This allows enough recovery time for optimum development.

2. As a warmup, do some aerobics and stretching and perform one set of 6 to 10 repetitions with a light to moderate load. This minimizes the chances of a muscle strain or pull during the subsequent training period.

3. After you have completed the warmup, find a starting load that is difficult to lift 6 times. This may take some experimenting on your first day.

After you have identified that load, that's the amount of weight that you will use until it becomes too easy.

Complete one set of 6 repetitions for each exercise listed in the routine you've chosen. Perform the positive phase (also known as the concentric or lifting phase) of each exercise as quickly as possible while maintaining proper form. Perform the negative (or eccentric or lowering) phase much more slowly, to a count of four.

4. After a few sessions, 6 reps will seem easier. Add repetitions, following proper form, up to 10 reps.

5. When you are able to perform 10 repetitions, make a note to add weight the next session.

6. With the added weight, drop back to 6 repetitions. Then repeat steps 3 to 5 above until you have completed 12 weeks of the program. Then, if you still need to focus on arm workouts, you may move on to the intermediate level. Remember, we recommend that you do the balanced, full-body workouts rather than work on individual muscle groups.

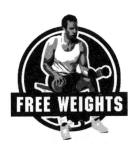

FREE WEIGHTS

1. HAMMER CURL (PAGE 68)
2. LYING TRICEPS EXTENSION (PAGE 73)
3. FOREARM CURL (PAGE 74)
4. REVERSE FOREARM CURL (PAGE 75)

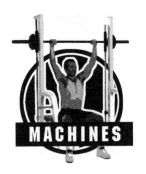

MACHINES

1. CABLE CURL (PAGE 77)
2. CABLE PUSHDOWN (PAGE 79)
3. FOREARM CABLE CURL (PAGE 81)
4. REVERSE FOREARM CABLE CURL (PAGE 82)

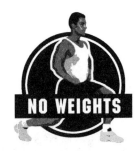

NO WEIGHTS

1. BICEPS CURL WITH TUBING (PAGE 82)
2. DESK DIP (PAGE 83)
3. FOREARM CURL WITH TUBING (PAGE 85)
4. REVERSE FOREARM CURL WITH TUBING (PAGE 85)

POWERFUL ARMS
INTERMEDIATE WORKOUT

We recommend that you train with the balanced, full-body plan on page 52. But if you need to concentrate specifically on arm work, this program will produce quick gains. Choose one exercise routine to follow: free weights, machines, or no weights.

INSTRUCTIONS

1. Train 3 days a week. To allow sufficient recovery, wait at least 48 hours between sessions.

2. Always warm up with some aerobics and stretching, plus one set of 6 to 10 repetitions using a light to moderate load. This minimizes the chances of a muscle strain or pull during the subsequent training period.

3. Your standard intermediate workout is three sets of 6 to 10 repetitions for each exercise listed in the routine you've chosen. The warmup set is your first set. The starting load for the second and third sets should be one that is difficult to lift 6 times. As your strength increases, increase the repetitions per set until you can do 10 repetitions while maintaining proper form. Then, for your next session, increase the load and drop back to 6 repetitions.

Perform the positive phase (also known as the concentric or lifting phase) of each exercise as quickly as possible while maintaining proper form. Perform the negative (or eccentric or lowering) phase much more slowly, to a count of four.

4. Vary your routines. Instead of some of the separate exercises, do combo lifts, or supersets, two exercises in succession (one rep of each) without a rest. You can do many of the exercises this way. Combo lifts increase the intensity of a workout, create some variety, and can shorten your workout sessions.

Another variation is to use a lighter load than usual and do 15 to 20 repetitions, and/or to increase the load on successive sets and reduce the number of repetitions (this last variation is called pyramids). So, for example, in set 1, you might do 10 repetitions with 200 pounds; in set 2, you might do 7 repetitions with 250 pounds; and in set 3, you might do 4 repetitions with 300 pounds.

5. As you gain training experience, you might try doing 1 or 2 partial repetitions at the end of each set, when you can no longer complete a full repetition. This is called going to muscle failure, and it may enhance muscle development. *Note:* If you try this, you will need a partner to spot you, especially with free weights.

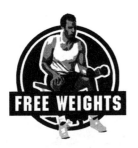

FREE WEIGHTS

1. CONCENTRATION CURL (PAGE 68)
2. SEATED OVERHEAD TRICEPS EXTENSION (PAGE 71)
3. PREACHER CURL (PAGE 71)
4. LYING CROSS-SHOULDER TRICEPS EXTENSION (PAGE 72)
5. REVERSE-GRIP BARBELL CURL (PAGE 69)
6. FOREARM CURL (PAGE 74)
7. REVERSE FOREARM CURL (PAGE 75)

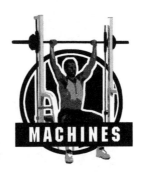

MACHINES

1. CONCENTRATION CABLE CURL (PAGE 78)
2. CABLE PUSHDOWN (PAGE 79)
3. CABLE CURL (PAGE 77)
4. CABLE PULLDOWN (PAGE 79)
5. REVERSE-GRIP CABLE CURL (PAGE 77)
6. FOREARM CABLE CURL (PAGE 81)
7. REVERSE FOREARM CABLE CURL (PAGE 82)

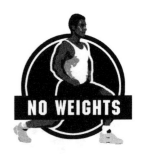

NO WEIGHTS

1. BICEPS CURL WITH TUBING (PAGE 82)
2. DESK DIP (PAGE 83)
3. INCLINE CURL WITH TUBING (PAGE 83)
4. FRENCH CURL WITH TUBING (PAGE 84)
5. TRICEPS PRESS WITH TUBING (PAGE 84)
6. FOREARM CURL WITH TUBING (PAGE 85)
7. REVERSE FOREARM CURL WITH TUBING (PAGE 85)

POWERFUL ARMS
ADVANCED WORKOUT

We recommend that you train with the balanced, full-body plan on page 56. If you need to concentrate specifically on arm work, however, this program will produce quick gains. Choose one exercise routine to follow: free weights, machines, or no weights.

INSTRUCTIONS

1. Train 3 days a week. Allow sufficient recovery by waiting at least 48 hours between sessions.

2. Your standard advanced workout is three sets of 6 to 10 repetitions for each exercise in the routine you've chosen. The first set, after your aerobics and stretching, is a warmup with a lighter-than-normal weight. The starting load for the second and third sets should be one that is difficult to lift 6 times. As your strength increases, increase the number of repetitions per set until you can do 10 repetitions. Then, for your next session, increase the load and drop back to 6 repetitions.

Perform the positive phase (also known as the concentric or lifting phase) of each exercise as quickly as possible while maintaining proper form. Perform the negative (or eccentric or lowering) phase of the exercise much more slowly, to a count of four.

3. Vary your workouts as at the intermediate level, and try replacing some of the exercises with tri-sets and giant sets. Tri-sets are like combo lifts except that you add another exercise so that you're doing three in succession without rest. With giant sets, you do four exercises in succession without resting between them.

4. Do 1 or 2 partial repetitions at the end of each set when you reach the point where you can no longer complete a full repetition. This is called going to muscle failure, and it may enhance muscle development. *Note:* At the advanced level, you always need the assistance of a partner for safety when doing partial reps with free weights.

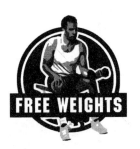

FREE WEIGHTS

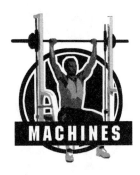

MACHINES

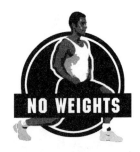

NO WEIGHTS

1. FRENCH CURL (PAGE 73)
2. PREACHER CURL (PAGE 71)
3. LYING TRICEPS EXTENSION (PAGE 73)
4. INCLINE DUMBBELL CURL (PAGE 70)
5. SEATED OVERHEAD TRICEPS EXTENSION (PAGE 71)
6. REVERSE-GRIP BARBELL CURL (PAGE 69)
7. LYING CROSS-SHOULDER TRICEPS EXTENSION (PAGE 72)
8. FOREARM CURL (PAGE 74)
9. REVERSE FOREARM CURL (PAGE 75)
10. WRIST RAISE (PAGE 76)
11. REVERSE WRIST RAISE (PAGE 76)

1. FRENCH CABLE CURL (PAGE 80)
2. CONCENTRATION CABLE CURL (PAGE 78)
3. CABLE PUSHDOWN (PAGE 79)
4. CABLE CURL (PAGE 77)
5. CABLE PUSH (PAGE 80)
6. LYING CABLE CURL (PAGE 78)
7. CABLE PULLDOWN (PAGE 79)
8. LYING CROSS-SHOULDER TRICEPS CABLE EXTENSION (PAGE 81)
9. FOREARM CABLE CURL (PAGE 81)
10. REVERSE FOREARM CABLE CURL (PAGE 82)

1. BICEPS CURL WITH TUBING (PAGE 82)
2. DESK DIP (PAGE 83)
3. INCLINE CURL WITH TUBING (PAGE 83)
4. FRENCH CURL WITH TUBING (PAGE 84)
5. TRICEPS PRESS WITH TUBING (PAGE 84)
6. FOREARM CURL WITH TUBING (PAGE 85)
7. REVERSE FOREARM CURL WITH TUBING (PAGE 85)
8. WRIST ROLLER WITH TUBING (PAGE 86)

QUICK-SET PATH TO
POWERFUL SHOULDERS

STRONG SHOULDERS ARE AN ASSET IN NEARLY EVERY ACTIVITY
IN WHICH YOU USE YOUR ARMS. BUT IN THE ZEAL TO BUILD THEM
UP, MANY MEN OVEREXTEND THEIR SHOULDERS AND END UP
INJURING THEM.

Does any part of the body so define a man as his shoulders? Is anything more synonymous with strength, both physical and mental? Consider: When Carl Sandburg described Chicago as a city of slaughterhouses, tool makers, and railroads, he called it "city of the big shoulders." And when we say that a man shouldered the load, we mean that he had the strength to assume a burden or responsibility.

Brawny shoulders are practical too. You need them to lift your son over your head (especially now that he's 18), to push your car when it's stuck in the snow, and to pull the other team into the mud at the tug-of-war contest at the company picnic. Plus, almost every upper body training exercise involves your shoulder muscles, so by strengthening them you will be able to lift heavier weights for your chest and back routines.

"Everything you do with your arms pretty much involves the shoulders," says Joe Sumrell, a five-time national champion professional bodybuilder and personal trainer in Boston.

Broad shoulders fairly scream one word: *stud!* People notice you. "If you get that V-shaped back that is accented with broad shoulders, it tapers the waistline," says John Abdo, a trainer of personal trainers in Santa Barbara, California.

"You'll get compliments both ways: 'Wow, your shoulders are getting bigger.' 'Look how skinny your waist is getting,'" says Abdo.

DAZZLING DELTOIDS

Your shoulder muscles are called deltoids, or delts in gym jargon. The deltoids are two large muscles whose name means "triangular in outline." There is one deltoid muscle in each of your shoulders, extending from your collarbone and shoulder blade to the humerus, the large bone in your upper arm.

The deltoids enable you to lift, rotate, and extend your arms. They can be broken down into anterior, lateral, and posterior, meaning the front, side, and back "heads" of the muscle.

Each area of the deltoids can and should be exercised individually. Doing so provides muscular balance and reduces your chance of injury.

"You get guys who just do bench presses—they're primarily working the front or anterior of the deltoids and some of the lateral, but they're certainly not getting the rear [back] head," Abdo says.

Beneath each deltoid is the rotator cuff: four muscles and tendons that keep your arm from popping out of the socket. Pitchers occasionally hurt their rotator cuffs, often jeopardizing their careers.

TRAIN THE TRAPEZIUS

This muscle raises your shoulder, rotates your shoulder blades, and helps you turn your head. The trapezius extends out and down from the neck and down between the shoulder blades. It's that big muscle you see bulging on each side of a bodybuilder's neck, like some concealed alien creature ready to explode from the skin.

Some guys have hunched shoulders because they give their trapezius less thought than their smelly gym gear. But for better-looking, less-injury-prone shoulders, the trapezius is worth working individually, says Sumrell.

It's not hard. "There is no way you can work your back without working your trapezius," he says.

THE BIG HURT

Shoulders are particularly prone to injuries during workouts. Here are some reasons why.

• **Overtraining.** Either a guy is doing an exercise (say, the bench press) too often or he's lifting too much weight. Or both.

HARD-BODY MOMENT

He's about the same height as those diminutive Olympic girl gymnasts, but Naim Suleymanoglu is no pixie. The 4-foot-11 Turk made history at the Olympic games in Atlanta in 1996 when he won his third gold medal in weight lifting—the most ever in the sport.

Dubbed the Pocket Hercules, Suleymanoglu set two world records in the 141-pound division: 413¼ pounds in the clean-and-jerk and 738½ pounds in total weight.

• **Unbalanced workouts.** Shoulder injuries may occur because this is a joint with a wide range of motion. "The tendency is not to do exercises that support that much range of motion," says Joe Ogilvie, a fitness instructor in Massachusetts and New York. That's why the Hard-Body Plan gives you plenty of shoulder exercises that work the whole range of motion.

• **Poor technique.** Many men have poor form when doing chest and overhead shoulder presses, stretching muscle tissue too much in the process, says Sumrell.

When you do shoulder exercises on an incline bench, be careful not to arch your back. Doing so gives you extra leverage to lift heavier weights but also exposes your lower back to injury.

As with other muscle groups, you should do simple stretches not only before you work the shoulders but also after, in order to minimize the risk of injury and remain flexible, Ogilvie says.

During your shoulder workouts, alternate between higher weight with fewer repetitions and lighter weight with more repetitions, Abdo advises. This enables you to exercise a variety of muscle fibers. "If you train the same way all the time, you're only going to develop one form of strength," he says.

To illustrate his point, Abdo tells the joke about the power lifter who can press 500 pounds but argues with his wife over who will take out the garbage. He doesn't want to because he lacks the endurance to carry the garbage can to the curb. A stereotypical marathon runner, by contrast, has the stamina to take out the garbage but lacks the power to pick up the can.

DELTOIDS ▶ FREE WEIGHTS

FRONT DELTOID RAISE

This move also works your pectoral, trapezius, and inner upper arm muscles.

[**A**] Stand straight with your feet shoulder-width apart, your knees slightly bent. Hold a dumbbell in each hand and let your arms hang at your sides, with your elbows slightly bent. Your palms should face your upper thighs. Lean forward slightly at the waist, keeping your elbows back, your chest out, and your lower back straight.

[**B**] Slowly raise your left arm in front of you until it's at shoulder height. The palm of that hand should face downward. Don't rock your hips or swing your arms for momentum. Hold for a second, then slowly return to the starting position.

Finish the set, then switch arms.

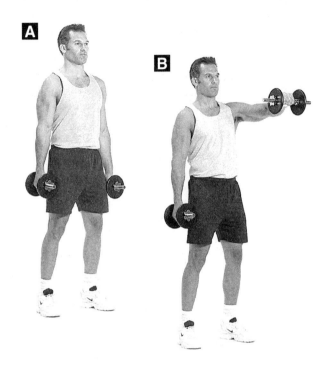

SIDE DELTOID RAISE

This exercise targets your side deltoids.

[**A**] Stand upright, arms at your sides, holding a dumbbell in each hand, with your palms facing your body and your elbows slightly bent. Keep your shoulders back, your chest out, and your lower back straight with a slight forward lean. Your feet should be shoulder-width apart.

[**B**] Slowly raise both dumbbells in unison in a straight line until they're at shoulder level. Make sure that your elbows are slightly bent, and keep your arms in the same plane as your torso. Hold for a second, then slowly lower your arms to the starting position.

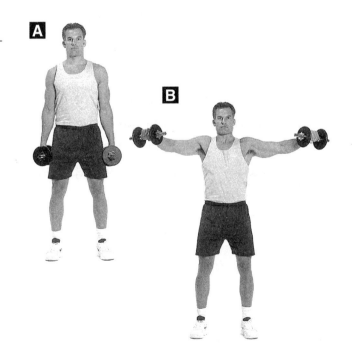

BENT-OVER LATERAL RAISE

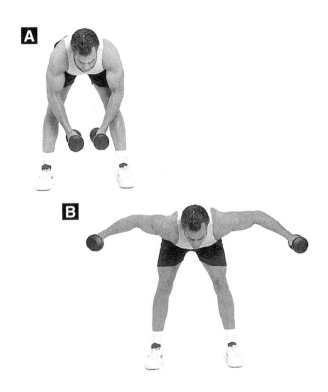

This exercise emphasizes your back deltoids.

[**A**] Bend over at the waist with a dumbbell in each hand, your arms before you and your elbows slightly bent. Your palms should face each other. Place your feet slightly farther than shoulder-width apart, and keep your back straight and roughly parallel to the floor.

[**B**] Slowly raise the dumbbells in unison out toward your sides as if you were flapping your arms. Raise your arms until they're parallel to the floor, keeping your back straight. Hold for a second, then slowly return to the starting position.

BEHIND-THE-NECK PRESS WITH BARBELL

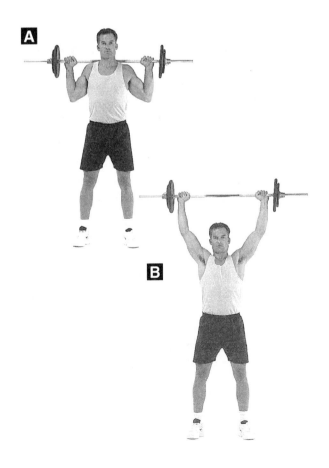

This all-purpose exercise targets not only your front and back deltoids but also your pectoral, upper back, triceps, and rib cage muscles. It is equally effective when done in front of the neck, which some experts consider a safer variation. Caution: Use lighter-than-usual weights to start.

[**A**] Stand with your back straight, your feet shoulder-width apart, and your knees slightly bent. Hold a barbell behind your neck across the top of your shoulders. Your hands should be slightly more than shoulder-width apart, palms facing forward. Keep your elbows pointing down and your chest high.

[**B**] Slowly raise the barbell straight up, keeping your elbows pointed outward. Pull your head slightly forward to allow space for the bar to move. Hold for a second, then slowly lower the bar to the starting position.

OVERHEAD PRESS WITH BARBELL

This move targets your front and side deltoids.

Stand with your back straight, your feet shoulder-width apart, and your knees slightly bent. Hold a barbell overhand, with your hands shoulder-width or slightly farther apart.

[A] Bend your elbows and raise the bar to shoulder level. Keep your elbows pointing down and your chest high.

[B] Slowly lift the barbell straight over your head. Hold for a second, then slowly lower it to chest level and repeat.

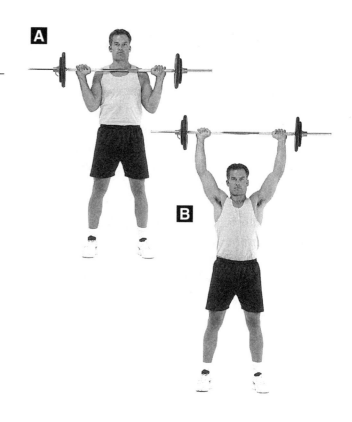

LYING SIDE DELTOID RAISE

This exercise also works your trapezius and shoulder blade muscles.

[A] Stand facing an incline bench, your chest against the incline. Your legs should be shoulder-width apart, feet on the floor, with your chin just above the top of the bench. Hold a dumbbell in each hand, with your arms dangling below the bench. Keep your elbows slightly bent and your palms facing each other.

[B] Slowly raise your arms to the sides until they're at about shoulder height, keeping your elbows relaxed. Hold for a second, then slowly lower to the starting position.

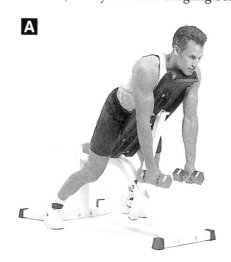

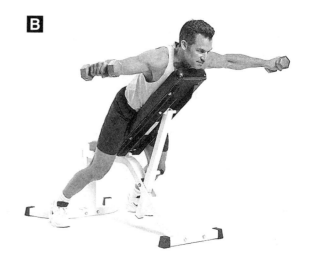

DUMBBELL MILITARY PRESS

This exercise works your front and side deltoids as well as your trapezius and triceps. Note: Since your arms must work alone, use less weight than for an overhead press.

[**A**] Sit on the end of a bench with your back straight. With your palms facing your body at shoulder height, hold a dumbbell in each hand.

[**B**] Slowly raise both dumbbells overhead until they almost touch. Extend your arms fully, but don't let your elbows lock. Pause for a second, then slowly lower the dumbbells to the starting position.

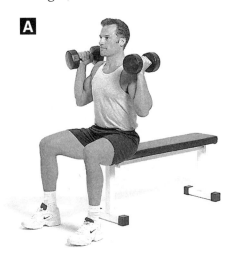

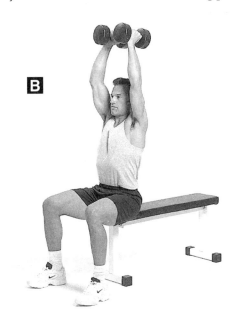

TRAPEZIUS ► FREE WEIGHTS

SHRUG

This exercise also strengthens your rhomboids, which lie between your spine and your shoulder blades.

[**A**] Stand straight with your feet shoulder-width apart and your knees slightly bent. Hold a dumbbell in each hand, letting your arms hang alongside your body. Your palms should face your body. Make sure your shoulders are back and relaxed.

[**B**] Slowly shrug your shoulders as high as they'll go, keeping your head still and your chin slightly tucked. Hold for a second, then slowly return to the starting position.

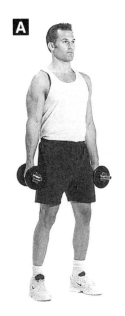

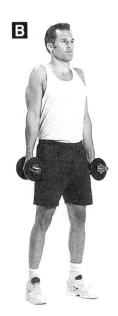

DELTOIDS AND TRAPEZIUS ► FREE WEIGHTS

UPRIGHT ROW

This exercise also strengthens your biceps and fore-arms.

[**A**] Stand upright holding a barbell in both hands, your palms down in a narrow grip. Your arms should be fully extended in front of you, with the barbell at your upper thighs. Allow your shoulders to relax slightly, but keep your back straight.

[**B**] Slowly pull the barbell straight up and tuck it under your chin. Your elbows should be pointing up and out. Hold briefly, then slowly lower the weight.

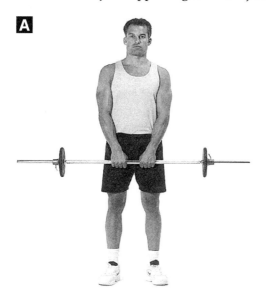

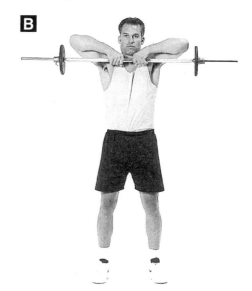

DUMBBELL RAISE

In addition to working your side deltoids and trapezius, this exercise builds your rhomboids, which lie between your spine and your shoulder blades, as well as your pecs and biceps.

[**A**] Stand with your back straight, your legs shoulder-width apart, and your knees slightly bent. Hold a dumbbell in each hand, with your arms hanging down and your palms facing your body.

[**B**] Slowly raise the weights as far as you can toward your armpits without jerking at the top of the lift. Keep your elbows pointing out and the weights close to your body. Hold for a second, then slowly lower your arms to the starting position.

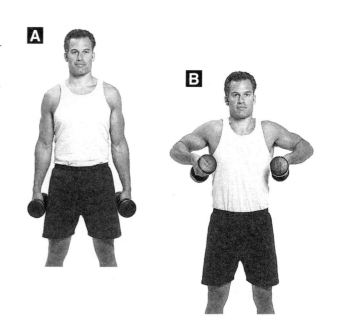

DELTOIDS ► MACHINES

OVERHEAD PRESS

This move strengthens your front and side deltoids.

Sit at a bench-press machine, legs a bit more than hip-width apart and feet flat on the floor. Pick up the weight bar and grip it overhand, with your hands shoulder-width or slightly farther apart.

[**A**] Bend your elbows and raise the bar to shoulder level. Keep your elbows pointed down and your chest high.

[**B**] Slowly lift the bar straight over your head. Hold for a second, then slowly lower it to chest level.

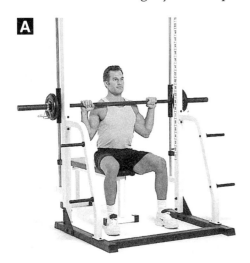

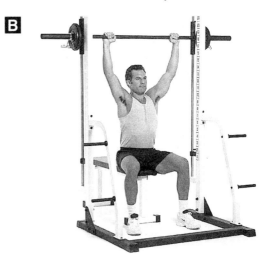

PULLEY RAISE

This exercise also works your trapezius and your rhomboid muscles, which lie between your spine and your shoulder blades.

[**A**] Stand sideways in front of a low pulley with a D handle on the cable. Your right shoulder should be closest to the machine—the closer you are, the better the resistance will be. Spread your legs shoulder-width apart and bend your knees slightly, keeping your back straight. Grip the handle with your right hand, your arms hanging down and your palms facing your body.

[**B**] Slowly raise the handle as far as you can toward your armpit without jerking at the top of the movement. Keep your right elbow pointing outward and the handle close to your body. Hold for a second, then slowly return to the starting position.

Finish the set, then turn around and switch arms.

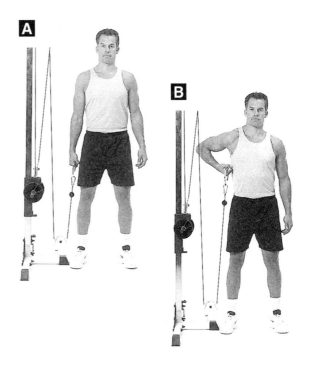

FRONT DELTOID PULLEY RAISE

This exercise works your shoulder flexors, the front portion of your deltoids.

Stand in front of a low pulley with a T handle on the cable. Keep your back straight, your feet shoulder-width apart, and your knees slightly bent.

[A] Grip the handle overhand with your hands about shoulder-width apart, your arms at your sides and your elbows slightly bent. Your palms should face your upper thighs. Lean forward slightly at the waist, keeping your elbows back, your chest out, and your lower back straight.

[B] Slowly raise the handle in front of you with arms extended until it is at shoulder height. Your palms should face down. Don't rock your hips or swing your arms for momentum. Hold for a second, then slowly return to the starting position.

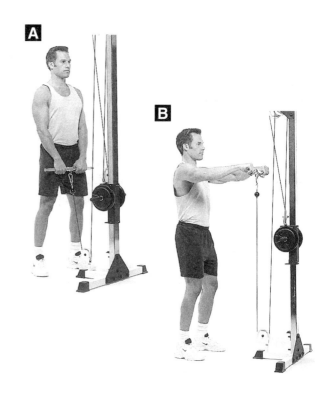

BEHIND-THE-NECK PRESS

This exercise also works your trapezius, pectoral muscles, and triceps as well as your rib cage muscles. It is equally effective when done in front of the neck, which some experts consider a safer variation.

Sit at a bench-press machine with your legs shoulder-width or farther apart and your feet flat on the floor.

[A] Grip the bar overhand. Keep your elbows pointing down and your chest high.

[B] Slowly push the bar straight up, keeping your elbows pointed outward, until your arms are fully extended but not locked. Hold for a second, then slowly return to the starting position.

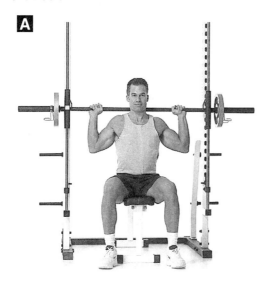

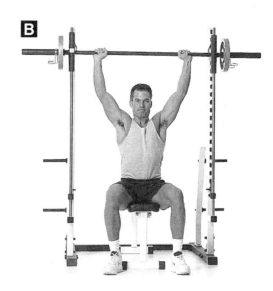

BENT-OVER CABLE LATERAL RAISE

As well as targeting your side and back deltoids, this exercise works your trapezius and your rhomboids, which lie between your spine and your shoulder blades.

Stand between two low pulleys with your feet shoulder-width apart and your knees slightly bent. With both hands, reach across your body to grasp the D handles on the opposite sides. Allow your arms to hang down, your elbows slightly bent and your forearms crossed. [A] Bend forward at the waist, keeping your back slightly arched but not rounded, until your upper body is parallel to the floor.

[B] Slowly raise your arms outward and upward as high as you can. Hold for a second, then slowly lower to the starting position.

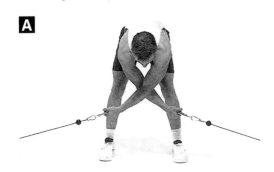

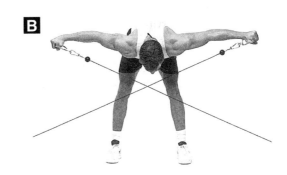

TRAPEZIUS ► MACHINES

PULLEY SHRUG

This exercise also works your rhomboids, which lie between your spine and your shoulder blades, and your levator scapulae, which lies under the trapezius.

Stand sideways in front of a low pulley with a D handle on the cable. Your right shoulder should be closest to the machine—the closer you are, the better the resistance will be. Position your legs shoulder-width apart and bend your knees slightly.

[A] Grip the handle with your right hand, both arms hanging down and both palms facing your body. Keep your shoulders back and relaxed.

[B] Slowly shrug your right shoulder as high as it will go, keeping your head still and your chin slightly tucked. Hold for a second, then slowly return to the starting position.

Finish the set, then turn around and switch arms.

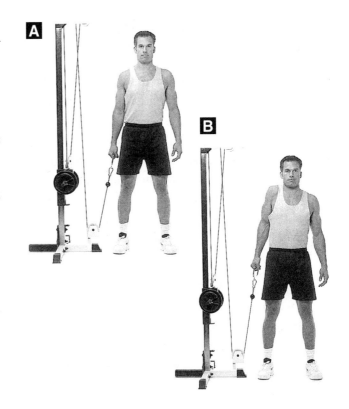

DELTOIDS AND TRAPEZIUS ► MACHINES

UPRIGHT PULLEY ROW

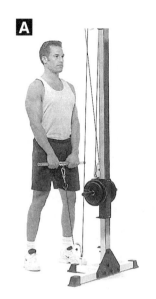
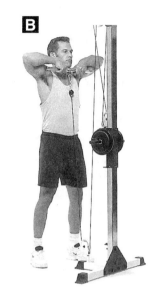

This exercise also strengthens your chest, biceps, and forearms.

Stand in front of a low pulley with a T handle on the cable. Keep your back straight, your knees slightly bent, and your feet shoulder-width apart.

[**A**] Grip the bar overhand with your hands 4 to 6 inches apart and your arms extended so that the bar touches your upper thighs. Allow your shoulders to relax slightly, but don't slouch.

[**B**] Pull the bar straight up and tuck it under your chin. Your elbows should point up and out. Hold briefly, then lower the weight to the starting position.

DELTOIDS ► NO WEIGHTS

FRONT DELTOID RAISE WITH BOOKS

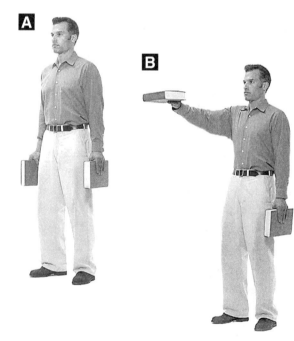

In addition to working key shoulder muscles, this exercise builds your trapezius, chest, and inner upper arm muscles.

[**A**] Stand straight with your feet shoulder-width apart and your knees slightly bent. Hold a book in each hand and let your arms hang at your sides, with your elbows slightly bent. Your palms should face your upper thighs. Lean forward slightly at the waist, keeping your elbows back, your chest out, and your lower back straight.

[**B**] Slowly raise your right arm in front of you until it's at shoulder height. The palm of your hand should face down. Don't rock your hips or swing your arms for momentum. Hold for a second, then slowly return to the starting position. Repeat once with your left arm. That's one repetition total.

LATERAL RAISE WITH BOOKS

This exercise works your side deltoids.

[**A**] Hold a book in each hand while you stand straight with your feet slightly apart and your knees unlocked. Place your hands at your sides with your palms facing your body.

[**B**] Slowly raise both arms outward as if they were wings flapping, keeping your elbows slightly bent and making sure that your thumbs are higher than your pinkies as you lift. Bring both arms up to shoulder height, hold for a second, and then slowly lower them back toward your sides. If you can't keep your wrists straight as you lift your arms, use lighter books that you can lift without bending at the wrists.

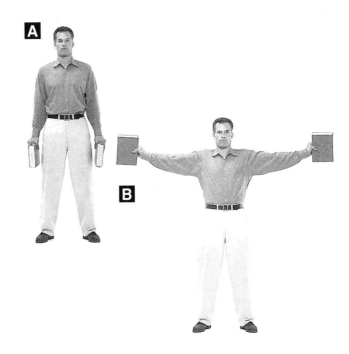

SHRUG WITH TUBING

This exercise also works your biceps, triceps, and forearms.

[**A**] Hook rubber exercise tubing taut under each foot and stand upright, grasping the handles of the tubing with your palms facing your body and your arms just in front of you.

[**B**] Slowly shrug your shoulders as high as they'll go, keeping your head still and your chin tucked. Hold for a second, then return to the starting position.

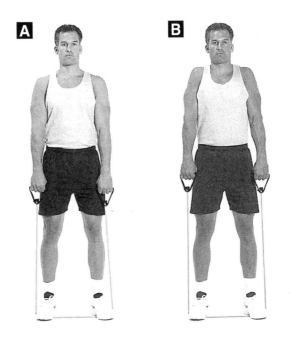

SHOULDER PRESS WITH BRIEFCASE

This exercise also works your upper back.

[**A**] Sit comfortably in a chair with your back straight, your knees bent, and your feet flat on the floor. Hold your briefcase by the bottom corners with your palms facing each other, and lift the briefcase directly in front of your face with your elbows bent and in at your sides.

[**B**] Slowly press the briefcase straight up toward the ceiling until your arms are fully extended above your head. Then slowly lower the briefcase back to the starting position in front of your face.

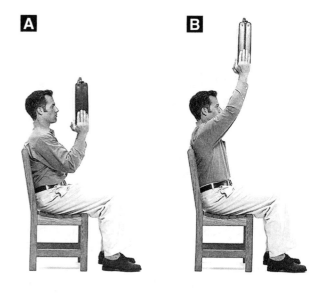

FOREARM RAISE WITH TUBING

This multipurpose upper-body exercise also works your biceps, your chest, and your rhomboid muscles (which lie between your spine and your shoulder blades).

[**A**] With your feet spread shoulder-width apart, hook some exercise tubing under each foot. Grasp the handles with your arms extended and facing your outer thighs. Let your shoulders relax slightly, but keep your back straight.

[**B**] Slowly raise the handles as far as you can toward your armpits without jerking at the top of the lift. Keep your back straight, your elbows pointing outward, and the handles close to your body. Hold for a second, then slowly lower your arms to the starting position.

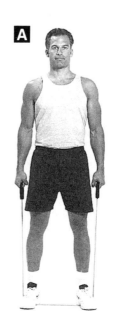
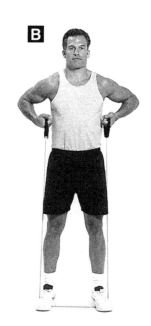

TRAPEZIUS ► NO WEIGHTS

PULLUP

This exercise is also a great workout for your rhomboids (between your spine and your shoulder blades) and for the latissimus dorsi muscles in your back.

[**A**] Stand at a chinning bar, grasping the bar overhand with your hands 18 to 20 inches apart. Your feet shouldn't touch the ground.

[**B**] With a slow, steady motion, pull yourself up until your chin is higher than the bar. Hold for a second, then slowly lower yourself to the starting position. Exhale on your way up, and inhale on your way down. Don't let your body swing.

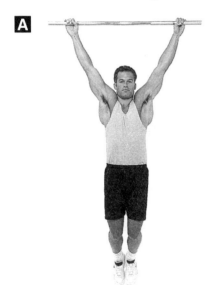

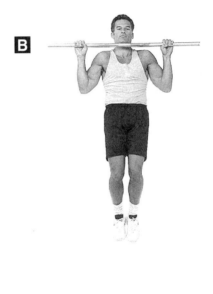

UPRIGHT ROW WITH TUBING

This exercise also strengthens your biceps, your entire back, and your rhomboids, which lie between your spine and your shoulder blades.

[**A**] Hook rubber exercise tubing under each foot and stand upright, grasping the handles with your arms fully extended and the tubing handles at your upper thighs. Grip the handles palms-down. Let your shoulders relax slightly, but keep your back straight.

[**B**] Slowly pull the handles straight up toward your chin, as high as you can. Your elbows should be pointing up and out. Hold briefly, then slowly return to the starting position.

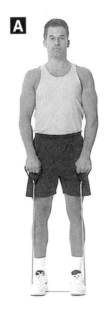

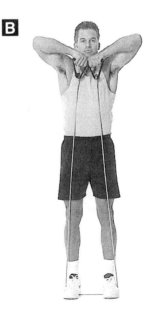

POWERFUL SHOULDERS
BEGINNER WORKOUT

We recommend that you train with the balanced, full-body plan on page 48. But if you need to concentrate specifically on shoulder work, however, this program will produce quick gains. Choose one exercise routine to follow: free weights, machines, or no weights.

INSTRUCTIONS

1. Do the complete exercise routine 2 or 3 days a week. Wait at least 48 hours between sessions to allow sufficient recovery time for optimum development.

2. Get warmed up by doing some aerobics and stretching and performing one set of 6 to 10 repetitions with a light to moderate load. This minimizes the chances of a muscle strain or pull during the subsequent training period.

3. After the warmup, find a starting load that is difficult to lift 6 times. This may take some experimenting on your first day. Once you have iden-

tified that load, that's what you will use until it becomes too easy.

Complete one set of 6 repetitions for each exercise listed in the routine you've chosen. Perform the positive phase (also known as the concentric or lifting phase) of each exercise as quickly as possible while maintaining proper form. Perform the negative (or eccentric or lowering) phase much more slowly, to a count of four.

4. After a few sessions, you will find that completing the 6 repetitions is easier. At that point, add repetitions, following proper form, up to 10 reps.

5. When you are able to perform 10 repetitions, make a note to add weight on the next session.

6. With the added weight, drop back to 6 repetitions. Then repeat steps 3 to 5 until you have completed 12 weeks of the program. Then, if you still need to focus on shoulder workouts, you may move on to the intermediate level. Remember, we recommend that you do the balanced, full-body workouts rather than working on individual muscle groups.

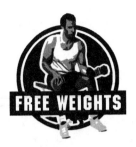

FREE WEIGHTS

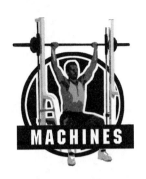

MACHINES

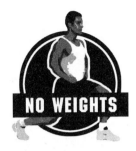

NO WEIGHTS

1. UPRIGHT ROW
   (PAGE 100)

2. SIDE DELTOID RAISE
   (PAGE 96)

3. FRONT DELTOID RAISE
   (PAGE 96)

4. OVERHEAD PRESS
   WITH BARBELL
   (PAGE 98)

1. UPRIGHT PULLEY ROW
   (PAGE 104)

2. BENT-OVER CABLE
   LATERAL RAISE
   (PAGE 103)

3. FRONT DELTOID
   PULLEY RAISE
   (PAGE 102)

4. OVERHEAD PRESS
   (PAGE 101)

1. UPRIGHT ROW WITH
   TUBING (PAGE 107)

2. LATERAL RAISE WITH
   BOOKS (PAGE 105)

3. FRONT DELTOID RAISE
   WITH BOOKS
   (PAGE 104)

4. SHOULDER PRESS
   WITH BRIEFCASE
   (PAGE 106)

POWERFUL SHOULDERS
INTERMEDIATE WORKOUT

INTERMEDIATE WORKOUT

We recommend that you train with the balanced, full-body plan on page 52. If you need to concentrate specifically on shoulder work, though, this program will give you quick gains. Choose one exercise routine to follow: free weights, machines, or no weights.

INSTRUCTIONS

1. Train 3 days a week. Allow enough recovery by waiting at least 48 hours between sessions.

2. Always warm up by doing some aerobics and stretching and performing one set of 6 to 10 repetitions with a light to moderate load. This minimizes the chances of a muscle strain or pull during the subsequent training period.

3. Your standard intermediate workout is three sets of 6 to 10 repetitions for each exercise listed in the routine you've chosen. The warmup set is your first set. The starting load for the second and third sets should be one that is difficult to lift 6 times. As your strength increases, increase the repetitions per set until you can do 10 repetitions while maintaining proper form. Then, for your next session, increase the load and drop back to 6 repetitions.

Perform the positive phase (also known as the concentric or lifting phase) of each exercise as quickly as possible while maintaining proper form. Perform the negative (or eccentric or lowering) phase much more slowly, to a count of four.

4. Vary your routines. Instead of some of the individual exercises, do combo lifts, or supersets, two exercises in succession (one rep of each) without a rest. You can do almost any two exercises this way. Combo lifts increase the intensity of a workout, create some variety, and can shorten your workout session.

Another variation is to use a lighter load than usual and do 15 to 20 repetitions, and/or to increase the load on successive sets and reduce the number of repetitions (this last variation is called pyramids). So, for example, in set 1, you might do 10 repetitions with 200 pounds; in set 2, you might do 7 repetitions with 250 pounds; and in set 3, you might do 4 repetitions with 300 pounds.

5. As you gain training experience, you might try experimenting with 1 or 2 partial repetitions at the end of each set at the point where you can no longer complete a full repetition. This is called going to muscle failure, and it may enhance muscle development. *Note:* If you try this, you will need a partner to spot you, especially when you're using free weights.

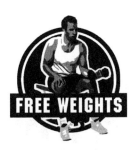

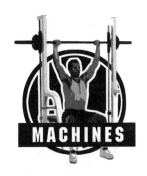

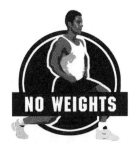

1. UPRIGHT ROW
   (PAGE 100)
2. SIDE DELTOID RAISE
   (PAGE 96)
3. BEHIND-THE-NECK
   PRESS WITH BARBELL
   (PAGE 97)
4. FRONT DELTOID RAISE
   (PAGE 96)
5. OVERHEAD PRESS
   WITH BARBELL
   (PAGE 98)
6. SHRUG (PAGE 99)

1. UPRIGHT PULLEY ROW
   (PAGE 104)
2. BENT-OVER CABLE
   LATERAL RAISE
   (PAGE 103)
3. BEHIND-THE-NECK
   PRESS (PAGE 102)
4. FRONT DELTOID
   PULLEY RAISE
   (PAGE 102)
5. OVERHEAD PRESS
   (PAGE 101)
6. PULLEY SHRUG
   (PAGE 103)

1. UPRIGHT ROW WITH
   TUBING (PAGE 107)
2. LATERAL RAISE WITH
   BOOKS (PAGE 105)
3. SHOULDER PRESS
   WITH BRIEFCASE
   (PAGE 106)
4. FRONT DELTOID RAISE
   WITH BOOKS
   (PAGE 104)
5. PULLUP (PAGE 107)
6. SHRUG WITH TUBING
   (PAGE 105)

POWERFUL SHOULDERS
ADVANCED WORKOUT

We recommend that you train with the balanced, full-body plan on page 56. If you need to concentrate specifically on shoulder work, however, this program will produce quick gains. Pick one exercise routine to follow: free weights, machines, or no weights.

INSTRUCTIONS

1. Train 3 days a week. Allow sufficient recovery time by waiting at least 48 hours between sessions.

2. Your standard advanced workout is three sets of 6 to 10 repetitions for each exercise in the routine you've chosen. After you do your aerobics and stretching, the first set is a warmup with a lighter-than-normal weight. The starting load for the second and third sets should be one that is difficult to lift 6 times. As your strength increases, increase the repetitions per set until you can do 10 repetitions. Then, for your next session, increase the load and drop back to 6 repetitions.

Perform the positive phase (also known as the concentric or lifting phase) of each exercise as quickly as possible while maintaining proper form. Perform the negative (or eccentric or lowering) phase much more slowly, to a count of four.

3. Vary your workouts as at the intermediate level, and try replacing some of the exercises with tri-sets and giant sets. Tri-sets are like combo lifts except that you add another exercise so that you're doing three in succession without rest. With giant sets, you do four exercises in succession without resting between them.

4. Do 1 or 2 partial repetitions at the end of each set when you reach the point where you can no longer complete a full repetition. This is called going to muscle failure, and it may enhance muscle development. *Note:* At the advanced level, you always need the assistance of a partner for safety when doing partial reps with free weights.

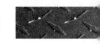

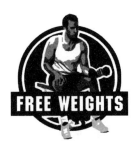

FREE WEIGHTS

1. UPRIGHT ROW (PAGE 100)
2. OVERHEAD PRESS WITH BARBELL (PAGE 98)
3. DUMBBELL RAISE (PAGE 100)
4. SIDE DELTOID RAISE (PAGE 96)
5. BEHIND-THE-NECK PRESS WITH BARBELL (PAGE 97)
6. FRONT DELTOID RAISE (PAGE 96)
7. SHRUG (PAGE 99)
8. BENT-OVER LATERAL RAISE (PAGE 97)
9. DUMBBELL MILITARY PRESS (PAGE 99)

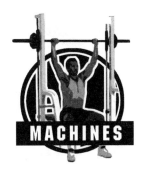

MACHINES

1. UPRIGHT PULLEY ROW (PAGE 104)
2. OVERHEAD PRESS (PAGE 101)
3. PULLEY RAISE (PAGE 101)
4. BENT-OVER CABLE LATERAL RAISE (PAGE 103)
5. BEHIND-THE-NECK PRESS (PAGE 102)
6. FRONT DELTOID PULLEY RAISE (PAGE 102)
7. PULLEY SHRUG (PAGE 103)

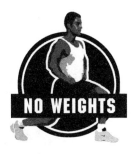

NO WEIGHTS

1. UPRIGHT ROW WITH TUBING (PAGE 107)
2. SHOULDER PRESS WITH BRIEFCASE (PAGE 106)
3. FOREARM RAISE WITH TUBING (PAGE 106)
4. LATERAL RAISE WITH BOOKS (PAGE 105)
5. SHRUG WITH TUBING (PAGE 105)
6. FRONT DELTOID RAISE WITH BOOKS (PAGE 104)
7. PULLUP (PAGE 107)

QUICK-SET PATH TO A
POWERFUL CHEST

A WELL-DEVELOPED CHEST EVOKES A POWERFUL IMAGE.
TO ACHIEVE ONE, INCORPORATE SEVERAL EXERCISES AND DO
CHEST PRESSES AT MANY DIFFERENT ANGLES TO WORK AS MANY
MUSCLE FIBERS AS POSSIBLE. DEVELOPING STRONG TRICEPS
AND DELTOIDS ALSO WILL HELP YOU BUILD YOUR CHEST.

Bigger than Arnold Schwarzenegger. Larger than Dolly Parton. That would be Isaac Nesser's chest. At a tad more than 74 inches, the Pennsylvania man's trunk is bigger than a coffee table. Make that a picnic table. Nesser's workout routine includes bench-pressing 560 pounds and curling 300-pound barbells.

PECS APPEAL

Nesser is a bit extreme, of course, but men do like developing their chests. And women like them to, too. It's a fact. In an experiment, 30 female undergraduates at Newcastle University in England ranked color photos of 50 men (faces weren't visible). The men with the best chest-to-waist ratios were ranked the most attractive.

Women prefer men whose torsos have an inverted triangle shape—a broad chest and shoulders and a narrow waist—researchers concluded.

A lot of guys have figured this out, of course, without the help of science. That's why some of them are willing to pay more for silicone pectoral implants than for a penis enlargement. Really.

Also, as with strong shoulders, a well-muscled chest gives you the power to push, whether it be a pit bull off your leg or an irate coworker at your throat.

And a colossal chest conveys strength and power. "A barrel-chested person just seems impervious to harm," says Michael Youssouf, manager of trainer education at Chelsea Piers Sports Center in New York City.

Read on and you'll learn how to develop your chest the old-fashioned way: by lifting weights.

IMPECCABLE PECS

Your chest muscles are called the pectorals, or more commonly pecs. The *pectoralis major* is by far the biggest. A thick, triangular muscle, it spans most of your collarbone and breastbone and connects to your upper arm.

The *pectoralis minor* is located beneath its big brother. You may also hear discussions of upper and lower pecs and clavicular (upper) and sternal (lower) chest fibers.

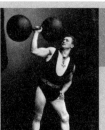

HARD-BODY FACT

If you're vacationing or on a business trip and can't hit the weight room, pushups are a tried and true alternative for working your pectoral muscles. To extend yourself to the max, try doing them with a chair or a low table that is about 18 inches high, suggests Joe Ogilvie, a fitness instructor in New York City and Lenox, Massachusetts. To do a decline pushup, you need to kneel on the floor in front of the chair or table with your hands shoulder-width apart and under your shoulders. Place your feet on the chair or table behind you. With your back straight and head in line with your spine, lower yourself until your chest almost touches the floor. (See the photos on page 125.) Pause in this position, then press back to the starting position. "If you can do 25 decline or standard pushups or two sets of 12, you're fairly strong," Ogilvie says.

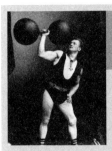

HARD-BODY FACT

The bench press is a long-standing favorite among guys who are working their chest muscle fibers. Since this exercise usually entails lifting quite a bit of weight, use a spotter, or make sure that somebody is nearby who can assist you in completing the repetition or the set should you become trapped underneath the bar.

Most men have success building up their chest muscles for the same reason they do their arms and shoulders, says John Abdo, a trainer of personal trainers in Santa Barbara, California. "I always say that the muscles closest to your head are the easiest to develop," he says. "You think about them more often because they are the first thing you look at in the mirror and what others tend to notice first about you."

Developing a muscled chest requires that you also build up your triceps and front deltoids, says Joe Sumrell, a fitness trainer in Boston who has won five national bodybuilding titles. The three work as a unit. Sometimes Sumrell has a client who has hit a plateau in his chest presses due to a deficiency in one of these other muscle groups.

"I strengthen those two muscle groups and all of a sudden, boom, his chest starts growing again," he says.

You can build up your chest muscles by doing chest presses on an incline bench, a flat bench, or a decline bench.

These angles will target your upper, middle, and lower pectoral muscles, respectively.

You don't need endless exercises at countless angles during every workout to develop your chest, but do try for variety over the course of a week or a month, Youssouf advises. "You need a multitude of tools to get the best chest development," he says.

A CHEST, NOT BREASTS

And now let's take a moment to address a concern that some of you have. You don't want to become anybody's bosom buddy. You're afraid that if you quit lifting weights after you have developed pec power, you'll have more jiggle than Jenny McCarthy . . . that, in profile, you'll look more like Pamela Anderson than baseball's Brady Anderson.

"That's a bunch of malarkey," Sumrell says, laughing. If you get fat once you stop lifting weights, you'll get fat everywhere, not just in your chest, he says.

"If a guy's chest turned into breasts, I'm pretty sure he'd have a big gut and a big butt, too," Sumrell says.

PECTORALS ► FREE WEIGHTS

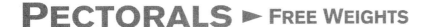

BARBELL OVERHEAD PULL

This exercise also works the latissimus dorsi in your back, as well as your rhomboids and your shoulder blade muscles. Use light weights.

[**A**] Lie flat on a bench with one foot to each side on the floor. With your palms facing your

feet, lift the barbell above your chest until your arms are perpendicular to the floor, keeping your elbows unlocked and slightly bent.

[**B**] Slowly lower the barbell behind your head in a semicircular motion until your upper arms are parallel to the bench or lower. Don't let your elbows form less than a 90-degree angle. Hold for a second, then slowly pull the barbell back over your head to the starting position.

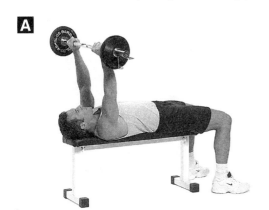

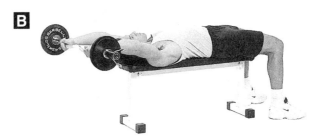

DUMBBELL FLY

This move also works your shoulder adductors, from your chest to inner arm, and flexors, across the front of your shoulders.

[**A**] Lie on your back on a bench with your legs parted and your feet firmly on the floor. Hold two dumbbells above you, your palms facing each other.

The dumbbells should nearly touch each other above your chest. Your back should be straight and firm against the bench. Don't lock your elbows.

[**B**] Slowly lower the dumbbells out and away from each other in a semicircular motion to chest level. Keep your wrists locked, your elbows bent at roughly 90 degrees, and your back straight. Hold for a second, then slowly raise the dumbbells to the starting position.

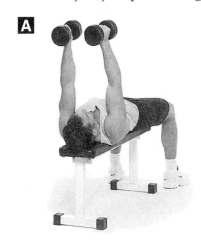

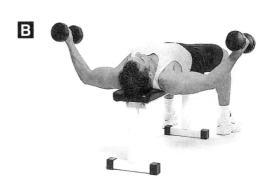

BENCH PRESS

This classic exercise also works your deltoids and triceps. Use a spotter for all bench-press exercises.

[**A**] Lie on a bench-press bench with a barbell above your chest. Grasp the barbell with your hands about shoulder-width or slightly farther apart. Your palms should face your legs, and your feet should rest on the floor. Keep your back straight and against the bench.

[**B**] Slowly lower the barbell to your nipple line. Your elbows should point down while the rest of your body remains in position. Don't arch your back or bounce the bar off your chest. Hold for a second, then slowly raise the barbell to the starting position.

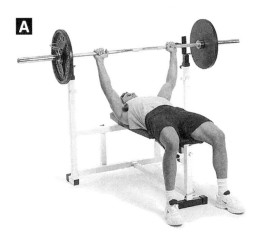

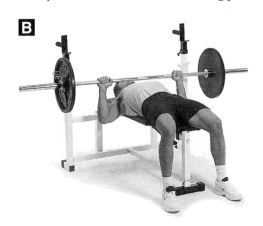

DUMBBELL BENCH PRESS

This exercise works your triceps slightly more than a barbell bench press does. As with the barbell version, use a spotter.

[**A**] Lie flat on a weight bench with a dumbbell in each hand, your arms fully extended and perpendicular to the floor. The ends of the dumbbells should almost touch. Your feet should be flat on the floor and your palms should face your feet. Keep your head and body in full contact with the bench.

[**B**] Slowly bend your elbows and lower your arms straight down until the weights are just above the sides of your chest. Your elbows should be no lower than your ears. Pause for a second, then slowly raise your arms back up again. Keep the weights under control: Don't arch your back or let the dumbbells bounce.

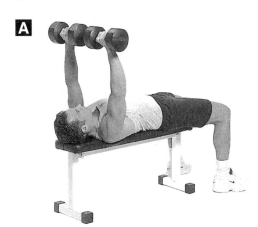

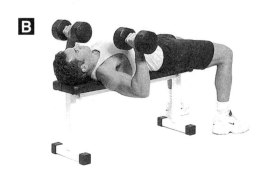

UPPER PECTORALS ► FREE WEIGHTS

INCLINE BENCH PRESS

This exercise builds your shoulders and rib cage muscles too. Use a spotter.

Lie on a 45-degree incline bench. Grasp the barbell with your arms shoulder-width apart and your palms facing your feet. Keep your back flat on the bench and your feet flat on the floor. [**A**] Press the weight off the barbell rack and completely extend your arms until they are perpendicular to the floor.

[**B**] Bend your elbows and slowly lower the barbell to just above your chest, between your shoulders and nipples. Pause for a second, then slowly raise the barbell over your chest again in a controlled movement. Try not to arch your back or bounce the bar off your chest.

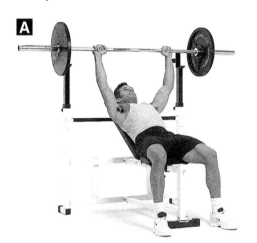

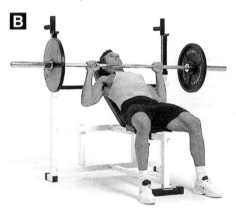

INCLINE DUMBBELL BENCH PRESS

This move builds your triceps. Use a spotter.

[**A**] Lie on a 45-degree incline bench with your arms fully extended and perpendicular to the ground. Hold a dumbbell overhand in each hand, your palms facing your feet, your arms shoulder-width apart, your back against the bench, and your feet flat on the floor.

[**B**] Slowly lower the weights to your shoulders, keeping your elbows pointing out. Pause for a second, then slowly extend your arms again in a controlled motion. Try not to arch your back or bounce the dumbbells off your chest at the bottom of the lift.

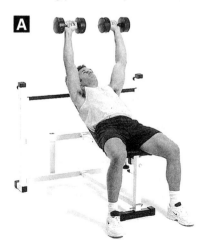

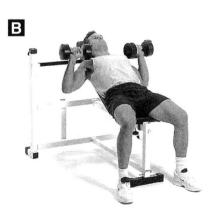

LOWER PECTORALS ► FREE WEIGHTS

DECLINE BENCH PRESS

This is similar to a regular bench press but stresses the lower portion of the pecs. Caution: This is a difficult and potentially dangerous move. Use lighter-than-usual weights and be sure to have a spotter. To avoid injury, use especially light weights until you master the movement.

Lie on a decline bench with your head under the barbell rack and your knees over the far end of the bench. Hook your feet under the support pads. With your arms shoulder-width apart, hold the bar using an overhand grip, palms facing your feet. [A] Lift the bar off the rack and hold it straight over your chest.

[B] Slowly bend your elbows, lowering the weight to just under your nipples, always keeping your elbows pointed out. Hold for a second, then slowly press the barbell back up in a controlled motion, extending it to arm's length.

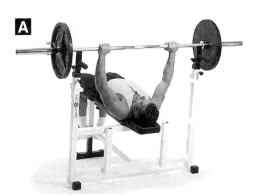

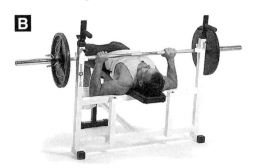

BENT-ARM PULLOVER

This move also strengthens the latissimus dorsi muscles of your back, as well as your triceps. Use lighter-than-normal weights until you get used to it. If the dumbbell's weight plates are removable, make sure the collars are tight before beginning.

[A] Lie crosswise on a bench with your head just off the end. Keep your torso straight and your feet flat on the floor. Hold a dumbbell by the end, palms up and thumbs around the bar. Your arms should be extended above your chest, your elbows slightly bent.

[B] Slowly lower the dumbbell backward over your head until your upper arms are parallel to the floor. Don't arch your back. Pause for a second, then slowly raise the dumbbell back to the starting position.

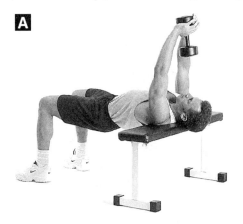

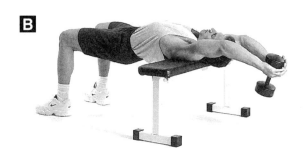

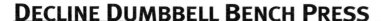

DECLINE DUMBBELL BENCH PRESS

Use a spotter for this exercise. Use especially light weights at first, to avoid injury.

[A] Lie on a decline bench with your knees over the far end of the bench. Hook your feet under the support pads. With your arms shoulder-width apart, hold a dumbbell overhand in each hand, your palms facing your feet. The dumbbells should extend straight over your chest at arm's length.

[B] Slowly bend your elbows, lowering the weights to just under your nipples, always keeping your elbows pointed out. Hold for a second, then slowly press the dumbbells back up in a controlled motion, extending them to arm's length.

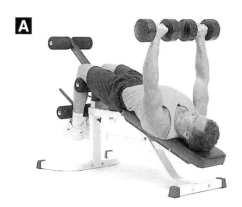

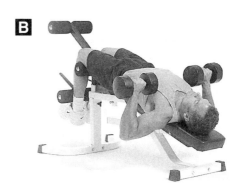

PECTORALS ► MACHINES

PEC DECK EXERCISE

This exercise also works your deltoid muscles.

[A] Sit at a pec deck machine with your feet flat on the floor and your back against the seat back. Keep your forearms against the pads and your arms in a straight line with your shoulders—no farther back.

[B] Use your elbows to slowly squeeze your arms together toward the center of your body until they can't go any farther. Keep your head up and your chest out as you squeeze. Hold for a second or two, then slowly return to the starting position.

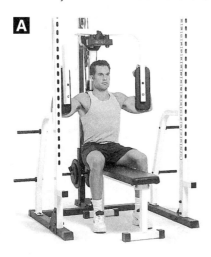

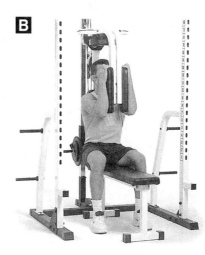

CABLE CROSSOVER

This move also strengthens your front deltoids. To avoid injury, start conservatively, with light weights, until you master the movement.

Stand between two overhead pulleys with D handles on the cables. Position your feet shoulder-width apart and grip the handles over-hand. Bend at the waist so that your upper body is parallel to the floor. [**A**] Keeping your elbows slightly bent and your wrists straight, pull the handles down until they are in line with your shoulders. This is the starting position.

[**B**] Slowly pull the handles down and in until they cross in front of your chest. Pause for a second, then slowly return to the starting position.

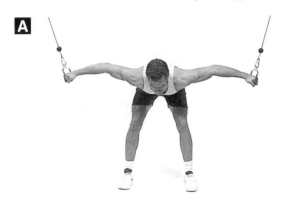

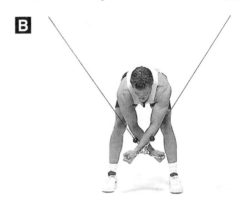

OVERHEAD PULLEY PULL

This exercise also works the latissimus dorsi muscles of your back, as well as your rhomboids and your shoulder blade muscles.

Position a weight bench so that one end is about 2 feet from a low pulley with a bar handle on the cable. Lie flat on the bench with your feet on the floor and your head pointing toward the pulley.

[**A**] Gripping the bar overhand, slowly lower it behind your head in a semicircular motion until your upper arms are almost parallel to the bench. Don't let your elbows form less than a 90-degree angle. This is the starting position.

[**B**] Slowly lift the bar above your chest until your arms are perpendicular to the floor, with your palms facing your feet. Keep your elbows unlocked and slightly bent. Hold for a second, then allow the bar to slowly return to the starting position.

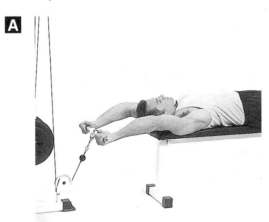

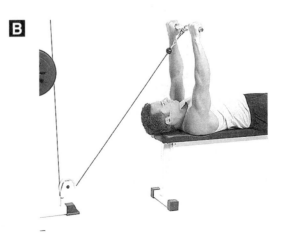

BENCH PRESS ON A MACHINE

This exercise also works your deltoids and triceps.

Lie on a flat bench at a machine with a bench-press station. The weight bar should be above your chest.

[A] Grasp the bar with your hands shoulder-width or slightly farther apart. Your palms should face your legs, and your feet should rest on the ground. Keep your back straight and against the bench.

[B] Slowly lower the bar to your nipple line. Your elbows should point out while the rest of your body stays in position. Don't arch your back or bounce the bar off your chest. Hold for a second, then slowly press the bar up again.

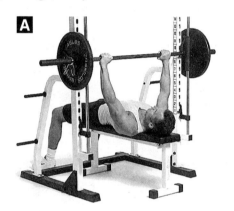

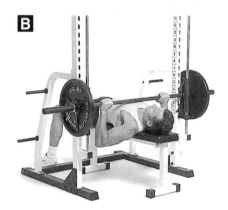

UPPER PECTORALS ▶ MACHINES

INCLINE BENCH PRESS ON A MACHINE

This move is similar to a bench press but places more emphasis on the upper portion of your pecs.

Lie on a 45-degree incline bench at a machine with a bench-press station. Grip the weight bar over-hand, your arms shoulder-width apart.

[A] Press the weight up until your arms are perpendicular to the floor, your elbows slightly bent.

[B] Slowly bend your elbows and lower the bar to just above your chest, between your shoulders and nipples. Keep your elbows pointing out, and keep your head and hips on the bench. Pause for a second, then slowly press the bar up again in a controlled movement, without arching your back or bouncing the bar off your chest.

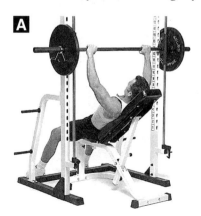

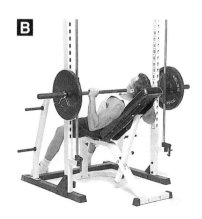

LOWER PECTORALS ► MACHINES

DECLINE BENCH PRESS ON A MACHINE

Caution: *This is a very difficult move. To avoid injury, use light weights until you've mastered the movement.*

Lie on a decline bench at a machine with a bench-press station. Your head should be under the weight rack and your knees over the far end of the bench. Hook your feet under the support pads.

With your arms shoulder-width apart, grip the weight bar overhand, your palms facing your feet.

[A] Lift the bar up and hold it straight over your chest. Your back, head, and shoulders should stay firmly on the bench.

[B] Slowly bend your elbows, lowering the bar to just under your nipples, always keeping your elbows pointed out. Hold for a second, then slowly press the bar up again with a controlled movement, extending it to arm's length.

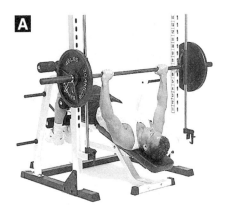
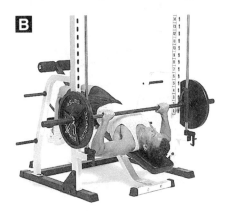

BENT-ARM PULLEY PULLOVER

This exercise also works your triceps and the latissimus dorsi muscles of your back. Use less weight than normal until you get the hang of it.

Position a weight bench 2 to 3 feet from a multi-station weight machine with a D-handle low pulley cable. The long edge of the bench should face the machine.

Lie crosswise on the bench with your head just off the end, gripping the pulley handle overhand with both hands. Keep your torso straight and your feet flat on the floor.

[A] Lower the handle backward over your head until your upper arms are parallel to the floor. This is the starting position.

[B] Slowly press the handle forward, extending your arms above your chest, with your elbows slightly bent. Don't arch your back. Pause, then slowly lower the bar back to the starting position.

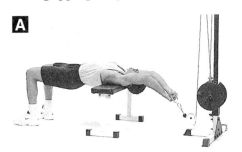
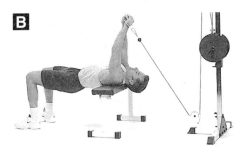

PECTORALS ► NO WEIGHTS

PUSHUP

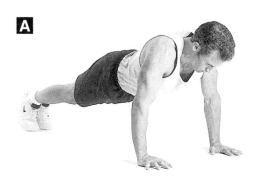

This classic exercise also strengthens your shoulders, arms, wrists, and upper back.

Lie facedown on the floor, balancing your weight on the balls of your feet and the palms of your hands.

[**A**] With your hands shoulder-width apart, extend your arms fully, but don't lock your elbows. Keep your legs together and fully extended and your fingers pointing forward. Make sure your legs, back, and neck are in a straight line, and keep your eyes on the floor.

[**B**] Slowly bend your arms, keeping your body straight and lowering yourself until your chest almost touches the floor. Hold for a second, then slowly return to the starting position.

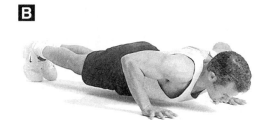

DECLINE PUSHUP

This is a more difficult variation on the standard pushup.

[**A**] Assume the standard position, with your legs together and your arms and legs extended. But instead of putting your feet on the ground, rest them on a weight bench. Keep your elbows slightly bent and your fingers pointing forward.

Keep your eyes on the floor and your legs, back, and neck in a straight line.

[**B**] Keeping your body straight, bend your arms, slowly lowering yourself until your chest almost touches the floor. Hold for a second, then slowly return to the starting position.

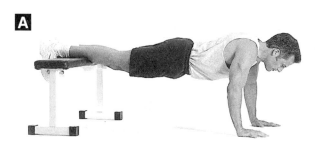

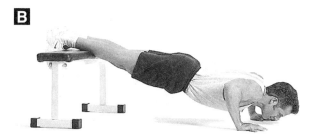

POWER PUSHUP

In this pushup variation, the emphasis is on speed (power) rather than strength.

Stand at the bottom of a flight of stairs.

[A] Let yourself fall forward, catching yourself with your hands by assuming a pushup position.

Your weight should rest on your palms and toes. Your legs and back should be straight.

[B] Immediately lower yourself and explosively push yourself back up to the starting position.

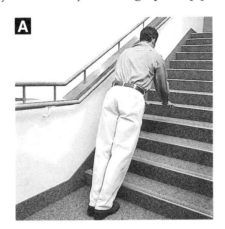

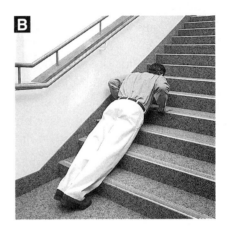

ONE-HANDED PUSHUP

This pushup variation works one side of the body at a time. One-handed pushups aren't for beginners. You need very strong arms and shoulders and good balance to avoid serious injury while doing this.

Place your right hand on the floor and twist your body sideways. Place your left hand behind your back. If you need to, put your left foot sideways on the floor for balance. Only the toes and ball of your right foot should touch the floor.

[A] Push yourself up with your arm—when it's straight and supporting your body weight, you're ready to begin.

[B] Slowly lower yourself until you're roughly 4 to 5 inches from the floor. As you go down, you may place your free hand on your hip for more balance. Hold for a second at the bottom, then push back up to the starting position.

Do 3 to 5 repetitions, then switch arms. Slowly work your way up to more repetitions.

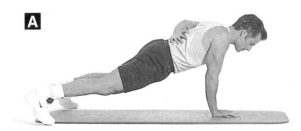

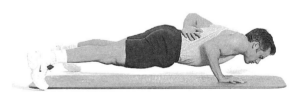

MILK JUG FLY

This exercise also works your shoulder adductors, from your chest to inner arm, and flexors, across the front of your shoulders. As you get stronger, add more water to the milk jugs.

[**A**] Lie on your back on a bench with your legs parted and your feet firmly on the floor. Hold two milk jugs above you, with your palms facing each

other. The jugs should nearly touch each other above your chest. Your back should be straight and firm against the bench, your elbows unlocked.

[**B**] Slowly lower the jugs out and away from each other in a semicircular motion to chest level. Keep your wrists locked, your elbows bent at roughly 90 degrees, and your back straight. Hold for a second, then slowly raise the jugs back to the starting position.

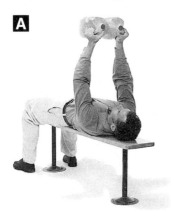

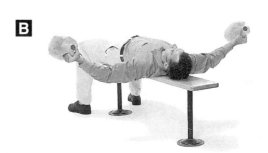

LOWER PECTORALS ► NO WEIGHTS

DIP

This versatile move also works your triceps, latissimus dorsi, and front deltoids.

[**A**] Raise yourself off the ground and onto parallel bars. Grip the bar handles with your fingers on the outsides. Keep your elbows close to your

sides, and slightly bend your legs if your feet drag on the floor.

[**B**] Slowly lower yourself until your upper arms are parallel to the floor. Keep your elbows close to your sides, and bend your legs slightly if your feet touch the ground. Then slowly raise yourself back to the starting position.

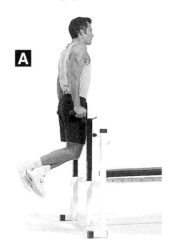

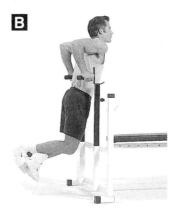

POWERFUL CHEST
BEGINNER WORKOUT

We recommend that you train with the balanced, full-body plan on page 48. If you need to concentrate specifically on chest work, however, this program will produce quick gains. Choose one exercise routine to follow: free weights, machines, or no weights.

INSTRUCTIONS

1. Do the complete exercise routine 2 or 3 days a week. Wait at least 48 hours between sessions to allow sufficient recovery time for optimum development.

2. To warm up, do some aerobics and stretching and perform one set of 6 to 10 repetitions with a light to moderate load. This minimizes the chances of a muscle strain or pull during the subsequent training period.

3. After the warmup, find a starting load that is difficult to lift 6 times. This may take some experimenting on your first day. After you identify that load, that's the amount of weight you will use until it becomes too easy.

Complete one set of 6 repetitions for each exercise listed in the routine you've chosen. Perform the positive phase (also known as the concentric or lifting phase) of each exercise as quickly as possible while maintaining proper form. Perform the negative (or eccentric or lowering) phase much more slowly, to a count of four.

4. After a few sessions, you'll find it easier to complete the 6 repetitions. At that point, add repetitions, following proper form, up to 10 reps.

5. When you are able to perform 10 repetitions, make a note to add weight on the next session.

6. With the added weight, drop back to 6 repetitions. Repeat steps 3 to 5 until you have completed 12 weeks of the program. Then, if you still need to focus on chest workouts, you may move on to the intermediate level. Remember, we recommend that you do the balanced, full-body workouts rather than working on individual muscle groups.

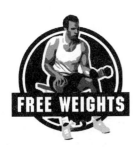

FREE WEIGHTS

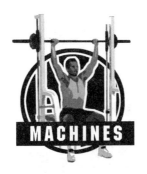

MACHINES

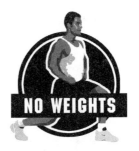

NO WEIGHTS

1. DUMBBELL BENCH PRESS (PAGE 118)
2. BENT-ARM PULLOVER (PAGE 120)
3. DUMBBELL FLY (PAGE 117)
4. BARBELL OVERHEAD PULL (PAGE 117)

1. BENCH PRESS ON A MACHINE (PAGE 123)
2. BENT-ARM PULLEY PULLOVER (PAGE 124)
3. PEC DECK EXERCISE (PAGE 121)
4. OVERHEAD PULLEY PULL (PAGE 122)

1. PUSHUP (PAGE 125)
2. MILK JUG FLY (PAGE 127)
3. DECLINE PUSHUP (PAGE 125)
4. POWER PUSHUP (PAGE 126)

POWERFUL CHEST
INTERMEDIATE WORKOUT

We recommend that you train with the balanced, full-body plan on page 52. But if you need to concentrate specifically on chest work, this program will produce quick gains. Choose one exercise routine to follow: free weights, machines, or no weights.

INSTRUCTIONS

1. Train 3 days a week. Allow enough recovery by waiting at least 48 hours between sessions .

2. Always warm up with aerobics and stretching, plus one set of 6 to 10 repetitions using a light to moderate load. This minimizes the chances of a muscle strain or pull during the subsequent training period.

3. Your standard intermediate workout is three sets of 6 to 10 repetitions for each exercise listed in the routine you've chosen. The warmup set is your first set. The starting load for the second and third sets should be one that is difficult to lift 6 times. As your strength increases, increase the repetitions per set until you can do 10 repetitions while maintaining proper form. Then, for your next session, increase the load and drop back to 6 repetitions.

Perform the positive phase (also known as the concentric or lifting phase) of each exercise as quickly as possible while maintaining proper form. Perform the negative (or eccentric or lowering) phase much more slowly, to a count of four.

4. Vary your routines. Instead of some of the individual exercises, do combo lifts, or supersets, two exercises in succession (one rep of each) without a rest. You can do almost any two exercises this way. Combo lifts increase the intensity of your workout, create some variety, and can shorten your workout session.

Another variation is to use a lighter load than usual and do 15 to 20 repetitions, and/or to increase the load on successive sets and reduce the number of repetitions (this last variation is called pyramids). So, for example, in set 1, you might do 10 repetitions with 200 pounds; in set 2, you might do 7 repetitions with 250 pounds; and in set 3, you might do 4 repetitions with 300 pounds.

5. As you gain training experience, you might try experimenting with 1 or 2 partial repetitions at the end of each set, at the point where you can no longer complete a full repetition. This is called going to muscle failure, and it may enhance muscle development. *Note:* If you try this, you will need a partner to spot you, especially when you're using free weights.

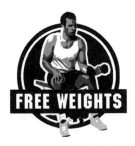

FREE WEIGHTS

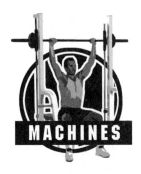

MACHINES

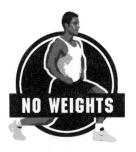

NO WEIGHTS

1. DUMBBELL BENCH PRESS (PAGE 118)
2. DUMBBELL FLY (PAGE 117)
3. INCLINE DUMBBELL BENCH PRESS (PAGE 119)
4. BENT-ARM PULLOVER (PAGE 120)
5. DECLINE DUMBBELL BENCH PRESS (PAGE 121)

1. BENCH PRESS ON A MACHINE (PAGE 123)
2. CABLE CROSSOVER (PAGE 122)
3. INCLINE BENCH PRESS ON A MACHINE (PAGE 123)
4. BENT-ARM PULLEY PULLOVER (PAGE 124)
5. DECLINE BENCH PRESS ON A MACHINE (PAGE 124)

1. PUSHUP (PAGE 125)
2. MILK JUG FLY (PAGE 127)
3. POWER PUSHUP (PAGE 126)
4. DIP (PAGE 127)
5. DECLINE PUSHUP (PAGE 125)

POWERFUL CHEST
ADVANCED WORKOUT

We recommend that you train with the balanced, full-body plan on page 56. If you need to concentrate specifically on chest work, however, this program will produce quick gains. Choose one exercise routine to follow: free weights, machines, or no weights.

INSTRUCTIONS

1. Train 3 days a week. Allow sufficient recovery by waiting at least 48 hours between sessions.

2. Your standard advanced workout is three sets of 6 to 10 repetitions for each exercise in the routine you've chosen. The first set, after your aerobics and stretching, is a warmup with a lighter-than-normal weight. The starting load for the second and third sets should be one that is difficult to lift 6 times. As your strength increases, increase the number of repetitions per set until you can do 10 repetitions. Then, for your next session, increase the load and drop back to 6 repetitions.

Perform the positive phase (also known as the concentric or lifting phase) of each exercise as quickly as possible while maintaining proper form. Perform the negative (or eccentric or lowering) phase of the exercise much more slowly, to a count of four.

3. Vary your workouts as at the intermediate level, and try replacing some of the exercises with tri-sets and giant sets. Tri-sets are like combo lifts except that you add another exercise so that you're doing three in succession without rest. With giant sets, you do four exercises in succession without resting between them.

4. Do 1 or 2 partial repetitions at the end of each set when you reach the point where you can no longer complete a full repetition. This is called going to muscle failure, and it may enhance muscle development. *Note:* At the advanced level, you always need the assistance of a partner for safety when doing partial reps with free weights.

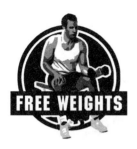

FREE WEIGHTS

1. DUMBBELL BENCH PRESS (PAGE 118)
2. DUMBBELL FLY (PAGE 117)
3. INCLINE DUMBBELL BENCH PRESS (PAGE 119)
4. BARBELL OVERHEAD PULL (PAGE 117)
5. DECLINE DUMBBELL BENCH PRESS (PAGE 121)

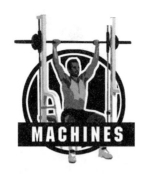

MACHINES

1. BENCH PRESS ON A MACHINE (PAGE 123)
2. PEC DECK EXERCISE (PAGE 121)
3. INCLINE BENCH PRESS ON A MACHINE (PAGE 123)
4. OVERHEAD PULLEY PULL (PAGE 122)
5. DECLINE BENCH PRESS ON A MACHINE (PAGE 124)
6. CABLE CROSSOVER (PAGE 122)

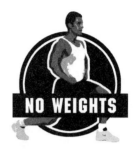

NO WEIGHTS

1. PUSHUP (PAGE 125)
2. MILK JUG FLY (PAGE 127)
3. ONE-HANDED PUSHUP (PAGE 126)
4. DIP (PAGE 127)
5. DECLINE PUSHUP (PAGE 125)
6. POWER PUSHUP (PAGE 126)

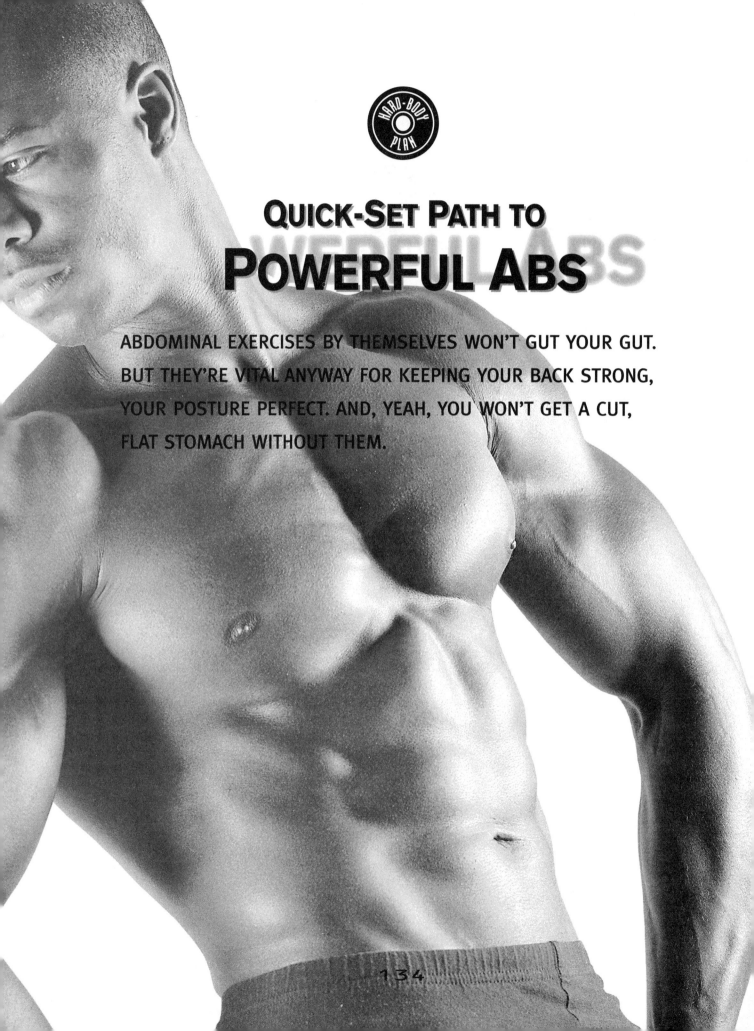

QUICK-SET PATH TO
POWERFUL ABS

ABDOMINAL EXERCISES BY THEMSELVES WON'T GUT YOUR GUT.
BUT THEY'RE VITAL ANYWAY FOR KEEPING YOUR BACK STRONG,
YOUR POSTURE PERFECT. AND, YEAH, YOU WON'T GET A CUT,
FLAT STOMACH WITHOUT THEM.

134

From Michelangelo's naked David to Calvin Klein's Marky Mark in briefs, men and women admire a guy with "washboard" abs. Achieving this look, however, can be as hard as squeezing a sumo wrestler into a Mazda Miata: difficult but doable.

BELLY BUSTERS

Hope you can stomach some bad news: Working your abdominal muscles will not by itself enable you to look like a cover model for *Men's Health*. Your belly could even get bigger. Here's why.

Men tend to store fat in their stomachs. So, "you can have the strongest abs, but if you have 3 inches of fat in front of them, you're still going to have 3 inches of fat. It's just going to be pushed out a little more," says Harvey Wallmann, a certified athletic trainer and strength conditioning specialist in Las Vegas.

Spot reducing—trying to lose weight in one part of your body by exercising that area—simply doesn't work.

In order to see those abdominal muscles rippling like plates of armor, you must combine aerobic exercise—walking, running, treadmill workouts, stairclimbing, and the like—with abdominal workouts and Hard-Body eating.

"It takes a lot of dedication and the proper mix of abdominal work and cardiovascular work to get that look," Wallmann says.

You supply the dedication. The Hard-Body Plan gives you the perfect mix.

The truth is, an overweight man who exercises them may have stronger abs than a slender fellow who doesn't. But is there any point to merely being a fitter fatty?

Well, yes. If your abdominal muscles are weak, you are more susceptible to having a weak back and poor posture. And a guy who slouches at staff meetings hardly evokes an image of vitality and power.

Strong abs are useful for staggering out of bed (something that's fun to do often and for about as many reasons as you can come up with), and they're good for rotating your body and for bending forward or leaning backward. Can you say "limbo"? *Cha, cha, cha.*

The abs actually consist of several muscle groups. Most notable is the *rectus abdominis*, which starts near the middle of the sternum and runs vertically to below your navel. It is this muscle group that, when well-developed, give guys that layered "washboard" or "six-pack" look.

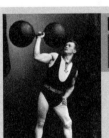

HARD-BODY FACT

You've seen those infomercials for gizmos and gadgets that claim that they'll take inches off your waistline and firm up your abs? Save your cash.

These products can't be classified as belly flops; some *are* helpful. But a study by researchers at California State University, Northridge, concluded that they aren't any better than your no-equipment-needed, basic, simple, time-tested crunch.

Beneath this muscle and out of sight is the *transversus abdominis*, which compresses and supports internal organs. Then there are the *obliques*, better known as love handles to those of us who have packed a few pounds around the middle. The external and internal obliques extend up and down your sides.

Abdominal muscles are amazingly useful when playing sports, Wallmann adds. When you're kicking a soccer ball, for example, they help you generate more power. And they assist you in weight training other muscle groups. "Think of the stomach as your core," suggests Brian Pfeufer, corporate program director at Sports Training Institute in New York City. "If the core is weak, then your extremities are weak. You want to be strong in the middle and work your way out."

CRUNCH TIME

You can crunch a lot of different exercises into an abs routine, but one popular move does the job and says it all: crunch. "Do a simple crunch and do it correctly, and you get a lot of benefit," Wallmann says.

The trouble is that a lot of guys do them wrong and do them too much.

Keep your knees bent and your feet on the ground and hip-width apart. Don't fling your body up or down, but move slowly and smoothly, Wallmann advises.

When you're lifting your body off the floor, it should be at 30 to 45 degrees to the floor. If you rise up all the way to your knees, you are exceeding 45 degrees, losing tension and working your hip flexor muscles, not your abs.

Remember the sadistic high school gym coach who made you do situps until you were sick? And how you laced your fingers behind your head when you did them? Well, don't do that. You're not in high school anymore. And if you were, you'd find that coaches nowadays know better. (You'd also get to work out with girls, in coed classes. They're doing a lot of things better now.)

Forget the interlaced fingers behind the head. Instead, place your fingertips near your temples or your ears. People have a tendency to yank their heads forward with their hands placed where the coach taught them, risking a neck injury in the process.

To put extra emphasis on your obliques during crunches, do a crossover crunch: Twist your torso to the right, with your left shoulder toward your right knee, then lower yourself and switch to the other side.

Learn to do the pelvic tilt.

Lie on your back with your knees bent, as if you were doing crunches. Keep your feet flat on the floor about hip-width apart. Place your arms wherever they feel most comfortable. Press your back down, pull your abs in, squeeze your butt, and tilt your hips until your butt curls an inch or two off the floor. Hold this position for a moment, then slowly lower your butt to the floor.

The pelvic tilt is a good abdominal exercise and it gets you in the habit of not arching your back during crunches, the bench press, and other exercises where doing so can injure your back, Pfeufer says. It also helps to strengthen your lower back.

Finally, don't get into a numbers crunch. Most guys wouldn't exercise their biceps or chest every day, doing dozens of repetitions in the process. But that's exactly what many of them do when it comes to abdominals, says Michael Youssouf, a trainer of fitness trainers in New York City. Exercise your abs just like other muscle groups, he advises.

ABS ► FREE WEIGHTS

HIP RAISE WITH ANKLE WEIGHTS

This move also works your gluteal (butt) muscles and the quadriceps muscles of your thighs.

Secure an ankle weight snugly around each ankle. [**A**] Lie flat on your back with your legs up in the air. Your knees should be unlocked and your toes pointed. Place your hands at your sides, palms down.

[**B**] Contracting your lower abdominal muscles and shifting your weight toward your shoulders, slowly lift your hips off the floor. Keep your legs in a vertical position throughout the exercise. Hold for a second, then slowly return to the starting position.

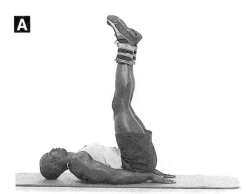

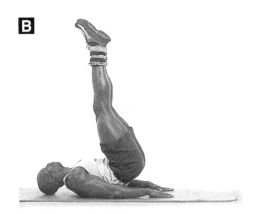

NEGATIVE SITUP WITH WEIGHT PLATE

This move works both your upper and lower abdominal muscles.

[**A**] Sit on the floor with your knees bent and your feet flat on the floor, shoulder-width apart. Place your feet under a support—the base of a weight machine, for example, or even your couch—to stabilize your lower body. Hold a weight plate to your chest. Begin with your upper body at slightly less than a 90-degree angle to the floor.

[**B**] Slowly lower your upper body toward the floor with your abdominal muscles contracted, curling your torso forward and rounding your lower back. When your body reaches a 45-degree angle to the floor, slowly return to the starting position.

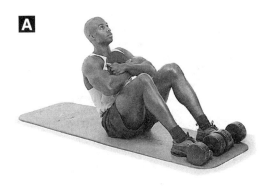

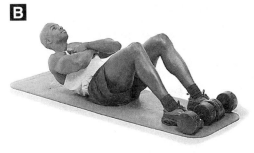

ABS AND OBLIQUES ► FREE WEIGHTS

OBLIQUE TRUNK ROTATION WITH WEIGHT PLATE

Do this exercise in one slow, continuous motion.

[**A**] Sit on the floor with your knees bent and your hands holding a weight plate against your chest. Place your feet under a support, such as the base of a weight machine, to stabilize your lower body. Hold your torso at a 45-degree angle to the floor.

[**B**] Start by slowly moving your torso to the left.

[**C**] Stay to the left as you lower to your back.

[**D**] Completing a clockwise rotation, slowly raise your torso to the right side.

Then repeat the exercise, this time moving down your right side and around to the left.

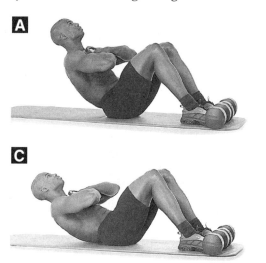

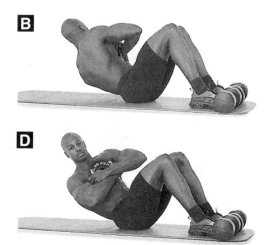

CURL-UP WITH WEIGHT PLATE

This move works both your upper and lower abs.

[**A**] Lie flat on your back, holding a weight plate behind your head with your elbows pointed out. Bend your knees about 45 degrees. Place your feet shoulder-width apart, about 6 inches from your butt. You may put them under a heavy object for stability.

[**B**] In a count of two, curl your upper torso in toward your knees, pressing your lower back to the floor and raising your shoulder blades as high off the ground as you can get them. Keep your knees in line with your feet, and don't pull your head with your hands. Then count to two again as you return to the starting position.

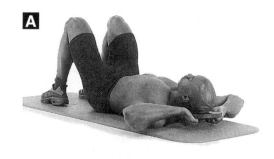

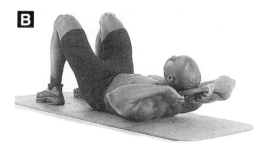

LEG RAISE WITH ANKLE WEIGHTS

This is a good general abdominal exercise.

Fasten an ankle weight around each ankle.

[**A**] Lie on your back on a bench with your hips near one end. Grasp the corners of the bench next to your hips and extend your legs straight out, your toes pointed.

[**B**] Keep your legs together with your knees unlocked, and slowly raise them to vertical, pressing your lower back into the bench. Then slowly lower your legs in a controlled motion until your body is completely horizontal.

Finish the set without resting between repetitions.

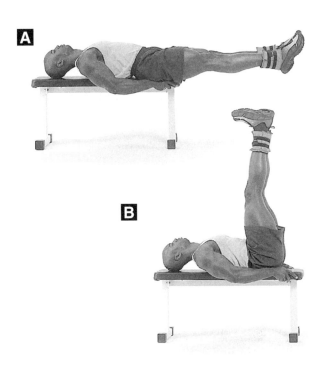

ROWING CRUNCH WITH ANKLE WEIGHTS

This move gives your abs a good overall workout.

Secure an ankle weight around each ankle. Sit on a bench with your knees bent and your feet flat on the floor. Grasp the sides of the bench for support and lean back to about a 45-degree angle.

[**A**] Keeping your knees slightly bent, extend your legs and raise them a few inches off the floor.

[**B**] While bringing your body to an upright positon, slowly pull your knees in to your chest as far as you can without losing your balance. Hold for a second, then simultaneously return your upper body and legs to the starting position, keeping your back straight as you go.

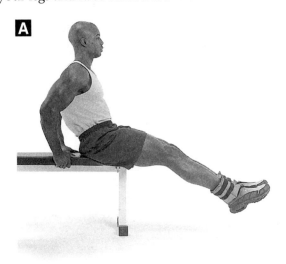

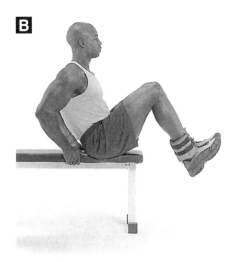

OBLIQUES ► FREE WEIGHTS

DUMBBELL SIDE BEND

This exercise strengthens the muscles responsible for side-to-side torso movement.

[**A**] Stand upright with a dumbbell in each hand. Your feet should be about shoulder-width apart, and your arms should rest at your sides with your palms facing in.

[**B**] Slowly bend to one side, allowing the dumbbell on that side to drop down your leg until you feel your obliques working. Keep your body facing front in the same plane—don't turn your torso into the side bend. Once you've gone as low as you can, slowly bring yourself upright to the starting position, keeping your abdominal muscles and obliques contracted.

Finish the set without resting between repetitions, then work the other side.

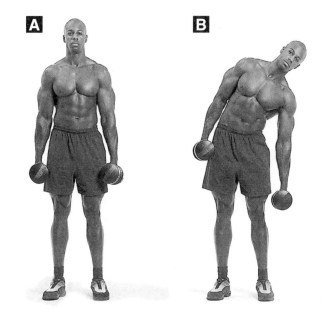

DUMBBELL TRUNK TWIST

This move also works your biceps and forearms.

[**A**] Sit at the edge of a bench with your feet flat on the floor. Keep your chest out and your head aligned with your torso. Hold a dumbbell in each hand, palms facing your body. Bend your arms and bring the weights close to your gut.

[**B**] Slowly and smoothly twist your torso to the right as far as you can comfortably go. When you reach the end of your range of motion, hold for a second, then slowly return to the starting position. Repeat to the left. Continue alternating right and left until your muscles are fatigued.

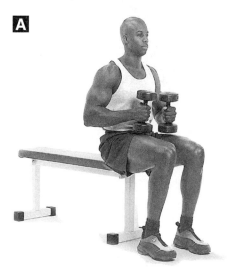
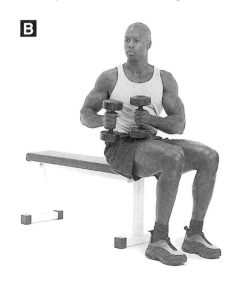

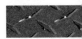

ABS AND OBLIQUES ► MACHINES

CABLE CRUNCH

This is a good general ab exercise.

[**A**] Kneel on the floor facing away from a high pulley with a rope handle on the cable. Bend your legs at a 45-degree angle. Grab the rope handle with both hands and hold it at the top of your forehead.

[**B**] Contract your abdominal muscles as you slowly curl your torso in and pull the handle forward. (Use only your abs, not your upper body.) Curl your body as far in as you can without moving the handle from your forehead. Hold for a second, then slowly return to the starting position.

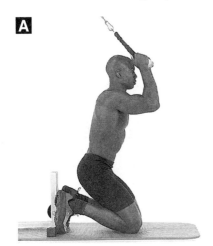

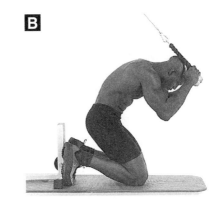

LYING CROSSOVER CABLE CRUNCH

This exercise strengthens all of your ab muscles.

[**A**] Lie in crunch position in front of a low pulley cable with a Y-shaped rope handle, your head pointing toward the pulley. Keep your feet flat on the floor about hip-width apart and bend your knees. Grip one end of the handle with each hand so the rope is behind your head with your hands a bit more than shoulder-width apart.

[**B**] Slowly lift your shoulders and shoulder blades off the ground. But instead of pausing at the top, slightly twist toward your right knee. Hold for a split second, then slowly lower yourself to the starting position.

[**C**] Immediately lift and twist toward your left knee. Don't relax between repetitions.

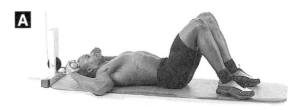

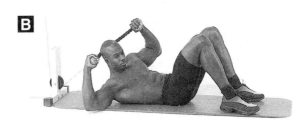

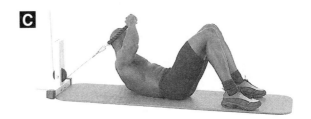

CABLE CURL-UP

This move works both the upper and lower abs.

[**A**] Lie flat on your back in crunch position in front of a low pulley cable with a Y-shaped rope handle. Your head should point toward the pulley. Keep your feet flat on the floor about shoulder-width apart, and bend your knees at about a 45-degree angle. Grip one end of the handle with each hand, with your hands just behind your ears.

[**B**] Curl your upper torso in toward your knees, raising your shoulder blades as high off the ground as you can and pressing your lower back to the floor. Keep your knees in line with your feet, and don't pull your head up with your hands. Move your torso all the way up in a count of two. Concentrate on contracting your abdominal muscles. Then count to two again as you return to the starting position.

Finish the set without resting between repetitions.

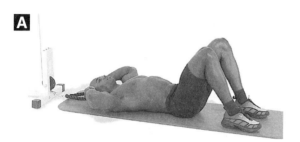

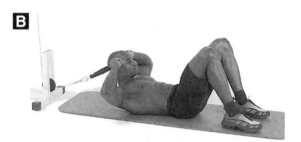

OBLIQUES ► MACHINES

CABLE SIDE CRUNCH

This gives your obliques a great workout.

Stand sideways under a D-handle overhead pulley cable. Your right side should be closest to the machine. Grip the handle underhand with your right hand, keeping your left hand on your hip.

[**A**] Pull the handle down until your right fist is roughly between your shoulder and your nose.

[**B**] Without moving your arm itself, slowly crunch toward the weight stack. You should feel your obliques contracting forcefully. If you use the proper form and crunch to the side rather than to the front, you'll move only a few inches. Hold for 2 seconds, then slowly return to the starting position.

Finish the set, then turn around and work your other side.

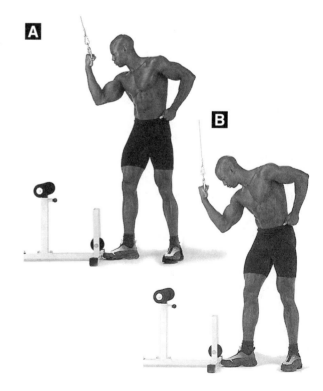

CABLE SIDE BEND

This exercise also works your upper and lower abs.

[**A**] Stand sideways next to a D-handle low pulley cable. Your right side should be closest to the machine. Grip the handle overhand with your right hand, your right palm at your side and facing in. Keep your left hand on your hip. Your feet should be about shoulder-width apart.

[**B**] Slowly bend to your right, letting the handle drop down your leg. Keep your body front—don't turn your torso into the bend. Go as low as you can, then slowly bring yourself upright. Don't rest between reps; keep your abs and obliques contracted.

Finish the set, then turn around and work your other side.

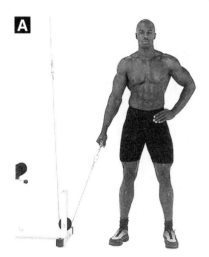

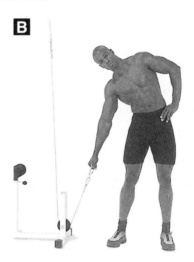

ABS ► NO WEIGHTS

HIP RAISE

In addition to strengthening your lower abs, this exercise works your butt and quadriceps.

[**A**] Lie flat on your back with your legs in the air, your knees unlocked, your toes pointed, and your hands at your sides, palms down.

[**B**] Using your lower abs and shifting your weight toward your shoulders, lift your hips off the floor. Keep your legs vertical throughout. Pause, then slowly return to the starting position.

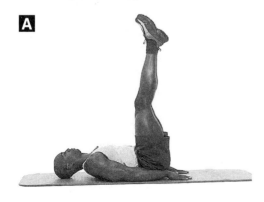

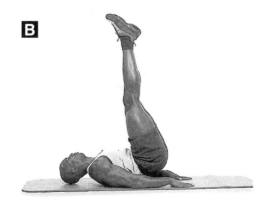

HANGING KNEE RAISE CROSSOVER

This exercise works not only your lower and upper abs but also your obliques.

[**A**] Hang fully extended from a chinning bar with your hands a little farther than shoulder-width apart. Your palms should face out and your feet should lightly touch the ground.

[**B**] Keeping your legs together, slowly lift your knees up toward your left shoulder as high as you can. Thrust your pelvis slightly forward, but don't rock or sway for momentum. Hold for a second at the top, then slowly lower your knees and repeat on your right side. Don't rest between repetitions. Keep your abdominal muscles tight.

For an even tougher variation, lift your legs instead of just your knees. Keep your feet together, and lift toward your left shoulder as high as you can. You'll need to tilt your pelvis slightly forward.

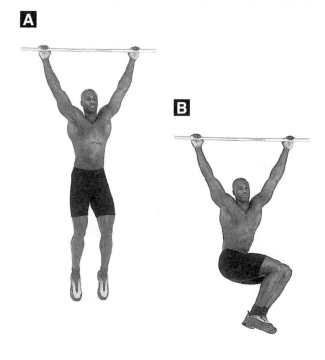

CURL-UP

This exercise works both your upper and lower abdominal muscles.

[**A**] Lie flat on your back with your hands cupped behind your ears and your elbows out. Bend your knees at about a 45-degree angle. Place your feet shoulder-width apart, about 6 inches from your butt.

[**B**] Curl your upper torso in toward your knees, pressing your lower back to the floor and raising your shoulder blades as high off the ground as you can get them. Keep your knees in line with your feet, and don't use your hands to pull your head up. Move your torso all the way up in a count of two. Concentrate on contracting your abdominal muscles. Hold for a second, then count to two again as you return to the starting position.

Finish the set without resting between repetitions.

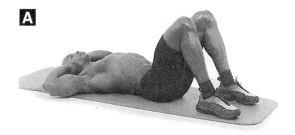

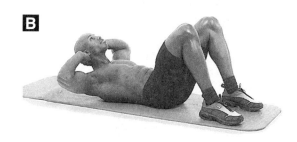

ROWING CRUNCH

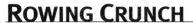

This exercise works both upper and lower abs.

Sit on a bench with your knees bent and your feet flat on the floor. Grasp the sides of the bench for support and lean back to about a 45-degree angle.

[**A**] Keeping your knees slightly bent, extend your legs and raise them a few inches off the floor.

[**B**] While bringing your upper body to an upright position, slowly pull your knees in to your chest. Hold for a second. Then, keeping your back straight, slowly and simultaneously return your upper body and legs to the starting position.

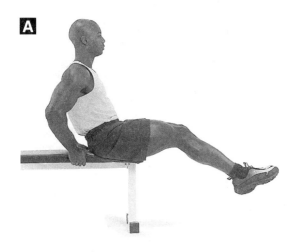

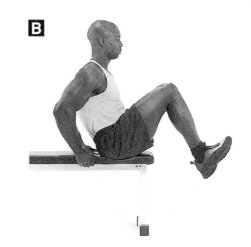

LEG RAISE

This exercise works both your upper and lower abs.

[**A**] Lie on your back on a bench with your hips near the edge. Grasp the corners of the bench by your hips and extend your legs straight out, with your toes pointed.

[**B**] Keep your legs together, knees unlocked, and slowly raise them to vertical. Hold for a second, then lower your legs in a controlled motion until your body is completely horizontal. Repeat without resting.

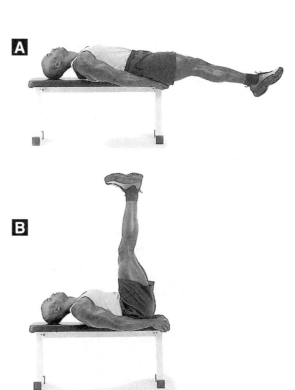

ABS AND OBLIQUES ► No Weights

FRONT HANGING KNEE RAISE

This exercise also works your quadriceps.

[**A**] Hang from a bar with your legs extended.

[**B**] Using your lower abdominal muscles, bend your knees and raise them as high as you can in a smooth, controlled movement. Your hips will naturally move forward slightly, but don't let the momentum swing your body. Hold for a second, then slowly return to the starting position.

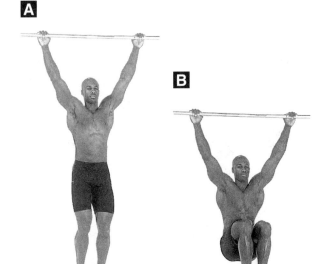

OBLIQUES ► No Weights

SEATED TWIST

This exercise also works your upper and lower abs.

Grab a stick or light bar about the length of a broomstick. [**A**] While seated, rest the bar behind your head, across your shoulders. Place your hands as close to the ends as you comfortably can with your elbows slightly bent.

[**B**] Use your oblique muscles to smoothly twist your torso as far to the right as you can while keeping your hips stationary. Your head should move with your torso. Repeat the same smooth movement to the left. Continue to rotate right and left, without pausing, until you have completed the set.

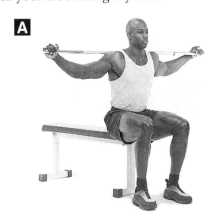

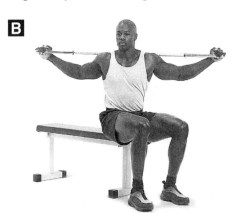

BRIEFCASE SIDE BEND

Maintain your zany office reputation and give your obliques a great workout at the same time.

[**A**] Stand upright with your briefcase in your right hand, palm facing in. Your feet should be shoulder-width apart.

[**B**] Bend to your right, allowing the briefcase to drop down your right leg until you feel your obliques working. Keep your body facing front in the same plane—don't turn your torso into the side bend. Once you've gone as low as possible, return to the starting position.

Finish the set, then switch sides.

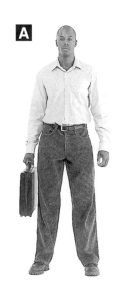
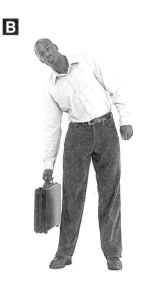

OBLIQUE TRUNK ROTATION

This exercise also works your upper and lower abs. Do it in one slow, continuous motion.

[**A**] Sit on the floor with your hands crossed over your chest and your knees bent. Place your feet under a support, such as the base of a weight machine or a heavy piece of furniture, to stabilize your lower body. Hold your torso at a 45-degree angle to the floor.

[**B**] Start by moving your torso to the left.

[**C**] Stay to the left as you lower to your back.

[**D**] Completing a clockwise rotation, raise your torso to the right side.

Then repeat the exercise, this time moving down your right side and around to the left.

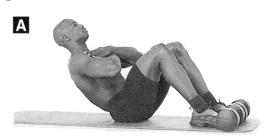
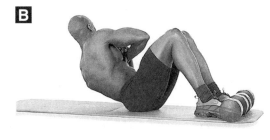

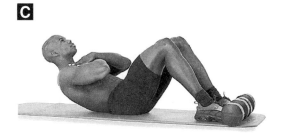
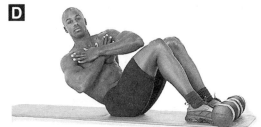

POWERFUL ABS
BEGINNER WORKOUT

We recommend that you train with the balanced, full-body plan on page 48. But if you need to concentrate specifically on ab work, this program will produce quick gains. Choose one routine to follow: free weights, machines, or no weights.

INSTRUCTIONS

1. Do the complete exercise routine 2 or 3 days a week. Wait at least 48 hours between sessions to allow enough recovery time for best development.

2. To warm up, do some aerobics and stretching and perform one set of 6 to 10 repetitions with a light to moderate load. This minimizes the chances of a muscle strain or pull during the subsequent training period.

3. After the warmup, find a starting load that is difficult to lift 6 times. This may take some experimenting on your first day. Once you have identified that load, that's what you will use until it becomes too easy.

Complete one set of 6 repetitions for each exercise listed in the routine you've chosen. Perform the positive phase (also known as the concentric or lifting phase) of each exercise as quickly as possible while maintaining proper form. Perform the negative (or eccentric or lowering) phase much more slowly, to a count of four.

4. After a few sessions, you will find that completing 6 repetitions is easier. At that point, add repetitions, following proper form, up to 10 repetitions.

5. When you are able to perform 10 repetitions, make a note to add weight at the next session.

6. With the added weight, drop back to 6 repetitions. Then repeat steps 3 to 5 until you have completed 12 weeks of the program. Then, if you still need to focus on ab workouts, you may move on to the intermediate level. Remember, we recommend that you do the balanced, full-body workouts rather than working on individual muscle groups.

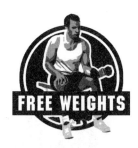

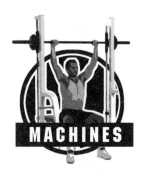

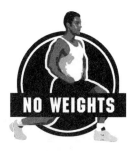

1. DUMBBELL TRUNK TWIST (PAGE 140)
2. CURL-UP WITH WEIGHT PLATE (PAGE 138)
3. OBLIQUE TRUNK ROTATION WITH WEIGHT PLATE (PAGE 138)
4. HIP RAISE WITH ANKLE WEIGHTS (PAGE 137)
5. DUMBBELL SIDE BEND (PAGE 140)

1. CABLE CRUNCH (PAGE 141)
2. CABLE SIDE CRUNCH (PAGE 142)
3. CABLE CURL-UP (PAGE 142)
4. LYING CROSSOVER CABLE CRUNCH (PAGE 141)
5. CABLE SIDE BEND (PAGE 143)

1. OBLIQUE TRUNK ROTATION (PAGE 147)
2. CURL-UP (PAGE 144)
3. LEG RAISE (PAGE 145)
4. BRIEFCASE SIDE BEND (PAGE 147)
5. HIP RAISE (PAGE 143)

POWERFUL ABS
INTERMEDIATE WORKOUT

We recommend that you train with the balanced, full-body plan on page 52. If you need to concentrate specifically on ab work, though, this program will produce quick gains. Choose one exercise routine to follow: free weights, machines, or no weights.

INSTRUCTIONS

1. Train 3 days a week. Allow enough recovery by waiting at least 48 hours between sessions.

2. Always warm up with aerobics and stretching, plus one set of 6 to 10 repetitions with a light to moderate load. This minimizes the chances of a muscle strain or pull during the subsequent training period.

3. Your standard intermediate workout is three sets of 6 to 10 repetitions for each exercise listed in the routine you've chosen. The warmup set is your first set. The starting load for the second and third sets should be one that is difficult to lift 6 times. As your strength increases, increase the repetitions per set until you can do 10 repetitions while maintaining proper form. Then, for your next session, increase the load and drop back to 6 repetitions.

Perform the positive phase (also known as the concentric or lifting phase) of each exercise as quickly as possible while maintaining proper form. Perform the negative (or eccentric or lowering) phase much more slowly, to a count of four.

4. Vary your routines. Instead of some of the individual exercises, do combo lifts, or supersets, two exercises in succession (one rep of each) without a rest. You can do almost any two exercises this way. Combo lifts increase the intensity of your workout, create some variety, and can shorten your workout session.

Another variation is to use a lighter load than usual and do 15 to 20 repetitions, and/or to increase the load on successive sets and reduce the number of repetitions (this last variation is called pyramids). So, for example, in set 1, you might do 10 repetitions with 200 pounds; in set 2, you might do 7 repetitions with 250 pounds; and in set 3, you might do 4 repetitions with 300 pounds.

5. As you gain training experience, you might try experimenting with 1 or 2 partial repetitions at the end of each set, at the point where you can no longer complete a full repetition. This is called going to muscle failure, and it may enhance muscle development. *Note:* If you try this, you will need a partner to spot you, especially when you're using free weights.

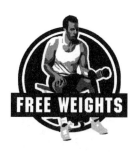

FREE WEIGHTS

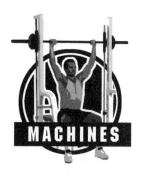

MACHINES

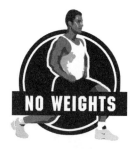

NO WEIGHTS

1. CURL-UP WITH WEIGHT PLATE (PAGE 138)
2. DUMBBELL TRUNK TWIST (PAGE 140)
3. HIP RAISE WITH ANKLE WEIGHTS (PAGE 137)
4. OBLIQUE TRUNK ROTATION WITH WEIGHT PLATE (PAGE 138)
5. DUMBBELL SIDE BEND (PAGE 140)
6. NEGATIVE SITUP WITH WEIGHT PLATE (PAGE 137)

1. CABLE CRUNCH (PAGE 141)
2. CABLE SIDE CRUNCH (PAGE 142)
3. CABLE CURL-UP (PAGE 142)
4. LYING CROSSOVER CABLE CRUNCH (PAGE 141)
5. CABLE SIDE BEND (PAGE 143)

1. OBLIQUE TRUNK ROTATION (PAGE 147)
2. CURL-UP (PAGE 144)
3. BRIEFCASE SIDE BEND (PAGE 147)
4. ROWING CRUNCH (PAGE 145)
5. HIP RAISE (PAGE 143)
6. FRONT HANGING KNEE RAISE (PAGE 146)
7. HANGING KNEE RAISE CROSSOVER (PAGE 144)

POWERFUL ABS
ADVANCED WORKOUT

We recommend that you train with the balanced, full-body plan on page 56. If you need to concentrate specifically on ab work, though, this program will produce quick gains. Choose one exercise routine to follow: free weights, machines, or no weights.

INSTRUCTIONS

1. Train 3 days a week. Allow sufficient recovery time by waiting at least 48 hours between sessions.

2. Your standard advanced workout is three sets of 6 to 10 repetitions for each exercise in the routine you've chosen. The first set, after your aerobics and stretching, is a warmup with a lighter-than-normal weight. The starting load for the second and third sets should be one that is difficult to lift 6 times. As your strength increases, increase the number of repetitions per set until you can do 10 repetitions. Then, for your next session, increase the load and drop back to 6 repetitions.

Perform the positive phase (also known as the concentric or lifting phase) of each exercise as quickly as possible while maintaining proper form. Perform the negative (or eccentric or lowering) phase of the exercise much more slowly, to a count of four.

3. Vary your workouts as at the intermediate level, and try replacing some of the exercises with tri-sets and giant sets. Tri-sets are like combo lifts except that you add another exercise so that you're doing three in succession without rest. With giant sets, you do four exercises in succession without resting between them.

4. Do 1 or 2 partial repetitions at the end of each set when you reach the point where you can no longer complete a full repetition. This is called going to muscle failure, and it may enhance muscle development. *Note:* At the advanced level, you always need the assistance of a partner for safety when doing partial reps with free weights.

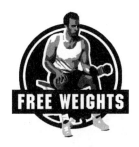

FREE WEIGHTS

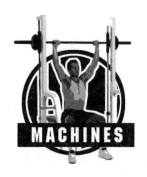

MACHINES

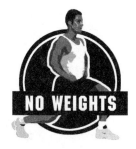

NO WEIGHTS

1. Dumbbell Trunk Twist (page 140)
2. Curl-Up with Weight Plate (page 138)
3. Oblique Trunk Rotation with Weight Plate (page 138)
4. Hip Raise with Ankle Weights (page 137)
5. Dumbbell Side Bend (page 140)
6. Rowing Crunch with Ankle Weights (page 139)
7. Negative Situp with Weight Plate (page 137)

1. Cable Crunch (page 141)
2. Cable Side Crunch (page 142)
3. Cable Curl-Up (page 142)
4. Lying Crossover Cable Crunch (page 141)
5. Cable Side Bend (page 143)

1. Oblique Trunk Rotation (page 147)
2. Curl-Up (page 144)
3. Leg Raise (page 145)
4. Briefcase Side Bend (page 147)
5. Rowing Crunch (page 145)
6. Hip Raise (page 143)
7. Front Hanging Knee Raise (page 146)
8. Hanging Knee Raise Crossover (page 144)

QUICK-SET PATH TO A
POWERFUL BACK

YOUR BACK ISN'T AS GLAMOROUS AS YOUR CHEST, BUT IT'S
AT LEAST AS IMPORTANT TO DEVELOP. TAKE CARE OF YOUR
BACK MUSCLES TO CURTAIL CHRONIC LOWER-BACK PAIN, REDUCE
INJURIES TO OTHER MUSCLES DURING WORKOUTS, IMPROVE
YOUR APPEARANCE, AND PERFECT YOUR POSTURE. IT'S EASY TO
BLOW OUT YOUR BACK WHILE LIFTING—ALL THE MORE REASON
TO STRENGTHEN IT.

If you're like a lot of men, you take your back for granted. It's hard to see, but you're pretty sure it likes you—it follows you everywhere.

You can't easily stand in front of a mirror admiring your back as you do your chest. You would if you could, we know. But no joke: You really do need to watch your backside.

If you develop your chest at the expense of your back, you cause a muscle imbalance that makes you prone to injury and also gives you really sloppy posture, says Brian Pfeufer, corporate program director at Sports Training Institute in New York City. You may have a champ's chest, but you'll walk around looking like a wimp.

Here's another good reason to be good to your back: Doing so will help ease the hurt. Eighty to 85 percent of us experience lower-back pain at some time in our lives.

Developing your back also pays off appearancewise. By beefing up your upper back, you can achieve the V shape that, among other things, makes your waist look smaller.

In this chapter, we'll give you lots of ways to strengthen your upper and lower back. Pay attention—the back is the most commonly injured part of the body among weight trainers.

LATS TALK (UPPER) BACK

Your back muscles enable you to pull with power. Develop your upper back and you'll be better able to effortlessly grab a heavy suitcase off the baggage claim carousel. You'll also benefit as you age: While your fellow geezers are brittle with osteoporosis and too weak to bend over and lift up the grandkids, you'll still be in fine form, bending over and picking up trophy girlfriends. See what a good, strong back can do for you?

The largest muscles in your entire upper body are the *latissimus dorsi*, or lats in gymspeak. You may remember seeing lats mentioned in some of the exercises in the chest chapter. Your lats extend from behind each armpit to the middle of your lower back. They pull your arms toward your body and provide that V-shaped look when properly developed.

Did you ever see a swimmer warming up by squeezing and rotating his shoulder blades? He's working his *rhomboideus* or rhomboid muscles, smaller muscles found between the shoulder blades and spine, along with the *trapezius* muscles that are discussed in the chapter on shoulders.

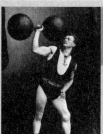

HARD-BODY FACT

Lat pulldowns are a great upper-back exercise, but fitness experts advise against pulling the bar down behind your head. Doing so can cause or exacerbate shoulder injuries. Instead, pull the bar down in front of your face to the top of your chest. Lean—but don't rock—back slightly so that you don't conk yourself in the head with the bar. And don't overdo the amount of weight you're lifting.

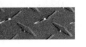

5-SECOND QUIZ

The backbone is a misnomer because it consists of more than one bone. How many little bones make up your backbone?

Answer: 33.

Much as you might like working on your chest, you should spend even more time on back exercises because the back is a bigger muscle.

That's advice from Todd Mattera, a competitive bodybuilder and fitness trainer in Foxboro, Massachusetts. "You need to hit it with a few more exercises than the chest," Mattera says.

Pfeufer agrees. "Your back should be stronger than your chest," he says.

THE LOWDOWN ON YOUR LOWER BACK

The primary muscles of your lower back are the *erector spinae*. They run along your spine and allow you to extend and flex it.

Think of the relationship between your lower-back muscles and abdominal muscles as a symbiotic one, akin to that of peanut butter and bread or Michael Douglas and young women. Each of these muscle groups works with the other to strengthen your lower back so that you are less apt to have back pain and more likely to have good posture.

Be especially careful not to employ too much weight in the gym and risk painful injury to your lower back. "Everyone goes into the gym and wants to lift more than the guy next to him," says Mattera. "Everyone wants to put on too much weight and try to impress. You need to check your ego and do the weight that your back can handle."

In doing the Romanian deadlift, for example, go easy on the pounds you pull, because you begin by holding the weighted bar rather than lifting it off the floor.

You might opt instead for a safer, weightless exercise such as a seated row using rubber tubing and both arms. Like the Romanian deadlift, this exercise works both your upper- and lower-back muscles, but it's easier on your lower back.

Another weightless variation is to use a stability ball. Place your body prone on the ball with your hips and abdominals positioned on its surface, your palms resting on the floor and toes touching for support. Shift your weight forward, draping your body over the ball until you feel no tension in your lower back. This exercise is both a stretch and a strengthener.

You can also lie on the floor with your arms extended to the sides and your heels resting on the ball. Slowly roll the ball to one side, keeping your arms extended to the sides and your chest open to the ceiling. Hold for a second, then roll the ball to the other side and hold again.

You can even stretch your lower back at work. While seated, bend down between your knees, reaching toward the floor. Reach as far as you can while keeping your palms flat. Hold briefly, then return slowly to the upright position. Repeat the sequence five times.

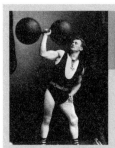

One thing you *don't* need to do to protect your lower back is wear a weight belt — unless you think that it makes a fashion statement. And if you do think that, we'd rather that you hang out with another group of guys when we're walking around town. Okay?

Studies show that weight belts don't reduce the risk of injury to your back; in fact, they inhibit the strengthening of lower-back and abdominal muscles. If you have already injured your back, however, a weight belt may have some value during lifting activities after the fact to help you *recover* faster from the injury.

ENTIRE BACK ► FREE WEIGHTS

ROMANIAN DEADLIFT

This all-purpose exercise strengthens not only your back but also your arms, shoulders, and legs. Use less weight than for a regular deadlift.

[**A**] Hold a lightly weighted barbell at midthigh level, your hands farther than shoulder-width apart and your palms facing your body. Keep the barbell against your legs with your arms fully extended, your back straight, your shoulders back, and your chest out. Pause for a second.

[**B**] Bend forward slowly at the hips, keeping the bar close to your thighs. Your back should stay straight and your knees should be slightly bent. Lower the bar slowly toward the floor, going as far as you comfortably can. With a slow, controlled movement and your back straight, return to the starting position.

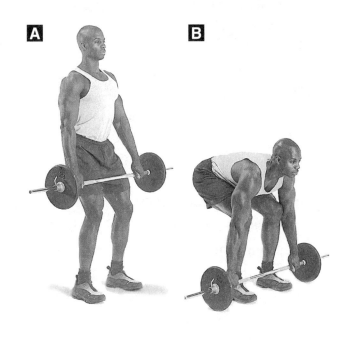

WIDE-GRIP ROW

This versatile move also works your back deltoids, butt, and abs.

Stand with your feet shoulder-width apart and your knees slightly bent. Bend at the waist until your upper body is parallel to the floor, without arching your back.

[**A**] Grab a barbell using a grip that's wider than shoulder-width, your palms facing your body.

[**B**] Raise the bar in a count of two until it touches your chest. Your elbows should be higher than your back. Hold for a second, then slowly lower the barbell to about the middle of your shins, and repeat.

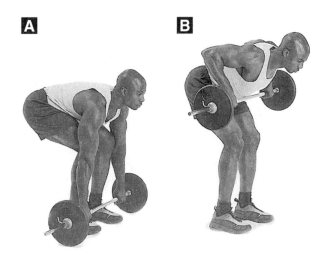

GOOD MORNING

This move especially strengthens your lower back, and it also works your hamstrings, abs, and glutes. But it's difficult, and not recommended for beginners. To avoid injury, use an empty bar at first, and pay close attention to your form. Then move on to light weights until you have mastered the movement.

[**A**] Stand with your legs shoulder-width apart and your knees unlocked. Hold a barbell across your shoulders, with your hands slightly farther than shoulder-width apart, palms facing out. Keep your upper body straight, your shoulders back, and your chest out. Lean forward slightly at the waist.

[**B**] Bend slowly at the waist, keeping your back straight, until your upper body is parallel to the floor. You should be looking forward, not down. Hold for a second, then slowly return to the starting position.

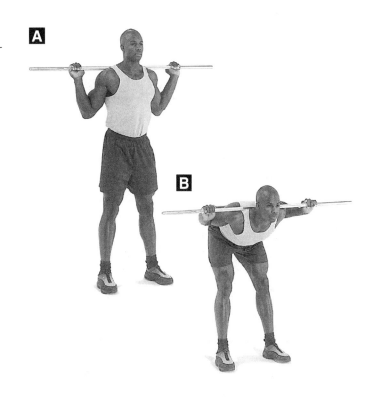

T-BAR ROW WITH BARBELL

This exercise also works your back deltoid muscles. To avoid injury, try to keep your lower back flat or, at most, slightly arched, but never curved.

Wedge one end of an Olympic-size (45-pound) barbell in the corner of a wall or between two weight plates, and place a weight plate on the other end. Put a V handle around the bar just below the weight, and hold it with both hands so that it doesn't slide or wobble.

[**A**] Straddle the bar, keeping your knees slightly bent. Your chin should be up, your chest out, your stomach in, your shoulders back, and your back flat.

[**B**] Slowly pull the bar to your chest, arching your back ever so slightly and letting your elbows rise above your chest. Hold for a second, then slowly lower the bar to arm's length and continue with the next repetition.

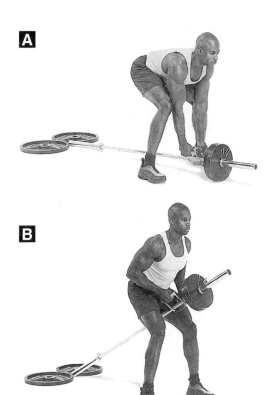

UPPER BACK ► FREE WEIGHTS

ONE-ARM DUMBBELL ROW

This exercise also works your trapezius muscles, which are part of your shoulders.

[A] With a dumbbell in your left hand, rest your right knee and right hand on the center line of a bench. Place your left foot firmly on the floor, your knee slightly bent. Keep your back straight and your eyes facing down. Let your left arm hang down; your left elbow should remain un-locked and your left palm should face your left side.

[B] Slowly pull the dumbbell up and in toward your torso, raising it as high toward your chest as possible. Your left elbow should point up toward the ceiling as you lift. Hold for a second, then re-turn to the starting position.

Finish the set, then switch sides.

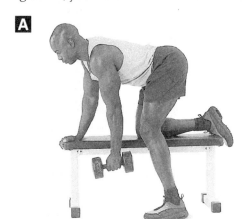

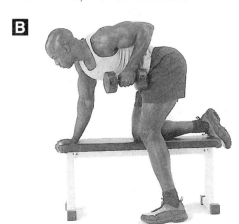

LOWER BACK ► FREE WEIGHTS

TOE TOUCH

This exercise also helps to strengthen your gluteal muscles and hamstrings.

[A] Hold a dumbbell in your left hand, your feet shoulder-width apart and your knees unlocked.

[B] Slowly bend forward and to the right, and touch the dumbbell to your right foot. Hold for a second, then slowly return to the starting position.

Finish the set, then switch sides.

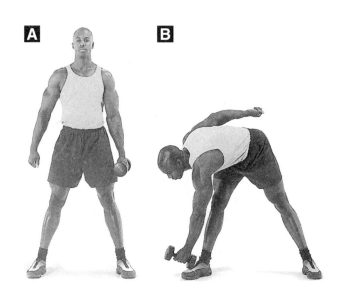

DUMBBELL SWING

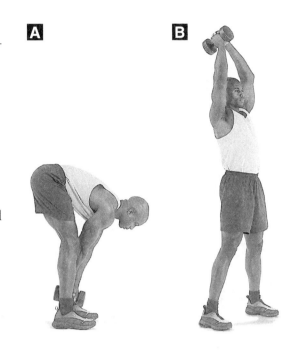

A   B

This move, which is great for strengthening your lower back, also strengthens your hamstrings, deltoids, and glutes. Unlike most weight exercises, it should be done with an explosive movement. Start with very light weights and high repetitions.

Hold a dumbbell with both hands. Stand with your feet farther than shoulder-width apart and your knees unlocked.

[A] Bend at the waist while holding the dumbbell between your shins, your arms fully extended and your back straight. Keep the weight off the floor.

[B] Swing the dumbbell until it's over your head, simultaneously standing upright with your back still straight. Hold the dumbbell over your head for a second, then bend at the waist as you return to the starting position.

DEADLIFT

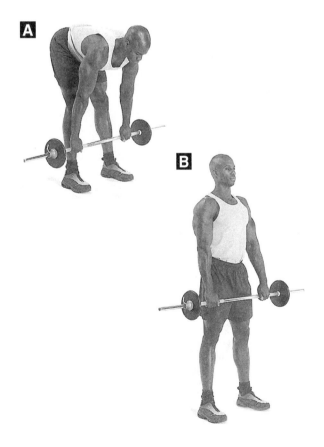

A   B

This versatile move also strengthens your legs, shoulders, and arms.

Stand upright with a lightly weighted barbell in front of you.

[A] Keeping your back straight, bend over the barbell and grasp it with your hands shoulder-width apart and palms down. Keep your legs stiff and fairly straight, but make sure your knees are unlocked. Keep your arms straight and your elbows unlocked.

[B] Slowly lift the barbell to upper-thigh level. Your back, arms, and legs should stay straight. Keep your knees unlocked. Hold for a second, then slowly lower the weight.

ENTIRE BACK ► MACHINES

WIDE-GRIP PULLEY ROW

This exercise also works your back deltoids.

Stand in front of a low pulley with a bar handle on the cable, your feet shoulder-width apart and your knees slightly bent.

[**A**] Bend at the waist until your back is flat and parallel to the floor. Grip the bar with your hands farther apart than shoulder width and your palms facing your body.

[**B**] Raise the bar in a count of two until it touches your chest. Your elbows should be higher than your back. Hold for a second, then slowly lower the bar to about the middle of your shins and repeat.

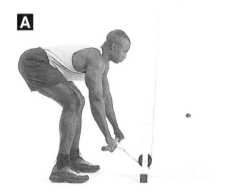

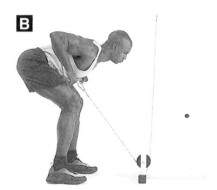

CABLE ROW

To avoid injury, keep your lower back flat or, at most, slightly arched, but never curved.

Stand in front of a low pulley with a V handle on the cable.

[**A**] Bend down as if to straddle the pulley, with your feet farther than shoulder-width apart. Keep your chin up, your chest out, your stomach in, your shoulders back, and your back flat. Grab the handle with both hands so that it points back between your legs.

[**B**] Slowly pull the handle to your chest, arching your back very slightly and letting your elbows rise to your sides. Hold for a second, then slowly lower the handle back to the starting position.

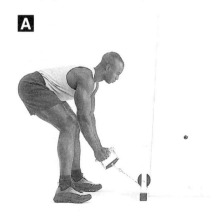

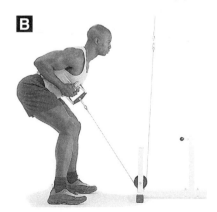

SEATED ROW

This exercise also works your shoulders.

[**A**] Sit at a pulley row machine. Anchor your feet against the foot platforms, with your knees slightly bent. Keep your back straight as you lean forward and grasp the handles with a narrow grip. Pull back until your arms are fully extended and you are leaning forward slightly.

[**B**] Pull the handles until they touch your chest, bringing your body into an upright position. Your elbows should point behind you. Don't lock your knees. Hold for a second, then return to the starting position.

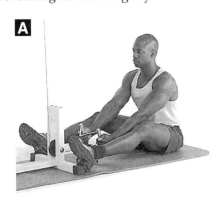

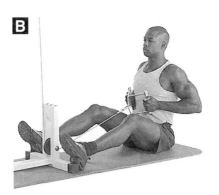

UPPER BACK ► MACHINES

ONE-ARM CABLE ROW

This exercise also works your trapezius.

[**A**] Stand facing a D-handle low pulley cable. Grip the handle underhand with your right hand, your arm fully extended. Lean forward with your knees slightly bent but your back straight. Brace your left hand against your left thigh.

[**B**] Slowly pull the handle toward your side. You should feel your right lats contracting as your elbow travels past your side, then makes a slight curve toward the middle of your lower back. Pause, then slowly return the handle to the starting position.

Finish the set, then switch sides.

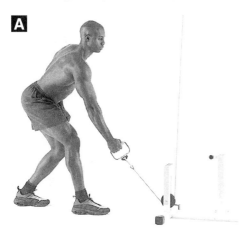

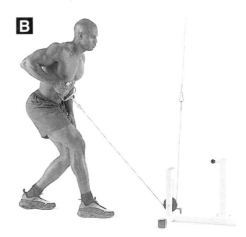

LAT PULLDOWN

This exercise also works your rhomboids, which lie between your spine and your shoulder blades. Don't overdo the amount of weight.

[**A**] Sit (or kneel if there isn't a seat) at a lat pull-down station. Grasp the bar overhead, placing your hands shoulder-width or farther apart. Your palms should face away from your body. Keep your upper body straight and your eyes forward.

[**B**] Slowly pull the bar down in front of your head until it reaches the top of your shoulders, keeping your upper body fairly upright throughout the movement. Hold for a second, then slowly return your arms to the starting position.

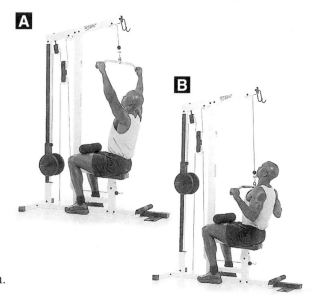

LOWER BACK ► MACHINES

PULLEY DEADLIFT

This move also works your gluteal (butt) muscles and hamstrings.

Stand in front of a low pulley with a bar handle on the cable.

[**A**] Keeping your back straight, bend over and grasp the handle overhand with your hands shoulder-width apart. Keep your legs stiff, but don't lock your knees—bend them slightly. Keep your arms straight and your elbows unlocked.

(You may need to stand on a step platform in order to maintain tension in the cable.)

[**B**] Slowly lift the bar handle to upper-thigh level. (Depending on the pulley design, if you're standing on a platform, you may have to be careful not to hit your head as you rise.) Keep your back, arms, and legs straight, but don't lock your knees. Hold for a second, then slowly lower the bar to the starting position.

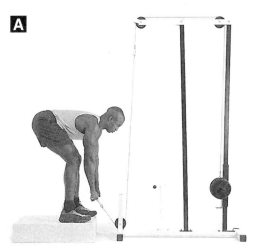

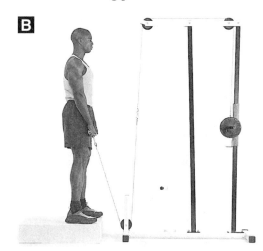

CABLE BACK EXTENSION

This is another move that strengthens your gluteal muscles and hamstrings.

Place a back extension machine in front of a low pulley with a bar handle on the cable. The padded ankle bars should be closest to the pulley.

[**A**] Position yourself in the back extension machine, your ankles under the padded bars and your groin and upper thighs resting on the padded platform. You can hold the cable handle in one hand as you do all this, or someone can hand it to you once you're in position. Fold your arms, holding the bar to your chest, and bend at the waist until your back is almost perpendicular to the floor.

[**B**] Slowly rise, straightening your torso until your back is parallel to the floor. Your arms should still be crossed over your chest and the rest of your body should stay in the starting position. Hold for a second, then slowly lower yourself to the starting position.

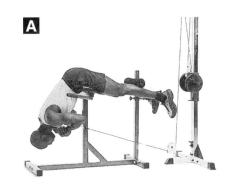

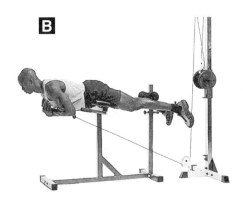

ENTIRE BACK ► NO WEIGHTS

SEATED ROW WITH TUBING

This exercise also strengthens your back deltoids, your trapezius muscles, and your biceps.

[**A**] Sit on the floor with your legs straight in front of you, your feet pointing up. Place a length of rubber exercise tubing around your feet and grasp it by the handles. Your arms should be ex-tended straight in front of you, and your back should be upright.

[**B**] Slowly pull the tubing toward your chest, squeezing your shoulder blades together as you move. Hold for a second, then slowly return your arms to the starting position.

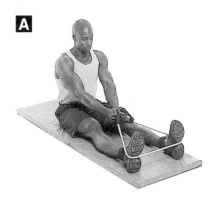

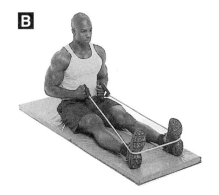

WIDE-GRIP ROW WITH TUBING

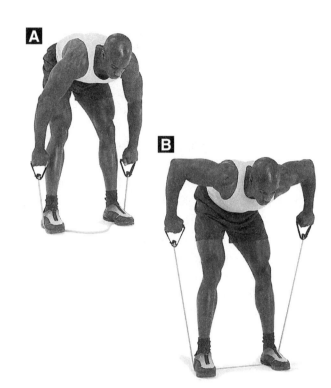

In addition to working your back, this exercise works your back deltoids and your hamstrings, gluteal muscles, and abs.

Stand with your feet shoulder-width apart and your knees slightly bent.

[**A**] Bend at the waist until your upper body is straight and parallel to the floor. Run a length of exercise tubing under your feet, and grab the tubing's handles with your hands farther than shoulder-width apart and your palms facing your body.

[**B**] Raise the handles in a count of two until your elbows are higher than your back. Your forearms should be perpendicular to the floor. Hold for a second, then slowly lower the handles to about mid-shin, and repeat.

T-BAR ROW WITH TUBING

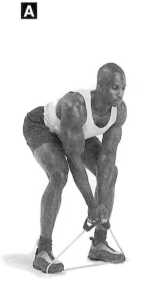
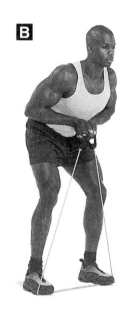

This exercise also builds your back deltoids. To avoid injury, try to keep your lower back flat or, at most, slightly arched, but never curved.

Stand with your feet farther than shoulder-width apart and your knees slightly bent.

[**A**] Run a length of exercise tubing under your feet and grab the handles with your hands together, palms facing each other. Your chin should be up, your chest out, your stomach in, your shoulders back, and your back flat.

[**B**] Slowly pull the handles to your chest, arching your back just slightly. Your upper body will become more upright, but your knees should not move. Hold for a second. Slowly lower the handles to arm's length, then return to the starting position.

ONE-ARM ROW WITH TUBING

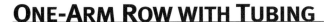

This move also works your trapezius and your rhomboids, which lie between your spine and your shoulder blades.

Wrap a length of exercise tubing around the foot of a weight bench, near the center of the foot. Keep wrapping until the tubing's handle is at bench height, with no slack in the tubing.

[**A**] Rest your left knee and left hand in the center of the bench. Plant your right foot firmly on the floor, your knee slightly bent. Keep your back straight and your eyes facing down. Hold the handle in your right hand, letting your right arm hang down with your elbow unlocked and your palm facing your side.

[**B**] Pull the handle up and in toward your torso, raising it as high as possible while keeping your right elbow close to your side. Your elbow should point toward the ceiling as you lift. Hold for a second, then slowly return to the starting position.

Finish the set, then switch sides.

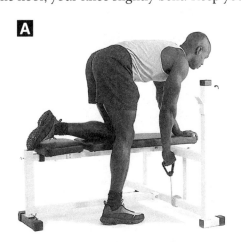

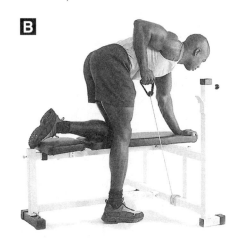

CLOSE-GRIP CHINUP

This exercise also works your arms and shoulders.

[**A**] Suspend a handle from a chinning bar and grasp it with both hands, your palms facing each other, so that you hang from the bar. Your knees should be slightly bent, and your feet should be about 6 inches off the floor when your arms are fully extended.

[**B**] Slowly pull yourself up, using your lat muscles and not your biceps, until your torso almost touches your hands. Then slowly lower yourself.

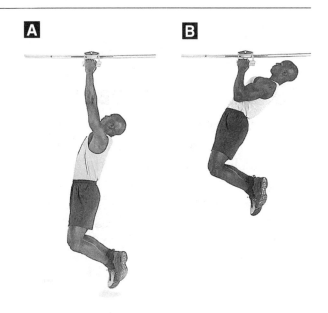

UPPER BACK ► NO WEIGHTS

LAT PULLDOWN WITH TUBING

This exercise also strengthens your rhomboids, which lie between your spine and your shoulder blades.

Run a length of exercise tubing over the top of an open door, and sit on a chair or bench in front of the door, with the door's leading edge in line with your spine.

[**A**] Grasp the tubing's handles overhead, your hands shoulder-width or farther apart. Your palms should face away from your body. Keep your upper body straight and your eyes forward.

[**B**] Slowly pull the handles so that your hands are in line with your neck and the handles are level with the top of your shoulders, keeping your upper body fairly upright throughout the movement. Hold for a second, then slowly return your arms to the starting position.

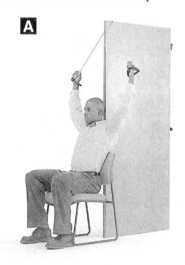

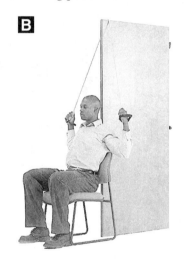

LOWER BACK ► NO WEIGHTS

DEADLIFT WITH TUBING

This move also works your legs, shoulders, and arms.

Run a length of exercise tubing under your feet.

[**A**] Keeping your back straight, bend over and grasp the handles overhand with your hands shoulder-width apart. Keep your legs stiff, but don't lock your knees; bend them very slightly. Keep your arms straight and your elbows unlocked.

[**B**] Slowly lift the handles to upper-thigh level, coming to a standing position. Your back, arms, and legs should stay straight. Keep your knees unlocked. Hold for a second, then slowly lower to the starting position.

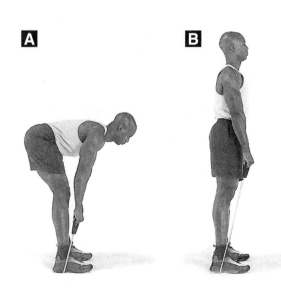

BACK EXTENSION WITH TUBING

This exercise also strengthens your gluteal muscles and hamstrings.

Secure a length of exercise tubing around the base of a back extension machine.

[A] Position yourself in the machine with your calves locked behind the padded bars and your groin and upper thighs resting on the padded platform. Your hips should be over the edge of the platform. Bend at the waist until your torso is just a few inches above being perpendicular to the floor. Grasp the tubing's handles in both hands, and fold your arms across your chest. This is the starting position.

[B] Slowly raise your torso until your back is parallel to the floor. Your arms should still be crossed over your chest and the rest of your body should stay in the starting position. Hold for a second, then slowly lower your torso back to the starting position.

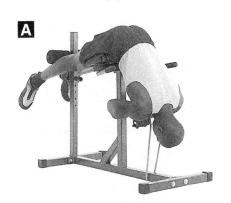

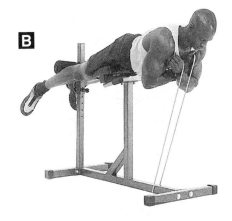

POWERFUL BACK
BEGINNER WORKOUT

We recommend that you train with the balanced, full-body plan on page 48. If you need to concentrate specifically on back work, however, this program will produce quick gains. Choose one exercise routine to follow: free weights, machines, or no weights.

INSTRUCTIONS

1. Do the complete exercise routine 2 or 3 days a week. Wait at least 48 hours between sessions to allow enough recovery time for best development.

2. To warm up, do some aerobics and stretching and perform one set of 6 to 10 repetitions with a light to moderate load. This minimizes the chances of a muscle strain or pull during the subsequent training period.

3. After the warmup, find a starting load that is hard to lift 6 times. This may take some experimenting on your first day. Once you have identified it, you'll use it until it becomes too easy.

Complete one set of 6 repetitions for each exercise listed in the routine you've chosen. Perform the positive phase (also known as the concentric or lifting phase) of each exercise as quickly as possible while maintaining proper form. Perform the negative (or eccentric or lowering) phase much more slowly, to a count of four.

4. After a few sessions, you will find that completing the 6 repetitions is easier. At that point, add repetitions, following proper form, up to 10 repetitions.

5. When you are able to perform 10 repetitions, make a note to add more weight on the next session.

6. With the added weight, drop back to 6 repetitions. Then repeat steps 3 to 5 until you have completed 12 weeks of the program. Then, if you still need to focus on back workouts, you may move on to the intermediate level. Remember, we recommend that you do the balanced, full-body workouts rather than working on individual muscle groups.

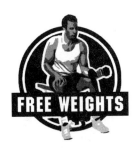

FREE WEIGHTS

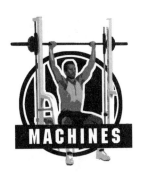

MACHINES

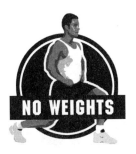

NO WEIGHTS

1. WIDE-GRIP ROW (PAGE 158)
2. ROMANIAN DEADLIFT (PAGE 158)
3. DUMBBELL SWING (PAGE 161)
4. ONE-ARM DUMBBELL ROW (PAGE 160)

1. CABLE ROW (PAGE 162)
2. PULLEY DEADLIFT (PAGE 164)
3. SEATED ROW (PAGE 163)
4. LAT PULLDOWN (PAGE 164)

1. T-BAR ROW WITH TUBING (PAGE 166)
2. DEADLIFT WITH TUBING (PAGE 168)
3. LAT PULLDOWN WITH TUBING (PAGE 168)
4. SEATED ROW WITH TUBING (PAGE 165)

POWERFUL BACK
INTERMEDIATE WORKOUT

We recommend that you train with the balanced, full-body plan on page 52. If you need to concentrate specifically on back work, though, this program will produce quick gains. Choose one exercise routine to follow: free weights, machines, or no weights.

INSTRUCTIONS

1. Train 3 days a week. Allow enough recovery by waiting at least 48 hours between sessions.

2. Always warm up with aerobics and stretching, plus one set of 6 to 10 repetitions using a light to moderate load. This minimizes the chances of a muscle strain or pull during the subsequent training period.

3. Your standard intermediate workout is three sets of 6 to 10 repetitions for each exercise listed in the routine you've chosen. The warmup set is your first set. The starting load for the second and third sets should be one that is difficult to lift 6 times. As your strength increases, increase the repetitions per set until you can do 10 repetitions while maintaining proper form. Then, for your next session, increase the load and drop back to 6 repetitions.

Perform the positive phase (also known as the concentric or lifting phase) of each exercise as quickly as possible while maintaining proper form. Perform the negative (or eccentric or lowering) phase much more slowly, to a count of four.

4. Vary your routines. Instead of some of the individual exercises, do combo lifts, or supersets, two exercises in succession (one rep of each) without a rest. You can do almost any two exercises this way. Combo lifts increase the intensity of a workout, create some variety, and can shorten your workout session.

Another variation is to use a lighter load than usual and do 15 to 20 repetitions, and/or to increase the load on successive sets and reduce the number of repetitions (this last variation is called pyramids). So, for example, in set 1, you might do 10 repetitions with 200 pounds; in set 2, you might do 7 repetitions with 250 pounds; and in set 3, you might do 4 repetitions with 300 pounds.

5. As you gain training experience, you might try experimenting with 1 or 2 partial repetitions at the end of each set, at the point where you can no longer complete a full repetition. This is called going to muscle failure, and it may enhance muscle development. *Note:* If you try this, you will need a partner to spot you, especially when you're using free weights.

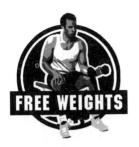

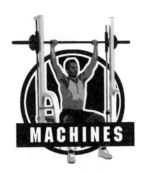

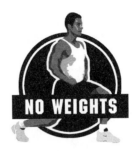

FREE WEIGHTS

1. WIDE-GRIP ROW (PAGE 158)
2. ROMANIAN DEADLIFT (PAGE 158)
3. DUMBBELL SWING (PAGE 161)
4. ONE-ARM DUMBBELL ROW (PAGE 160)
5. TOE TOUCH (PAGE 160)

MACHINES

1. CABLE ROW (PAGE 162)
2. PULLEY DEADLIFT (PAGE 164)
3. CABLE BACK EXTENSION (PAGE 165)
4. SEATED ROW (PAGE 163)
5. LAT PULLDOWN (PAGE 164)

NO WEIGHTS

1. T-BAR ROW WITH TUBING (PAGE 166)
2. DEADLIFT WITH TUBING (PAGE 168)
3. BACK EXTENSION WITH TUBING (PAGE 169)
4. SEATED ROW WITH TUBING (PAGE 165)
5. LAT PULLDOWN WITH TUBING (PAGE 168)

POWERFUL BACK
ADVANCED WORKOUT

We recommend that you train with the balanced, full-body plan on page 56. If you need to concentrate specifically on back work, though, this program will produce quick gains. Choose one exercise routine to follow: free weights, machines, or no weights.

INSTRUCTIONS

1. Train 3 days a week. Allow sufficient recovery by waiting at least 48 hours between sessions.

2. Your standard advanced workout is three sets of 6 to 10 repetitions for each exercise in the routine you've chosen. The first set, after your aerobics and stretching, is a warmup with a lighter-than-normal weight. The starting load for the second and third sets should be one that is difficult to lift 6 times. As your strength increases, increase the number of repetitions per set until you can do 10 repetitions. Then, for your next session, increase the load and drop back to 6 repetitions.

Perform the positive phase (also known as the concentric or lifting phase) of each exercise as quickly as possible while maintaining proper form. Perform the negative (or eccentric or lowering) phase of the exercise much more slowly, to a count of four.

3. Vary your workouts as at the intermediate level, and try replacing some of the exercises with tri-sets and giant sets. Tri-sets are like combo lifts except that you add another exercise so that you're doing three in succession without rest. With giant sets, you do four exercises in succession without resting between them.

4. Do 1 or 2 partial repetitions at the end of each set when you reach the point where you can no longer complete a full repetition. This is called going to muscle failure, and it may enhance muscle development. *Note:* At the advanced level, you always need the assistance of a partner for safety when doing partial reps with free weights.

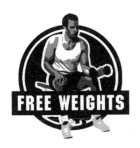

FREE WEIGHTS

1. WIDE-GRIP ROW (PAGE 158)
2. DEADLIFT (PAGE 161)
3. GOOD MORNING (PAGE 159)
4. ROMANIAN DEADLIFT (PAGE 158)
5. DUMBBELL SWING (PAGE 161)
6. ONE-ARM DUMBBELL ROW (PAGE 160)
7. TOE TOUCH (PAGE 160)

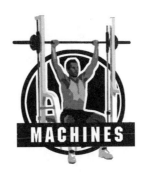

MACHINES

1. CABLE ROW (PAGE 162)
2. PULLEY DEADLIFT (PAGE 164)
3. CABLE BACK EXTENSION (PAGE 165)
4. SEATED ROW (PAGE 163)
5. ONE-ARM CABLE ROW (PAGE 163)
6. LAT PULLDOWN (PAGE 164)

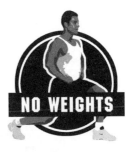

NO WEIGHTS

1. T-BAR ROW WITH TUBING (PAGE 166)
2. DEADLIFT WITH TUBING (PAGE 168)
3. BACK EXTENSION WITH TUBING (PAGE 169)
4. CLOSE-GRIP CHINUP (PAGE 167)
5. ONE-ARM ROW WITH TUBING (PAGE 167)
6. SEATED ROW WITH TUBING (PAGE 165)
7. LAT PULLDOWN WITH TUBING (PAGE 168)

QUICK-SET PATH TO A
POWERFUL BUTT

JUST BECAUSE YOU SIT ON THEM ALL DAY DOESN'T MEAN THAT THE MUSCLES IN YOUR BUTT AREN'T IMPORTANT. YOU USE THEM TO WALK, RUN, AND LIFT, AND THEY IMPROVE YOUR OVERALL APPEARANCE WHEN THEY'RE MAINTAINED.

Next time somebody says you're a big ass, just go with it, buddy. They're right—at least from a scientific standpoint. Basically that's what *gluteus maximus* means. *Gluteus maximus*—sounds like a theme hotel on the Vegas strip, doesn't it? Fact is, it's the most massive of all the 600-plus muscles in the human body.

And it's not like you've got just one of these glute things. You have three glutes, big guy. Beneath the meaty maximus are the daintier *gluteus medius* and the *gluteus minimus*. Derriere we say it? It's more accurate to call a weight lifter a muscle-butt than a musclehead.

Your glutes are good for more than providing a cushion when you fall off inline skates or slip on an icy sidewalk. They allow you to hoist a keg of beer or a sack of cement, go on an arduous hike, or pedal a bicycle.

BUTT BASICS

There's a good reason not to turn the other cheek on your cheeks in the gym. "That's the center of your body. It helps your balance," says fitness trainer and bodybuilding competitor Todd Mattera of Foxboro, Massachusetts.

Here's another reason not to ignore your butt: Women aren't ignoring it. A poll of women conducted for the book *Extraordinary Togetherness* uncovered this finding:

When they were asked what a man's most attractive physical feature is, women ranked the butt higher than all the other parts that you're going to be pumping up in the gym.

Sure, the butt got only 7 percent of the ballots, compared with 27 percent for eyes, 24 percent for face, and 22 percent for smile. But the butt ranked higher than chest, arms, legs, and abs.

Mattera is content to limit his own butt workout to one exercise: the squat. This exercise strengthens not only your quadriceps and hamstring muscles but also your butt muscles.

The lunge is another good all-around lower-body exercise.

You can perform several variations of the lunge. All are best attempted initially with light weight or no weight.

There is the standard stationary or front lunge, in which you step one foot forward a stride's length, bending both knees until your forward thigh is parallel to the floor and your stationary thigh is perpendicular to it, says Peter Lemon, Ph.D., designer of the Hard-Body exercise plan. Then you step back to the standing position from which you began.

You also might try lateral lunges, in which you step sideways rather than forward, or backward lunges, in which you step backward instead of forward.

TONING THE TUSH

Working your gluteal muscles, as with any other muscles, can make them bigger. Need you worry about having a big butt? Probably not; but if you already have a big behind, remember that you can't spot reduce any one ample area of the body. Here's what you can do, however, to keep your gluteus maximus to the minimum.

The bottom line is: If you have a big butt, don't do glute training exercises—such as squats and lunges—with heavy weight and few repetitions.

"That would definitely stimulate more muscle growth" and a larger behind, says Brian Pfeufer, a strength and conditioning specialist in New York City.

Instead, perform exercises that will tone and firm rather than add bulk, Pfeufer suggests. These can include routines where you use little or no weight. Example: Do lunges with only your body weight or holding light dumbbells.

Another such exercise is the kneeling kickback, in which you get on all fours and extend one foot toward the ceiling, then bring it back down and repeat. You can also do this with ankle weights or with somebody applying light pressure to your heel while you push upward against it. "That seems to target that area well," Pfeufer says.

More common than guys with big cabooses are men who seem to have no butts. Look in the back of certain men's magazines and you'll see ads for padded briefs that promise "eye-catching buttocks instantly!"

What can you do? Your genetic makeup only gives you so much to work with. If you want to

5-SECOND QUIZ

If you have a persistent pain in the butt, are you exercising it too hard?

Answer: Not necessarily. Sometimes butt pain or discomfort is due to nerve damage. This can occur from a fall on your butt, prolonged bicycle riding, or even doing a lot of sitting.

maximize your maximus, hoist heavy weight on the bar when you do squats and lunges. Place the bar somewhat lower on your back, not on your neck as you would with a standard squat or a lateral lunge.

"When you're coming up to the standing phase, concentrate on squeezing and pressing your glutes," Pfeufer says. "You may be able to add some muscle size to your butt."

GLUTEAL MUSCLES ▶ FREE WEIGHTS

STANDING KICKBACK WITH ANKLE WEIGHTS

This exercise also tones your hamstrings.

Fasten an ankle weight around your right ankle.

[**A**] Stand facing a wall, lightly holding on with your hands for balance. Lean slightly forward so that your whole body is in a straight line. Shift your weight onto your left leg.

[**B**] Slowly raise your right leg as far behind you as you can, feeling the contraction in your butt. Your knee should be slightly bent. Don't arch your back or overextend yourself. Hold for a second, then slowly lower your leg.

Finish the set, then weight your left leg and repeat.

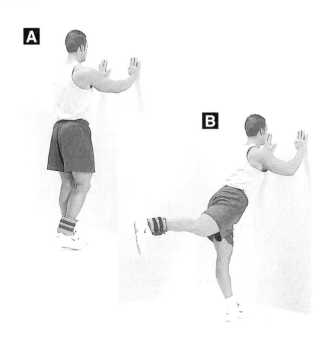

DUCK SQUAT WITH DUMBBELL

This move works your quadriceps and inner thigh muscles at an angle that's different from any other exercise.

[**A**] With your feet farther than shoulder-width apart, your knees unlocked, and your toes pointing out, hold a dumbbell by the end, using both hands with your arms extended. Your chest should be out, your shoulders back, your abs tight, and your back straight. Keep your head in line with your spine and look straight ahead. There will be a slight forward lean to your upper body, which is natural.

[**B**] Slowly squat until your thighs are parallel to the ground. Don't bounce, and don't let your knees turn in. Hold for a second. Then, keeping your feet flat on the floor, rise slowly with your hips slightly forward and your abs tight.

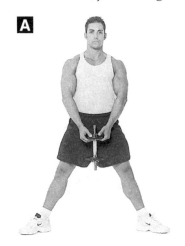

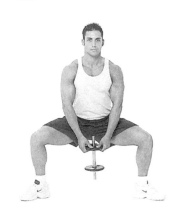

GLUTES AND HAMSTRINGS ► FREE WEIGHTS

REVERSE LEG EXTENSION WITH ANKLE WEIGHTS

This exercise also helps to strengthen your lower back.

[**A**] Wearing ankle weights, lie facedown on a bench or table with your hips at the edge, your legs together, your knees slightly bent, and your toes touching the floor. Grab the sides of the bench above your head to keep your upper body stable. Hold on firmly to avoid sliding off the bench.

[**B**] Raise your legs slowly, keeping your feet together, toes pointed, until your thighs are about parallel to your torso and no higher. Hold for a second, then slowly lower your legs to the starting position. Do not allow your feet to touch the floor until you have completed one set.

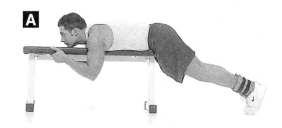

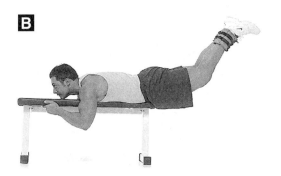

LATERAL LUNGE WITH BARBELL

This move also works your inner and outer thighs. To avoid injury, beginners should use a light weight until they master the movement.

[**A**] Balance a barbell behind your neck, resting it on your shoulders. Place your hands and feet slightly farther than shoulder-width apart. Keep your knees unlocked, your toes pointing out slightly, your chest out, your shoulders back, your stomach tight, and your back straight. Your head should be in line with your spine.

[**B**] Step to your right, landing heel to toe, pressing your hips down until your right thigh is parallel to the floor. Your right foot should point to the side; don't let your right knee extend past your toes. Keep your left leg extended and your left foot planted firmly on the floor, pointing forward. Your torso should face front. Hold for a second, then push with your right leg and return to the starting position.

Lunge to the right until you finish one set, then switch to the left.

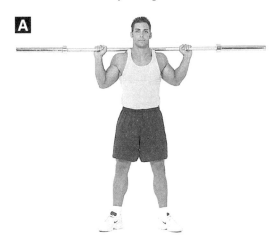

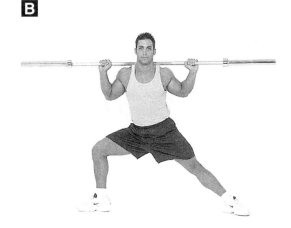

KNEELING KICKBACK WITH ANKLE WEIGHTS

This exercise will help improve your hip flexibility as well.

[**A**] Fasten ankle weights around both ankles, and get down on your hands and knees.

[**B**] Keeping your right knee slightly bent, slowly raise your right leg behind you until the thigh is parallel to your torso. Hold for a second, then slowly return almost to the starting position. Immediately raise the leg again before it touches the floor.

Finish the set, then switch legs.

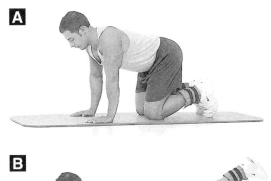

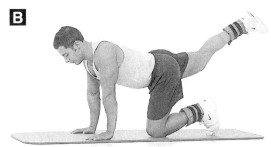

STATIONARY LUNGE WITH DUMBBELLS

This exercise gives the quadriceps muscles of your thighs a great workout, too.

[**A**] Stand with your head in line with your spine, your back straight, and your feet shoulder-width apart. Hold a dumbbell in each hand, with your arms hanging down and your palms facing your body.

[**B**] Take a long step forward with your right foot. Bend your leg until your right thigh is parallel to the floor. Your left leg should extend back with your left knee slightly bent and almost touching the floor. Hold this position for a second.

Keep your right foot stationary as you slowly straighten your right leg. Continue bending and straightening your right leg until you finish the set. Then switch legs.

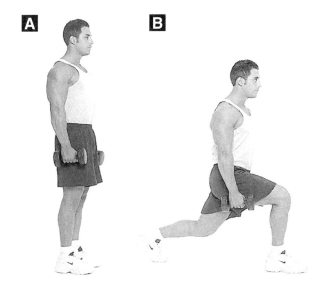

GLUTEAL MUSCLES ▶ MACHINES

REVERSE LEG EXTENSION WITH PULLEY

This exercise also works your lower back.

Place a weight bench far enough from a low pulley cable with ankle straps that you can extend your legs off one end without hitting the pulley.

[**A**] Put the ankle straps around your ankles and lie facedown with your hips at the edge of the bench, your legs together, your knees slightly bent, and your toes touching the floor. Grab the sides of the bench above your head to keep your upper body stable. Hold on firmly to avoid sliding off.

[**B**] Raise your legs slowly, keeping your feet together and your toes pointed, until your thighs are about parallel to your torso and no higher. Hold for a second, then slowly lower your legs almost to the starting position. Don't let your feet touch the floor until you have completed a set.

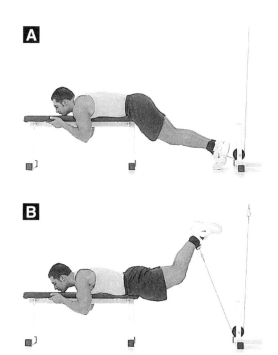

GLUTES AND HAMSTRINGS ▶ MACHINES

KNEELING KICKBACK WITH PULLEY

The downward resistance on your glutes and hamstrings in this exercise gives them a great workout.

Stand in front of a low pulley with an ankle strap on the cable. [**A**] Fasten the ankle strap around your right ankle, then get down on your hands and knees far enough from the pulley that you can extend your legs without hitting it.

[**B**] Keeping your right knee slightly bent, slowly raise that leg until your thigh is parallel to your torso. Hold for a second, then slowly return almost to the starting position. Immediately raise your right leg again before it touches the floor.

Finish the set, then put the strap on your left ankle and repeat.

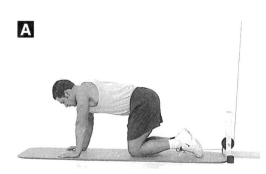

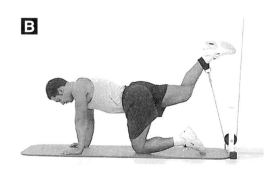

STANDING KICKBACK WITH PULLEY

This exercise is also good for your thighs.

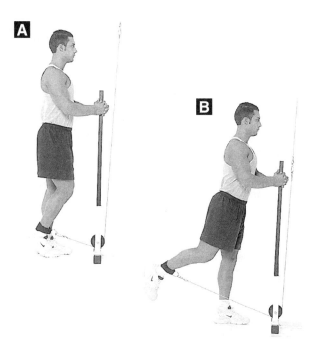

[**A**] Stand facing a low pulley with an ankle strap on the cable. Fasten the ankle strap around your right ankle. Use your hands for balance by holding on to the equipment at about waist height. Keep your head in line with your spine.

[**B**] Keep your right knee slightly bent as you slowly move your right leg straight back until you feel tightness in your butt. Do not overextend your leg to the point of discomfort. Slowly return to the starting position.

Finish the set, then put the strap on your left ankle and repeat.

GLUTEAL MUSCLES ► NO WEIGHTS

BENT-KICK CROSS

This exercise may look odd, but you'll feel the burn in your butt muscles.

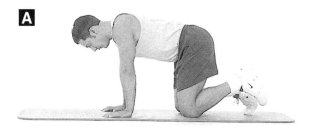

[**A**] Get down on your hands and knees and raise your left knee a few inches off the floor.

[**B**] Slowly push your left leg up and back, keeping it bent at about a 90-degree angle and forcing your heel to the ceiling. Feel your gluteal muscles contract as you push up. Don't let your thigh go beyond a position parallel to the floor. Hold for a second, then slowly lower your leg to the starting position.

Finish the set, then switch legs.

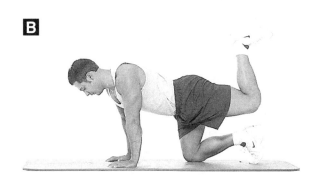

GLUTES AND HAMSTRINGS ▶ NO WEIGHTS

STANDING BACK LEG SWING

In addition to working your butt and back thigh muscles, this dynamic move loosens and strengthens your front hips and thighs and increases your legs' range of motion.

Stand with your left side to a stationary object, such as a ballet warmup bar or an exercise machine, and hold on to it with your left hand. Support your weight on your left leg, your right leg slightly bent. [A] Raise your right leg as high as possible in front of your body. Hold for a second.

[B] Allow your right leg to fall and swing as far behind your body as it will comfortably go. Hold for a second, then swing back to the starting position.

Finish the set, then switch sides.

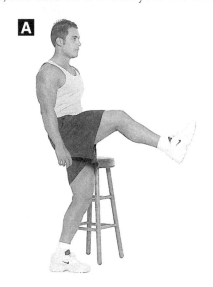

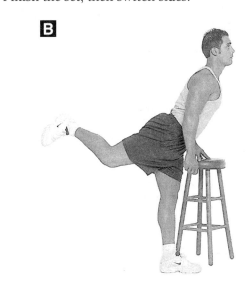

KNEELING KICKBACK

This exercise also increases your hip flexibility and will help improve your running time.

[A] Get down on your hands and knees.

[B] Keeping your right knee slightly bent, slowly raise your right leg behind you until your thigh is parallel to your torso. Hold for a second, then slowly return almost to the starting position. Immediately raise your leg again before it touches the floor.

Finish the set, then switch legs.

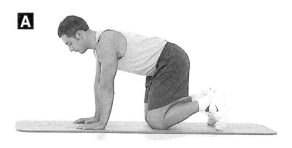

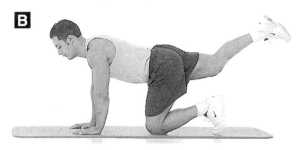

REVERSE LEG EXTENSION

This exercise is also great for your lower back, building strength without putting pressure on it.

[**A**] Lie facedown on a bench or table with your hips at the edge, your legs together, your knees slightly bent, and your toes touching the floor. Grab the sides of the bench above your head to keep your upper body stable as you move your legs. Hold on firmly to avoid sliding off the bench.

[**B**] Raise your legs slowly, keeping your feet together and your toes pointed, until your thighs are about parallel to your torso and no higher. Hold for a second, then slowly lower your legs until your feet almost touch the floor. (Don't let them touch the floor until you've finished the set.) Repeat.

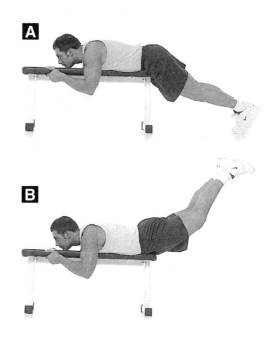

ALTERNATING LUNGE

This dynamic movement builds strength and coordination. It works your quadriceps muscles, too.

[**A**] Stand with your feet shoulder-width apart, your hands on your hips. Keep your upper body upright and your head in line with your spine.

[**B**] Take a long step forward with your right foot. Plant that foot firmly on the floor and bend your knees until your right thigh is parallel to the floor. Don't let your right knee extend past your right foot. Your left leg should be extended behind you, the knee slightly bent and the heel raised.

Immediately step back with your right foot, pressing your left heel to the ground. Your feet should be shoulder-width apart. Repeat the exercise with your left foot. That makes one repetition.

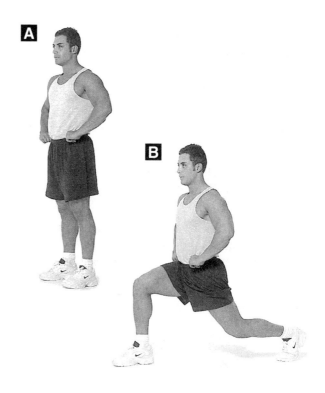

POWERFUL BUTT

BEGINNER WORKOUT

We recommend that you train with the balanced, full-body plan on page 48. If you need to concentrate specifically on your butt, however, this program will produce quick gains. Choose one exercise routine to follow: free weights, machines, or no weights.

INSTRUCTIONS

1. Do the complete exercise routine 2 or 3 days a week. Wait at least 48 hours between sessions to allow sufficient recovery time for optimum development.

2. To warm up, do some aerobics and stretching, and perform one set of 6 to 10 repetitions with a light to moderate load. This minimizes the chances of a muscle strain or pull during the subsequent training period.

3. After the warmup, find a starting load that is difficult to lift 6 times. This may take some experimenting on your first day. Once you have iden-

tified that load, that's what you will use until it becomes too easy.

Complete one set of 6 repetitions for each exercise listed in the routine you've chosen. Perform the positive phase (also known as the concentric or lifting phase) of each exercise as quickly as possible while maintaining proper form. Perform the negative (or eccentric or lowering) phase much more slowly, to a count of four.

4. After a few sessions, you'll find that completing the 6 repetitions is easier. At that point, add repetitions, following proper form, up to 10 repetitions.

5. When you are able to perform 10 reps, make a note to add weight on the next session.

6. With the added weight, drop back to 6 reps. Then repeat steps 3 to 5 until you have completed 12 weeks of the program. Then, if you still need to focus on butt workouts, you may move on to the intermediate level. Remember, we recommend that you do the balanced, full-body workouts rather than working on individual muscle groups.

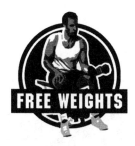

FREE WEIGHTS

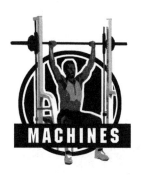

MACHINES

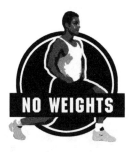

NO WEIGHTS

1. STATIONARY LUNGE WITH DUMBBELLS (PAGE 181)
2. LATERAL LUNGE WITH BARBELL (PAGE 180)
3. DUCK SQUAT WITH DUMBBELL (PAGE 179)
4. REVERSE LEG EXTENSION WITH ANKLE WEIGHTS (PAGE 180)

1. STANDING KICKBACK WITH PULLEY (PAGE 183)
2. REVERSE LEG EXTENSION WITH PULLEY (PAGE 182)
3. KNEELING KICKBACK WITH PULLEY (PAGE 182)

1. ALTERNATING LUNGE (PAGE 185)
2. REVERSE LEG EXTENSION (PAGE 185)
3. KNEELING KICKBACK (PAGE 184)
4. STANDING BACK LEG SWING (PAGE 184)

POWERFUL BUTT
INTERMEDIATE WORKOUT

We recommend that you train with the balanced, full-body plan on page 52. If you need to concentrate specifically on your butt, though, this program will produce quick gains. Choose one exercise routine to follow: free weights, machines, or no weights.

INSTRUCTIONS

1. Train 3 days a week. Allow enough recovery by waiting at least 48 hours between sessions.

2. Always warm up with aerobics and stretching, plus one set of 6 to 10 repetitions with a light to moderate load. This minimizes the chances of a muscle strain or pull during the subsequent training period.

3. Your standard intermediate workout is three sets of 6 to 10 repetitions for each exercise listed in the routine you've chosen. The warmup set is your first set. The starting load for the second and third sets should be one that is difficult to lift 6 times. As your strength increases, increase the repetitions per set until you can do 10 repetitions while maintaining proper form. Then, for your next session, increase the load and drop back to 6 reps.

Perform the positive phase (also known as the concentric or lifting phase) of each exercise as quickly as possible while maintaining proper form. Perform the negative (or eccentric or lowering) phase much more slowly, to a count of four.

4. Vary your routines. Instead of some of the individual exercises, do combo lifts, or supersets, two exercises in succession (one rep of each) without a rest. You can do almost any two exercises this way. Combo lifts increase the intensity of your workout, create some variety, and can shorten your workout session.

Another variation is to use a lighter load than usual and do 15 to 20 repetitions, and/or to increase the load on successive sets and reduce the number of repetitions (this last variation is called pyramids). So, for example, in set 1, you might do 10 repetitions with 200 pounds; in set 2, you might do 7 repetitions with 250 pounds; and in set 3, you might do 4 repetitions with 300 pounds.

5. As you gain training experience, you might try experimenting with 1 or 2 partial repetitions at the end of each set, at the point where you can no longer complete a full repetition. This is called going to muscle failure, and it may enhance muscle development. *Note:* If you try this, you will need a partner to spot you, especially when you're using free weights.

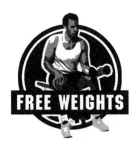

FREE WEIGHTS

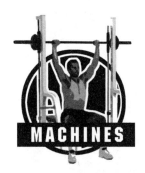

MACHINES

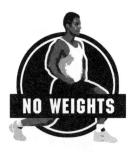

NO WEIGHTS

1. STATIONARY LUNGE WITH DUMBBELLS (PAGE 181)
2. LATERAL LUNGE WITH BARBELL (PAGE 180)
3. DUCK SQUAT WITH DUMBBELL (PAGE 179)
4. REVERSE LEG EXTENSION WITH ANKLE WEIGHTS (PAGE 180)
5. STANDING KICKBACK WITH ANKLE WEIGHTS (PAGE 179)

1. STANDING KICKBACK WITH PULLEY (PAGE 183)
2. REVERSE LEG EXTENSION WITH PULLEY (PAGE 182)
3. KNEELING KICKBACK WITH PULLEY (PAGE 182)

1. ALTERNATING LUNGE (PAGE 185)
2. REVERSE LEG EXTENSION (PAGE 185)
3. KNEELING KICKBACK (PAGE 184)
4. STANDING BACK LEG SWING (PAGE 184)
5. BENT-KICK CROSS (PAGE 183)

POWERFUL BUTT
ADVANCED WORKOUT

We recommend that you train with the balanced, full-body plan on page 56. If you need to concentrate specifically on your butt, however, this program will produce quick gains. Choose one exercise routine to follow: free weights, machines, or no weights.

INSTRUCTIONS

1. Train 3 days a week. Allow sufficient recovery time by waiting at least 48 hours between sessions.

2. Your standard advanced workout is three sets of 6 to 10 repetitions for each exercise in the routine you've chosen. The first set, after your aerobics and stretching, is a warmup with a lighter-than-normal weight. The starting load for the second and third sets should be one that is difficult to lift 6 times. As your strength increases, increase the number of repetitions per set until you can do 10 repetitions. Then, for

your next session, increase the load and drop back to 6 repetitions.

Perform the positive phase (also known as the concentric or lifting phase) of each exercise as quickly as possible while maintaining proper form. Perform the negative (or eccentric or lowering) phase of the exercise much more slowly, to a count of four.

3. Vary your workouts as at the intermediate level, and try replacing some of the exercises with tri-sets and giant sets. Tri-sets are like combo lifts except that you add another exercise so that you're doing three in succession without rest. With giant sets, you do four exercises in succession without resting between them.

4. Do 1 or 2 partial repetitions at the end of each set when you reach the point where you can no longer complete a full repetition. This is called going to muscle failure, and it may enhance muscle development. *Note:* At the advanced level, you always need the assistance of a partner for safety when doing partial reps with free weights.

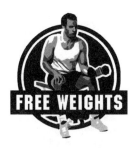

FREE WEIGHTS

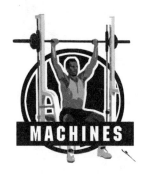

MACHINES

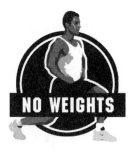

NO WEIGHTS

1. STATIONARY LUNGE WITH DUMBBELLS (PAGE 181)

2. LATERAL LUNGE WITH BARBELL (PAGE 180)

3. DUCK SQUAT WITH DUMBBELL (PAGE 179)

4. REVERSE LEG EXTENSION WITH ANKLE WEIGHTS (PAGE 180)

5. KNEELING KICKBACK WITH ANKLE WEIGHTS (PAGE 181)

6. STANDING KICKBACK WITH ANKLE WEIGHTS (PAGE 179)

1. STANDING KICKBACK WITH PULLEY (PAGE 183)

2. REVERSE LEG EXTENSION WITH PULLEY (PAGE 182)

3. KNEELING KICKBACK WITH PULLEY (PAGE 182)

1. ALTERNATING LUNGE (PAGE 185)

2. REVERSE LEG EXTENSION (PAGE 185)

3. KNEELING KICKBACK (PAGE 184)

4. STANDING BACK LEG SWING (PAGE 184)

5. BENT-KICK CROSS (PAGE 183)

QUICK-SET PATH TO
POWERFUL THIGHS

YOUR THIGH MUSCLE GROUPS ARE AMONG THE BIGGEST IN YOUR BODY. YOU USE THEM IN ALMOST ANY MANLY ENDEAVOR. CONDITION THEM IF YOU WANT TO RUN; PLAY SPORTS; PUSH, SHOVE, OR PULL ANYTHING; OR JUST WALK LIKE A MAN.

Every season, dozens of Major League Baseball players miss games—sometimes a lot of games—because of injuries to their thigh muscles. Thigh muscle injuries strike stars and benchwarmers with an equal vengeance. Among those who have missed playing time are big-name players such as Kenny Lofton, Omar Vizquel, and Nomar Garciaparra, and little-knowns like Cristian Guzman and Mickey Callaway.

Even if you don't make a living stealing bases or fielding flies, you need to keep your thigh muscles in shape. Doing so enables you to hike a mountain or merely climb stairs, pick up a barbell, or get up from your La-Z-Boy. As you age, your strong thighs will help you avoid falls that may result in broken bones.

And if you're a weekend jock, you have all the more reason to exercise your quadriceps and hamstrings—the two biggest muscles in your thighs—along with your butt muscles. "People with good glutes and quads are going to be better at almost any sport you can name," says Michael Youssouf, a trainer of fitness trainers in New York City. And that's another advantage of the Hard-Body Plan: It'll make you a better archer, golfer, pitcher, sprinter, slugger, quarterback. . . . A lot of the benefit comes from leg work.

Most of us, however, would just as soon shave our legs as exercise them. "Guys spend an hour in the gym, and they usually spend that hour doing upper-body exercises," says Brian Pfeufer of Sports Training Institute in New York City. You should, however, earmark about an equal amount of time for exercising your upper and lower body, he says.

"One of the reasons a lot of guys don't like lower-body work is that it just plain takes a lot of energy," says Tory Allman, an exercise physiologist in Solana Beach, California. "You do a set of squats, it's like flushing the gas tank on your oxygen and blood sugar levels."

Follow the mix of exercises in the Hard-Body Plan and you'll gain powerful thighs—but you'll *also* keep the "gas tank" topped off with proper Hard-Body eating for maximum energy.

QUALITY QUADRICEPS

The *quadriceps,* or quads, are a group of four large muscles at the front of each thigh. They allow you to extend your knee and flex your thigh at the hip.

Your quads should be stronger than your hamstrings, the muscles at the back of your thighs, because they are a bigger muscle group, Pfeufer says.

If you are lifting, say, 50 pounds on the leg curl machine to strengthen your hamstrings, try to use the same amount of weight on leg extensions for your quads, progressively increasing the weight or the number of reps with the latter while maintaining your hamstring strength.

Working big thigh muscles such as the quads also may protect you from knee injuries. That's because, as you build up muscle, you also strengthen connective tissue that stabilizes joints such as those in the knee. "Most of the stabilizing connective tissue around the leg is attached more to the quadriceps and the hamstrings," Allman says.

One of your quads is also part of the hip flexor muscle group, and some quad exercises also work these muscles. Developing the hip flexors enables you to climb stairs, kick a ball, and run better.

HELLACIOUS HAMSTRINGS

The hamstrings are a group of three muscles at the back of each thigh running from the knee to the hips. They allow you to bend your knee.

We told you that you should have stronger quads

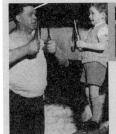

HARD-BODY MOMENT

Now this is a man with strong thighs: Paul Wai Man Chung did 4,289 squats in 1 hour in Hong Kong on April 5, 1993.

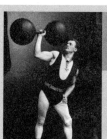

HARD-BODY FACT

Working your meaty thigh muscles may actually contribute to building your upper body as well. Here's how. Exercising massive muscle groups such as quads, hamstrings, and glutes stimulates protein assimilation, nitrogen retention, and the release of human growth hormone throughout your body. So your upper body may benefit too. By contrast, your bulging biceps are a comparatively tiny muscle group and release little of this muscle-building material.

than hamstrings, but don't ignore these important muscles in the backs of your thighs. Hamstrings are the most commonly injured thigh muscles. Hamstring injuries are slow to heal and often recur. And they can be debilitating, which is why the word *hamstring* also means "to make ineffective or powerless."

Fitness trainer John Abdo has worked with Olympic speed skaters who developed fantastic quadriceps but lacked hamstring development. That resulted in knee injuries. But "the injuries went away completely" once he added hamstring exercises to these athletes' training routines, he says.

Runners often have stronger hamstrings than quads. As with other muscle groups, achieving a balance is the key to avoiding injuries and even back pain, in the case of thigh muscles.

Don't drop down too quickly when doing the squat, an exercise that effectively works the butt, quadriceps, and hamstring muscles.

"You want to start out slowly. You want to control the weight," Pfeufer says. If you're performing this exercise for the first time, try it initially using just a barbell with no weights attached, or using dumbbells held at your sides to eliminate some of the strain on your back.

Don't arch your back, and concentrate on looking straight ahead. "If you look up, you throw your spine out of whack," Pfeufer says.

ENTIRE THIGHS ► FREE WEIGHTS

SQUAT

This is a great all-purpose exercise that conditions large muscle groups (specifically, your thighs and gluteal muscles) while also working your shoulders, back, arms, and legs. Beginners should practice with an unweighted bar.

Place a barbell at shoulder level on a squat rack. Grip the bar with your hands slightly farther than shoulder-width apart, palms facing forward. Step under the bar so that it is positioned evenly across your upper back and shoulders.

[**A**] Stand up straight with your feet hip-width apart, toes pointing slightly out. Don't drop your head; it should be in line with your torso, with your eyes looking ahead.

[**B**] Keeping your feet flat and your torso straight, bend your knees slightly and slowly squat down. Don't arch your back or let your knees extend past your toes. Squat until your thighs are almost parallel to the floor. Pause, then slowly rise to the starting position.

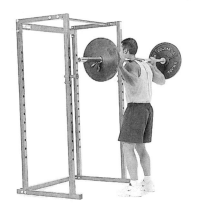

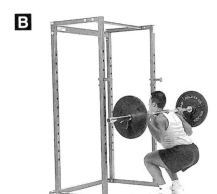

HACK SQUAT

This variation puts less pressure on your knees and lower back than the regular squat does, but it requires more balance. To avoid injury, start with an unweighted bar, and slowly work up to less weight than for a regular squat as you master the movement.

With your feet hip-width apart, stand with a barbell placed directly behind your heels. Squat down and grip the bar with your palms facing away from your body. Your hands should be slightly farther than shoulder-width apart.

[**A**] Stand up, holding the bar at arm's length behind your thighs. Keep your head in line with your body.

[**B**] Slowly squat down until your thighs are close

to parallel with the floor. Do not allow your knees to extend over your toes. Hold for a second, then slowly rise, keeping your arms fully extended.

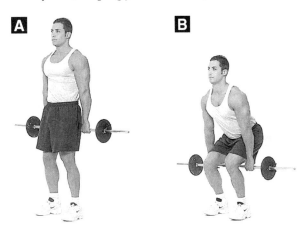

STEPUP WITH DUMBBELLS

This exercise also increases strength and flexibility in your gluteal muscles.

[**A**] Stand about 1 foot from a step platform or box that's between 12 and 18 inches high. Hold a dumbbell in each hand, arms down at your sides, palms facing your body. Stand upright with your shoulders back and your chest out.

[**B**] Keeping the dumbbells at your sides and your upper body straight, step forward with your left foot, placing it on the center of the step.

[**C**] Complete the step by bringing your right foot next to your right.

[**D**] Step backward with your left foot so that your left leg is about where you started. Then step down with your right foot to bring it back to the starting position.

Repeat the sequence of steps, this time leading with your right foot. That makes one repetition.

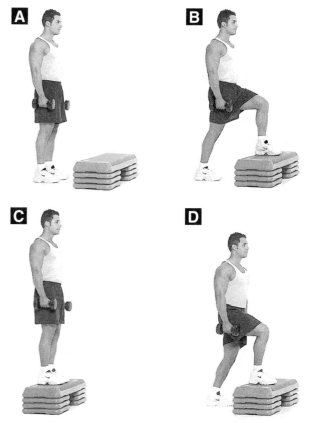

BENCH LATERAL STEPUP WITH DUMBBELLS

To avoid injury, beginners should use especially light weights until they master this movement.

Place two benches slightly farther than shoulder-width apart. Hold a dumbbell in each hand and stand between the benches with your arms down, your palms facing your sides, and your feet shoulder-width apart.

[**A**] Step up with your right leg, placing your foot to the far right on the width of the bench and leaving room for your left foot.

[**B**] Step up with your left leg, shifting your weight from your left to your right, and place your left foot on the bench next to your right.

[**C**] Step down, slowly extending your left leg toward the floor. When your weight is on your left leg, bring your right foot back to the starting position. Then repeat the exercise, this time leading with your left leg. That makes one repetition.

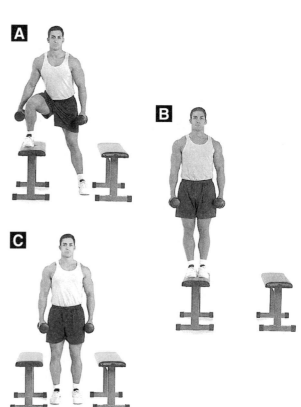

FRONT SQUAT

This move also strengthens your knees, hips, and lower back to help prevent sports injuries. It's difficult, though, so use less weight than for a regular squat.

Place the barbell at midchest level on a squat rack. Walk in toward the bar until it rests on top of the front of your shoulders. Cross your arms, using your right hand to grip the bar at your left shoulder and your left hand to grip it on the right.

[A] Stand up straight until the bar is fully supported by your shoulders and arms, keeping your elbows high. Take one step back away from the rack. Your feet should be flat on the floor and shoulder-width apart. Keep your upper body straight and your head in line with your body.

[B] Slowly squat down until your thighs are parallel to the floor. Don't let your knees extend over your toes. Keep your torso straight and your eyes looking ahead. Hold for a second, then slowly rise to the starting position.

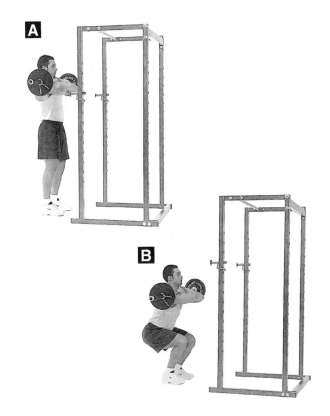

QUADRICEPS ► FREE WEIGHTS

DUMBBELL POWER LUNGE

This advanced exercise also works your gluteal and hamstring muscles. Begin with light weights.

[A] Stand upright with a dumbbell held firmly in each hand. Your arms should be fully extended at your sides, palms in. Keep your feet about hip-width apart and your torso upright. Maintain a natural curve in your lower back.

[B] With your left leg, step forward slightly farther than you would in a normal step. Keep your upper body upright with your arms at your sides and the dumbbells roughly in the centerline of your body. Bend your left leg 90 degrees so that you can still see your toes if you look down at them. Bend your right leg slightly at the knee. Your right heel will rise slightly, but the foot should remain in the same position.

Explosively jump up and switch legs in the air so that on landing your right leg is forward and your leg is back. That's one rep. As soon as you land, push off again, switching legs again.

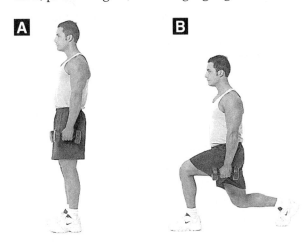

LEG EXTENSION WITH ANKLE WEIGHTS

In this exercise, foot positioning can change the way the muscles are worked. Try pointing your toes back toward you or straight out to work different parts of your quads.

Fasten ankle weights around your ankles.

[**A**] Sit on a bench, grasping its sides with your hands. Your knees should be bent 90 degrees or slightly more, your toes pointing in front of you.

[**B**] Using the sides of the bench for support, slowly straighten your legs by lifting with your ankles and contracting your quadriceps. Don't lock your knees at full extension. Your toes should point up and out at about a 45-degree angle to the floor. Hold for a second, then slowly lower your legs to the starting position.

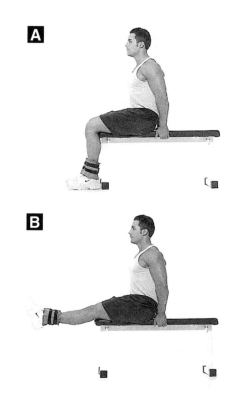

LATERAL SQUAT

This exercise also works your gluteal muscles as well as the sides of your thighs. Beginners may use dumbbells instead of a barbell.

[**A**] Stand straight and grip a barbell evenly across your upper back and shoulders, with your hands slightly farther than shoulder-width apart and your palms facing away from your body. Place your feet in a wide stance, toes pointed out, and keep your head in line with your body.

[**B**] Drop down by slowly bending your right leg until your right thigh is parallel to the floor. Don't let your right knee turn in or extend over your toes. Put most of your weight on your right leg, keeping your left leg extended, knee slightly bent. Hold for a second, then return to the starting position by slowly extending your right leg and bringing your torso back to the center. Repeat on your left side without resting. That makes one repetition.

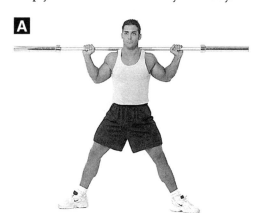

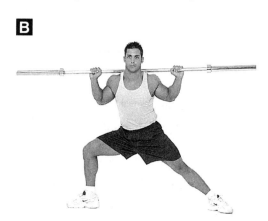

HAMSTRINGS ► FREE WEIGHTS

LEG CURL
WITH ANKLE WEIGHTS

This exercise also works the erector spinae muscles of your lower back.

[**A**] Lie on your stomach on a bench with both legs straight out and an ankle weight on each ankle. Your knees should be just past the bench's edge so you can bend your legs up. If necessary, hold on to the bench's legs for support.

[**B**] Keeping your feet together and pointed out, slowly curl the weights in a semicircular motion toward your butt until your legs are at about a 90-degree angle. Point your toes up, and don't arch your pelvis or back. Your body should remain flush with the bench. Hold for a second, then slowly lower your legs to the starting position.

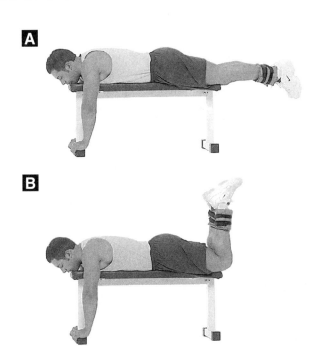

ENTIRE THIGHS ► MACHINES

HACK SQUAT
WITH SMITH MACHINE

This exercise also works your glutes. To avoid injury, start with an unweighted bar. Slowly work up to less weight than for a regular squat as you master the movement.

[**A**] Stand at a Smith machine with the weight bar set about butt-high. Back yourself up to the bar until you can grip it with your arms at your sides and your palms facing behind you. Your hands should be slightly more than shoulder-width apart. Keep your head in line with your body.

[**B**] Slowly squat down until your thighs are almost parallel to the floor. Do not allow your knees to extend over your toes. Hold for a second, then slowly rise without bending your arms.

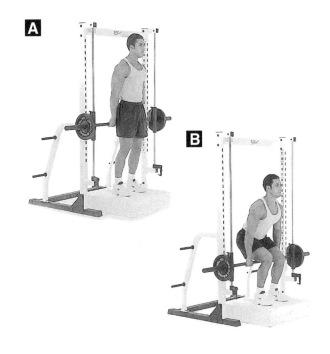

VERTICAL LEG PRESS

This machine exercise gives your hamstrings and quads a great workout.

[**A**] Sit in a vertical leg-press machine with the seat adjusted so that your knees are bent at a 90-degree angle or slightly less. Place your feet shoulder-width apart and turn your toes out slightly. Grip the handlebars and press your lower back to the pad.

[**B**] Slowly push forward on the foot plate to straighten your legs, keeping your knees un-locked. Hold for a second, then slowly return to the starting position.

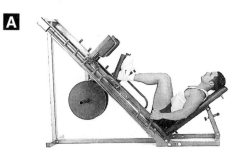

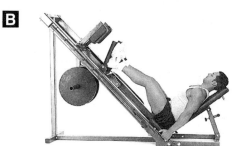

QUADRICEPS ► MACHINES

LEG EXTENSION

This exercise is a great way to build your quads. Foot positioning changes the way that your muscles are worked, so try pointing your toes back or straight to work different parts of your quadriceps.

[**A**] Sit in a leg extension machine with your legs behind the padded lifting bars and your hands grasping the machine's handles or the sides of the bench. Your knees should be bent 90 de-grees or slightly more, with your toes pointing in front of you.

[**B**] Using the machine's handles or the sides of the bench for support, slowly straighten your legs by lifting with your ankles and contracting your quadriceps. Don't lock your knees at full extension; keep them slightly bent. Your toes should point up and out at about a 45-degree angle. Hold for a second, then slowly return to the starting position.

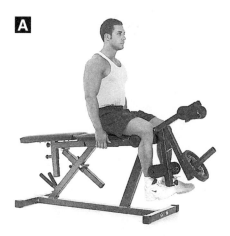

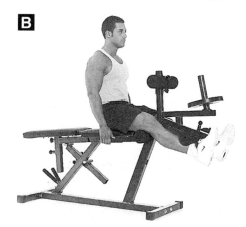

FORWARD CABLE KICK

This exercise is an excellent way to build your quads.

[**A**] Stand facing away from a low pulley, with an ankle strap attached to your left ankle and to the cable. Grab a support to one side—something waist-high, such as a chair—so you won't have to bend over.

[**B**] Slowly raise your left leg in front of you until your thigh is parallel to the floor. Keep your leg and back straight; don't bend forward or backward. Hold for a second, then slowly lower your leg to the starting position.

Finish the set, then switch legs.

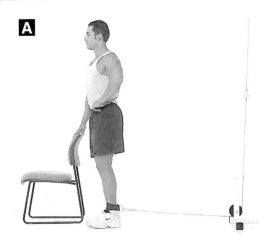

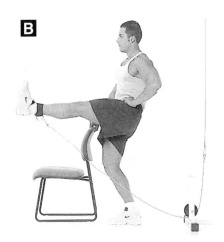

HAMSTRINGS ► MACHINES

LEG CURL

Use less weight on this hamstring exercise than you would for a leg extension.

[**A**] Lie facedown on a leg curl machine with your ankles hooked behind the lifting pads and your knees just over the bench's edge. Hold on to the machine's handlebars, if any, for support. Your legs should be fully extended with some natural bend at the knees, and your toes should point down.

[**B**] Keeping your pelvis flush against the bench, slowly raise your heels toward your butt so that your legs bend to about a 90-degree angle. Use the handlebars for support, and keep your feet pointing away from your body. Hold for a second, then slowly lower your heels to the starting position.

Note: Some leg curl machines are bent slightly at the end to relieve pressure from your pelvis. If yours is not, put a small pillow under your pelvis.

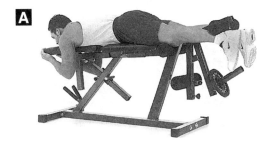

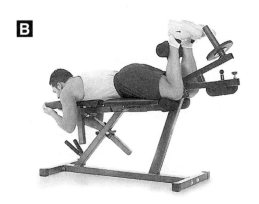

ENTIRE THIGHS ► NO WEIGHTS

BENCH LATERAL STEPUP WITH TUBING

This skiers' exercise works not only your front and back thighs but also the sides of your thighs. To avoid injury, beginners should use light resistance until they have mastered the movement.

Place two benches slightly farther than shoulder-width apart. Wrap exercise tubing securely under and around the nearest foot of each weight bench.

[**A**] Grasp the tubing's handles and stand between the benches, your arms down, your palms facing your sides, and your feet shoulder-width apart.

[**B**] Step up with your right foot on the right bench. Leave room for your left foot. Bring it up so that both feet are on the bench. Then step down slowly, leading with your left leg.

[**C**] Repeat the basics, but step up onto the left bench, leading with your left foot. That's one rep.

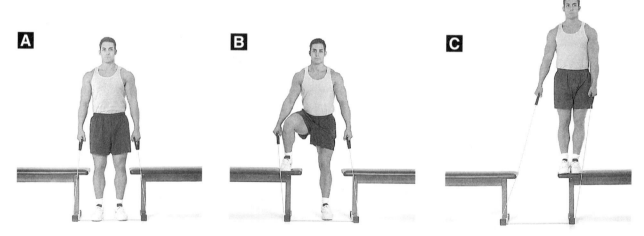

SINGLE-LEG SQUAT

This exercise also strengthens your gluteal muscles, hips, and back.

[**A**] Stand upright with your feet shoulder-width apart and your knees slightly bent. Position a sturdy chair or a piece of exercise equipment to your right so you can rest your right hand on it for balance. Keep your back straight and put your left hand on your hip for balance.

[**B**] Slowly begin to squat on your right leg while extending your left leg in front of you. Keep your back straight. As soon as your right thigh is parallel to the floor, slowly press yourself back up to the starting position. Don't pause between repetitions; you should look like a piston pumping up and down.

Finish the set, then switch legs.

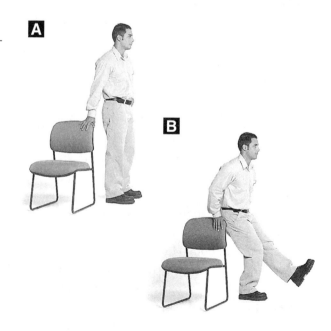

ALTERNATING JUMP LUNGE

This explosive move also works your gluteal muscles.

[**A**] Stand with your feet shoulder-width apart and your back straight.

[**B**] Take a long step forward with your right foot. Firmly plant that foot on the floor and bend your knees until your right thigh is parallel to the floor. Don't let your right knee extend past your right foot. Your left leg should be extended behind you, knee slightly bent, heel raised. Keep your upper body upright and your head in line with your spine.

Quickly and explosively push off your right foot, extending your left leg in front of you. You should end up in much the same lunging position as before, only with your left foot forward and your right foot behind you. Immediately push off your left foot, extending your right leg forward again. That's one repetition. Repeat without resting until you've finished the set.

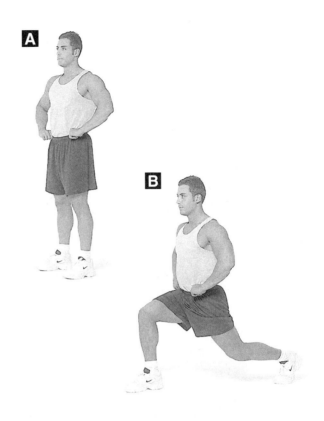

PHANTOM CHAIR

This exercise also works your gluteal muscles.

[**A**] Stand leaning with your back flat against a wall and your knees slightly bent. Your feet should be a little farther than shoulder-width apart, 1½ feet from the wall, and your toes should point out slightly. Keep your shoulders back and your chest out.

[**B**] Slowly bend your knees farther, lowering yourself until the tops of your thighs are parallel to the ground. Don't go so far down that your knees extend over your toes. Hold until your muscles are fatigued, then slowly straighten your legs and return to the starting position.

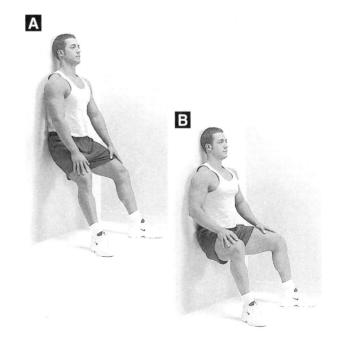

DOUBLE LEG POWER JUMP

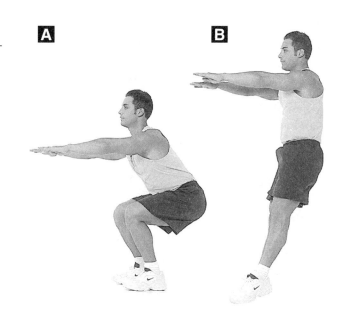

This exercise also works the gastrocnemius muscles of your leg.

Stand with your feet about shoulder-width apart and your knees bent.

[**A**] Lean forward in a half-squatting position, with your arms out in front of you for balance and your head and back in a straight line.

[**B**] Quickly and explosively push up off both feet, propelling yourself forward as if you were doing a long jump. Try to cover as much horizontal distance as possible. Your arms may swing behind you as you jump, but keep your feet together. The moment that you land, push off again. Do 6 to 10 repetitions without rest.

QUADRICEPS ► NO WEIGHTS

LEG EXTENSION WITH BRIEFCASE

This is a great quad exercise you can do in your office.

Sit on the edge of a chair with your knees slightly bent and your legs together.

[**A**] Place your briefcase or a big book on top of your shins, bending your feet upward so that it doesn't fall off. Stabilize yourself by holding the sides of your chair with your hands.

[**B**] Slowly lift your ankles to raise your legs. Don't lock your knees at full extension; keep them slightly bent. Your toes should point up and out at a 45-degree angle. Hold the extension for 2 or 3 seconds, then slowly lower your legs to the starting position.

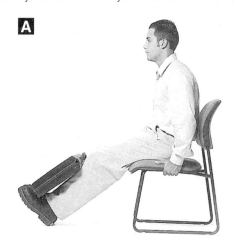

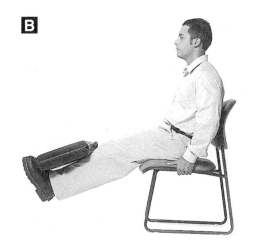

DOUBLE LEG SQUAT JUMP

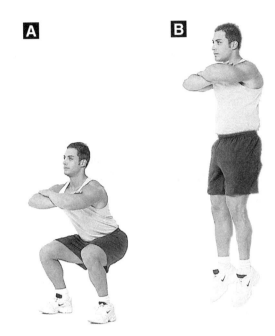

This exercise also works your butt muscles and hamstrings.

Stand with your feet slightly farther than shoulder-width apart and your arms crossed in front of you.

[**A**] Keeping your head up and your back straight, squat until your thighs are almost parallel to the floor.

[**B**] Jump straight up in an explosive movement. But don't let your lower legs provide all the power—make your butt, thighs, and hips do the work. As soon as you land, squat and jump again without resting.

HAMSTRINGS ► NO WEIGHTS

LEG CURL WITH TUBING

This simple exercise is very effective at building your hamstrings. Try to use less resistance for this move than you would for a leg extension.

Wrap a length of exercise tubing around the bottom of one foot of a weight bench, and put the tubing's handles around your ankles.

[**A**] Lie facedown on the bench with your knees just over the edge of the bench. Hold on to the bench's legs for balance. Your legs should be fully extended, your knees slightly bent.

[**B**] Keeping your pelvis against the bench and your feet flat, slowly raise your heels toward your butt until your legs are at about a 90-degree angle. Hold for a second, then slowly return to the starting position. The goal is to keep your hamstrings tense through the entire range of motion.

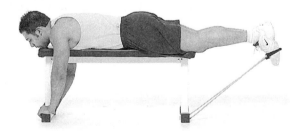

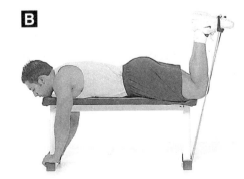

POWERFUL THIGHS
BEGINNER WORKOUT

We recommend that you train with the balanced, full-body plan on page 48. If you need to concentrate specifically on thigh work, however, this program will produce quick gains. Choose one exercise routine to follow: free weights, machines, or no weights.

INSTRUCTIONS

1. Do the complete exercise routine 2 or 3 days a week. Wait at least 48 hours between sessions to allow sufficient recovery time for optimum development.

2. To warm up, do some aerobics and stretching, and perform one set of 6 to 10 repetitions with a light to moderate load. This minimizes the chances of a muscle strain or pull during the subsequent training period.

3. After the warmup, find a starting load that is difficult to lift 6 times. This may take some experimenting on your first day. Once you have iden-

tified that load, that's what you will use until it becomes too easy.

Complete one set of 6 repetitions for each exercise in the routine you've chosen. Perform the positive phase (also known as the concentric or lifting phase) of each exercise as quickly as possible while maintaining proper form. Perform the negative (or eccentric or lowering) phase much more slowly, to a count of four.

4. After a few sessions, you will find that completing the 6 repetitions is easier. At that point, add repetitions, following proper form, up to 10 repetitions.

5. When you are able to perform 10 reps, make a note to add weight at the next session.

6. With the added weight, drop back to 6 reps. Then repeat steps 3 to 5 until you have completed 12 weeks of the program. Then, if you still need to focus on thigh workouts, you may move on to the intermediate level. Remember, we recommend that you do the balanced, full-body workouts rather than working on individual muscle groups.

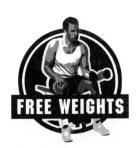

FREE WEIGHTS

1. HACK SQUAT (PAGE 195)
2. STATIONARY LUNGE WITH DUMBBELLS (PAGE 181)
3. LEG CURL WITH ANKLE WEIGHTS (PAGE 199)
4. LEG EXTENSION WITH ANKLE WEIGHTS (PAGE 198)

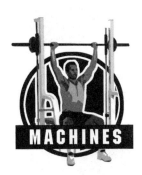

MACHINES

1. VERTICAL LEG PRESS (PAGE 200)
2. LEG CURL (PAGE 201)
3. LEG EXTENSION (PAGE 200)

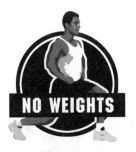

NO WEIGHTS

1. SINGLE-LEG SQUAT (PAGE 202)
2. PHANTOM CHAIR (PAGE 203)
3. LEG EXTENSION WITH BRIEFCASE (PAGE 204)
4. LEG CURL WITH TUBING (PAGE 205)

POWERFUL THIGHS
INTERMEDIATE WORKOUT

We recommend that you train with the balanced, full-body plan on page 52. If you need to concentrate specifically on thigh work, though, this program will produce quick gains. Choose one exercise routine to follow: free weights, machines, or no weights.

INSTRUCTIONS

1. Train 3 days a week. Allow enough recovery by waiting at least 48 hours between sessions.

2. Always warm up with aerobics and stretching, plus one set of 6 to 10 repetitions using a light to moderate load. This minimizes the chances of a muscle strain or pull during the subsequent training period.

3. Your standard intermediate workout is three sets of 6 to 10 repetitions for each exercise listed in the routine you've chosen. The warmup set is your first set. The starting load for the second and third sets should be one that is difficult to lift 6 times. As your strength increases, increase the repetitions per set until you can do 10 repetitions while maintaining proper form. Then, for your next session, increase the load and drop back to 6 reps.

Perform the positive phase (also known as the concentric or lifting phase) of each exercise as quickly as possible while maintaining proper form. Perform the negative (or eccentric or lowering) phase much more slowly, to a count of four.

4. Vary your routines. Instead of some of the individual exercises, do combo lifts, or supersets, two exercises in succession (one rep of each) without a rest. You can do almost any two exercises this way. Combo lifts increase the intensity of your workout, create some variety, and can shorten your workout session.

Another variation is to use a lighter load than usual and do 15 to 20 repetitions, and/or to increase the load on successive sets and reduce the number of repetitions (this last variation is called pyramids). So, for example, in set 1, you might do 10 repetitions with 200 pounds; in set 2, you might do 7 repetitions with 250 pounds; and in set 3, you might do 4 repetitions with 300 pounds.

5. As you gain training experience, you might try experimenting with 1 or 2 partial repetitions at the end of each set, at the point where you can no longer complete a full repetition. This is called going to muscle failure, and it may enhance muscle development. *Note:* If you try this, you will need a partner to spot you, especially when you're using free weights.

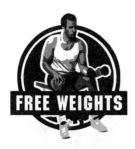

FREE WEIGHTS

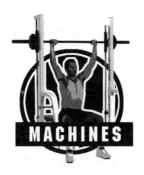

MACHINES

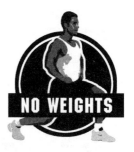

NO WEIGHTS

1. SQUAT (PAGE 195)
2. STATIONARY LUNGE WITH DUMBBELLS (PAGE 181)
3. STEPUP WITH DUMBBELLS (PAGE 196)
4. LEG CURL WITH ANKLE WEIGHTS (PAGE 199)
5. BENCH LATERAL STEPUP WITH DUMBBELLS (PAGE 196)
6. LEG EXTENSION WITH ANKLE WEIGHTS (PAGE 198)

1. VERTICAL LEG PRESS (PAGE 200)
2. LEG CURL (PAGE 201)
3. LEG EXTENSION (PAGE 200)
4. FORWARD CABLE KICK (PAGE 201)

1. SINGLE-LEG SQUAT (PAGE 202)
2. PHANTOM CHAIR (PAGE 203)
3. LEG EXTENSION WITH BRIEFCASE (PAGE 204)
4. BENCH LATERAL STEPUP WITH TUBING (PAGE 202)
5. LEG CURL WITH TUBING (PAGE 205)

POWERFUL THIGHS
ADVANCED WORKOUT

We recommend that you train with the balanced, full-body plan on page 56. If you need to concentrate specifically on thigh work, though, this program will produce quick gains. Choose one exercise routine to follow: free weights, machines, or no weights.

INSTRUCTIONS

1. Train 3 days a week. Allow sufficient recovery by waiting at least 48 hours between sessions.

2. Your standard advanced workout is three sets of 6 to 10 repetitions for each exercise in the routine you've chosen. The first set, after your aerobics and stretching, is a warmup with a lighter-than-normal weight. The starting load for the second and third sets should be one that is difficult to lift 6 times. As your strength increases, increase the number of repetitions per set until you can do 10 repetitions. Then, for

your next session, increase the load and drop back to 6 repetitions.

Perform the positive phase (also known as the concentric or lifting phase) of each exercise as quickly as possible while maintaining proper form. Perform the negative (or eccentric or lowering) phase of the exercise much more slowly, to a count of four.

3. Vary your workouts as at the intermediate level, and try replacing some of the exercises with tri-sets and giant sets. Tri-sets are like combo lifts except that you add another exercise so that you're doing three in succession without rest. With giant sets, you do four exercises in succession without resting between them.

4. Do 1 or 2 partial repetitions at the end of each set when you reach the point where you can no longer complete a full repetition. This is called going to muscle failure, and it may enhance muscle development. *Note:* At the advanced level, you always need the assistance of a partner for safety when doing partial reps with free weights.

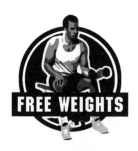

FREE WEIGHTS

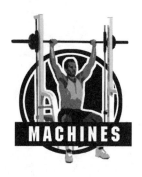

MACHINES

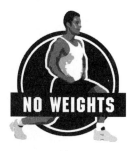

NO WEIGHTS

1. SQUAT (PAGE 195)
2. LATERAL SQUAT (PAGE 198)
3. FRONT SQUAT (PAGE 197)
4. DUMBBELL POWER LUNGE (PAGE 197)
5. STEPUP WITH DUMBBELLS (PAGE 196)
6. LEG CURL WITH ANKLE WEIGHTS (PAGE 199)
7. BENCH LATERAL STEPUP WITH DUMBBELLS (PAGE 196)
8. HACK SQUAT (PAGE 195)
9. LEG EXTENSION WITH ANKLE WEIGHTS (PAGE 198)

1. HACK SQUAT WITH SMITH MACHINE (PAGE 199)
2. VERTICAL LEG PRESS (PAGE 200)
3. LEG CURL (PAGE 201)
4. LEG EXTENSION (PAGE 200)
5. FORWARD CABLE KICK (PAGE 201)

1. SINGLE-LEG SQUAT (PAGE 202)
2. LEG EXTENSION WITH BRIEFCASE (PAGE 204)
3. DOUBLE LEG SQUAT JUMP (PAGE 205)
4. BENCH LATERAL STEPUP WITH TUBING (PAGE 202)
5. DOUBLE LEG POWER JUMP (PAGE 204)
6. LEG CURL WITH TUBING (PAGE 205)
7. ALTERNATING JUMP LUNGE (PAGE 203)
8. PHANTOM CHAIR (PAGE 203)

QUICK-SET PATH TO
POWERFUL LEGS

CALF MUSCLES ARE HARDER TO TRAIN THAN THIGH MUSCLES, BUT THEY'RE IMPORTANT FOR SUCH ACTIVITIES AS WALKING, JUMPING, AND STANDING ON YOUR TIPTOES. THE GOOD NEWS IS THAT THEY CAN BE EXERCISED MUCH FASTER THAN THIGH MUSCLES.

Perhaps you have seen this happen—maybe even to you: Weekend warrior accelerates quickly to snag a line drive in the gap or leaps high for a rebound in a pickup basketball game. He falls to the ground writhing in pain like a gunshot victim. Teammates help him off the field or court and haul him to the doc. Later you hear that he ripped his Achilles tendon. Had he kept his calf muscles—and, by extension, the corresponding tendons and ligaments—in better condition, our stricken athlete might still be on his feet. Since he didn't, the explosive, quick movement he made blew out the tendon, which connects the calf muscles to the heel bone.

This connective tissue is especially vulnerable to being ruptured when it loses some of its elasticity, which happens usually sometime after a man turns 40. Weight training exercises that involve a full range of motion, such as calf raises, not only work your calf muscles but also strengthen the connecting tendons and ligaments, making you less prone to injury.

Even if you aren't a weekend athlete, it behooves you to exercise your calves. As with other body parts, working all the muscles in your legs can give you a symmetrical look. "The old huge upper body and spindly legs doesn't look good any more," says Tory Allman, an exercise physiologist in Solana Beach, California.

"The thing you hear from guys is 'I don't do legs because I run a lot,'" says Brian Pfeufer, corporate program director at Sports Training Institute in New York City. But while running will maintain what leg strength you already have, it alone won't build on that strength, he says.

CALF SKINNY

The calf actually consists of two muscles, the *gastrocnemius* and the *soleus*. Look at the calves of a bodybuilder; they're shaped like diamonds. That's the gastrocnemius, which also has the practical function of enabling you to stand on your tiptoes to reach that bag of potato chips on the top shelf. The soleus is a broad, flat muscle below the gastrocnemius. It, too, helps you rise up on your toes, but it comes more into play when your knees are bent. Both muscles combine to help you walk, jump, or sprint.

Calves are odd muscles. They are hard to train, yet you don't need to spend a lot of time on them.

"What you've got to do is try and hit them again before they recover to enhance fiber recruitment," Allman says. Here's what he suggests.

Perform a set of calf or heel raises with a weight at which you can perform a fairly high number of repetitions—say, 15 to 20. Then rest for the same number of seconds as reps. In this example, you'd rest 15 to 20 seconds before doing the next set.

IT TAKES TWO

You can make an ass of yourself—or worse, get injured—if you aren't super careful when attempting the donkey calf raise.

In this exercise, you stand on a 2- to 4-inch platform, such as a block of wood, with your heels hanging off the edge. Your legs should be hip-width apart, toes pointed forward. Bend forward at the waist until your upper body is roughly parallel to the floor and extend your arms straight out while leaning on something sturdy with your knees bent slightly. Then have a friend who weighs no more than you sit atop your hips, and slowly lift yourself up as high as possible on the balls of your feet. Hold a second and slowly lower your heels. As this exercise becomes easier, you can increase resistance by choosing a heavier partner (or you can feed your current partner lots of pizzas and milkshakes).

To avoid a back injury, make sure your partner sits as far back as possible on your hips, below where your belt would be, advises exercise physiologist Tory Allman of Solana Beach, California.

If all this sounds like too much bother, take heart in the fact that weight machines now simulate this exercise. Or do the modified version in which you lift only your own weight, on page 218.

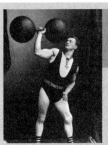

HARD-BODY FACT

If you want more challenge while building a Hard Body—say, 4 hours of sleep a week and lots of people shouting at you—then you might consider joining the Navy SEALs. Here are the physical screening requirements for entry into this military elite:

- 500-yard swim using breast and/or side stroke in 12.5 minutes
- At least 42 pushups in 2 minutes
- At least 50 situps in 2 minutes
- At least 6 pullups
- 1.5-mile run, wearing boots and pants, in 11.5 minutes

And, of course, you have to be 28 or younger and a U.S. citizen.

Since whatever muscle fibers your body recruited for the first set haven't fully recovered, your calves will recruit additional muscle fibers when you do the second set, the third set, and so on.

"By the third or fourth set, the burn is so deep into the muscle that you bring into play fibers that you normally don't even use," Allman says. "That's when you really begin to stimulate the gains and the growth."

SITTING AND STANDING

Calf exercises are generally done while either standing or seated. Calf exercises done in a seated position tend to work the soleus, or lower part of the calf, Allman says. When you straighten your leg out in a standing calf exercise, you hit more of the gastrocnemius, the diamond-shaped part of this muscle group.

The toe presses found in the Hard-Body Plan work both of the muscles that compose your calf.

Rise up on your toes when performing a squat if you want to hit your calf muscles in addition to your thigh and butt muscles.

That's Pfeufer's advice. And as with any calf muscle exercise, use slow, controlled movements.

"Don't bounce. That's how you tear a muscle or strain a knee ligament," Pfeufer says.

LEGS ► FREE WEIGHTS

HEEL RAISE WITH DUMBBELLS

This move specifically works the gastrocnemius muscles in your calves.

[**A**] Stand with a dumbbell in each hand. Your feet should be hip-width apart with your toes on a platform raised a couple of inches off the ground. Your heels should be on the floor, and your weight should be on the balls of your feet so that you're leaning forward slightly. Hold the dumbbells at your sides, with your arms extended down.

[**B**] Slowly rise all the way up onto your toes. Feel the contraction in your calves and pause briefly at the top. Your arms should remain in position, although your body will probably be more upright than it was at the start. Slowly lower yourself to the starting position.

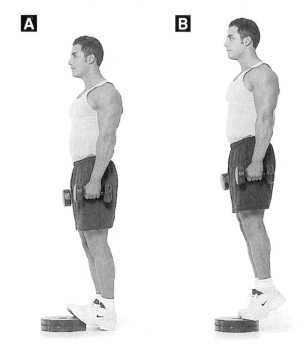

SEATED HEEL RAISE WITH BARBELL

This exercise especially works the soleus muscles in your calves.

[**A**] Sit on a stool or bench with the balls of your feet on a raised platform or footstool about a foot away from your seat. Your heels should be off the platform. Hold a barbell across your thighs, a few inches away from your knees.

[**B**] Slowly and deliberately raise your heels as high as possible by pressing your toes into the platform. Your hands should only steady the barbell in your lap—don't let them carry any of the weight. Hold for a moment, then relax and repeat.

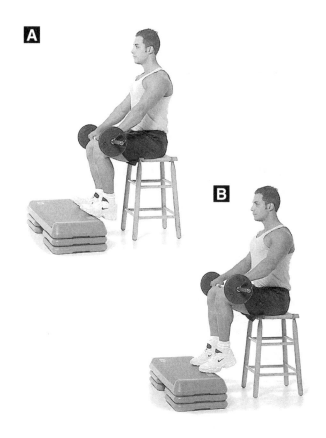

ANKLE FLEXION WITH WEIGHT PLATE

This exercise strengthens your feet's dorsiflexor muscles, which enable you to lift your foot and toes. Strong dorsiflexors are important in running and other aerobic sports.

[**A**] Sit on the end of a bench with your legs together and your feet flat on the floor. Your knees should be bent at a 90-degree angle. Keeping your back straight, lean forward slightly at the waist, holding in place a weight plate that rests across the base of your toes.

[**B**] Slowly and steadily lift your toes as high as you can, keeping the weight balanced and your back as straight as you can. Hold for a second, then slowly lower the weight to the starting position.

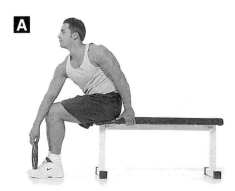

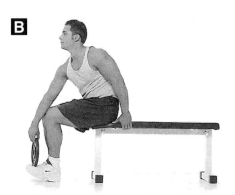

LEGS ► MACHINES

TOE PRESS

This exercise works both the gastrocnemius and the soleus muscles of your calves.

[**A**] Sit up straight on a leg-press machine, making sure that the small of your back is firmly against the back pad. Adjust the seat so that the balls of your feet rest comfortably on the foot plate, 4 to 6 inches apart, with your toes pointing up. Your legs should be slightly bent.

[**B**] Slowly push down with the balls of your feet, pointing your toes as much as you can. Hold for a second, then slowly allow your feet to return to the starting position.

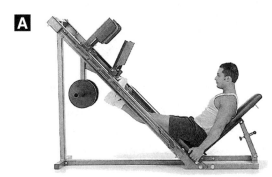

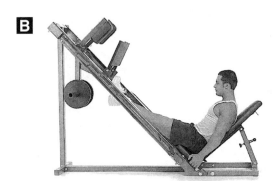

SEATED HEEL RAISE WITH BENCH-PRESS BAR

This move works your calves' soleus muscles.

[**A**] Sit on a bench at a bench-press station, with only the balls of your feet on a step about a foot away from your seat. The step should be low enough that your thighs are parallel to the floor. Hold the bar across your thighs, a few inches from your knees.

[**B**] Slowly and deliberately raise your heels as high as possible by pressing your toes into the step. Your hands should only steady the bar in your lap—don't let them carry any of the weight. Hold for a moment, then slowly return to the starting position.

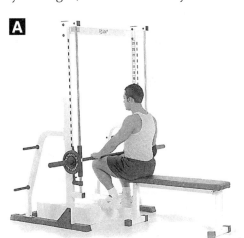

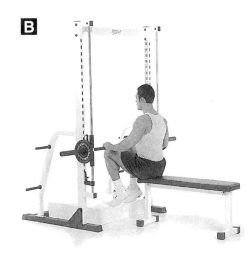

ANKLE FLEXION WITH PULLEY

This exercise works your dorsiflexors, foot muscles that help you lift your feet and toes.

[**A**] Position one end of a bench a few inches in front of a low pulley with an ankle strap. Stand to the left of the bench with your left knee slightly bent, and put your right heel on the edge of the bench closest to the pulley. The bottom of your foot should be level with or slightly below the

bench. Fasten the ankle strap snugly around the toes of your right foot.

[**B**] Slowly curl your toes as high as possible while keeping your heel planted firmly on the bench. Rest your arms on your right thigh for balance, if necessary, but keep your back straight. Pause, then slowly and deliberately return to the starting position.

Finish the set, then switch sides.

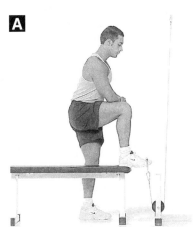

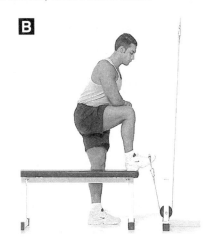

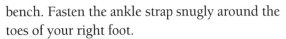

LEGS ► NO WEIGHTS

SINGLE-LEG HEEL RAISE

This exercise works the gastrocnemius muscles in your calves.

[**A**] Stand with your feet hip-width apart and put the toes of your left foot on a platform that's a couple of inches high. Keep that heel on the floor, and put your weight on the ball of that foot so that you lean forward slightly. Cross your right foot behind your left foot. Keep your arms out in front of you for balance.

[**B**] Slowly rise all the way up onto your toes. Feel the contraction in your calf and pause briefly at the top. Your arms should remain in the starting position, though your body will probably be more upright. Then slowly lower yourself to the starting position.

Finish the set, then switch legs.

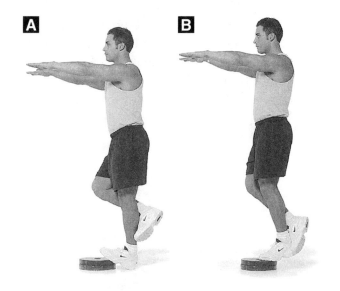

DONKEY CALF RAISE

This is another move that especially helps to strengthen your calves' gastrocnemius muscles.

[**A**] Stand on the edge of a 2- to 4-inch platform (a block of wood will work fine) with your heels hanging off the edge. Your legs should be hip-width apart, your toes pointed forward. Bend forward at the waist until your upper body is roughly parallel with the floor. Extend your arms out straight and lean on something in front of you (a bench will do nicely). Keep your knees slightly bent.

[**B**] Slowly lift yourself up as high as possible on the balls of your feet. Hold for a second, then slowly lower your heels as far as they will go.

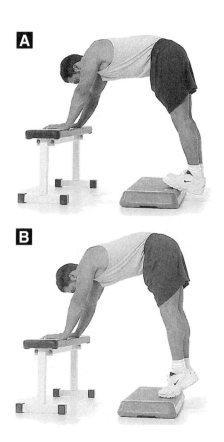

ANKLE FLEXION WITH BRIEFCASE

This exercise works your dorsiflexors, four foot muscles that help you lift your feet and toes. Strong dorsiflexors are important in running and other aerobic sports.

[**A**] Sit on a chair or the end of a bench with your legs together and your feet flat on the floor. Your knees should be bent at a 90-degree angle.

Keeping your back straight, lean forward slightly at the waist, holding in place a briefcase resting across the base of your toes.

[**B**] Slowly and steadily lift your toes as high as you can, keeping the briefcase balanced and your back as straight as you can. Hold for a second, then slowly lower the briefcase to the starting position.

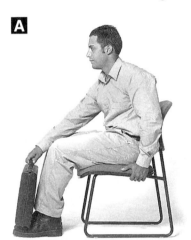

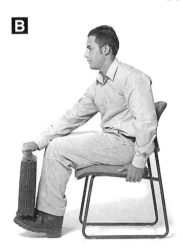

POWERFUL LEGS
BEGINNER WORKOUT

We recommend that you train with the balanced, full-body plan on page 48. But if you need to concentrate specifically on leg work, this program will produce quick gains. Choose one routine to follow: free weights, machines, or no weights.

INSTRUCTIONS

1. Do the complete exercise routine 2 or 3 days a week. Wait at least 48 hours between sessions to allow enough recovery time for best development.

2. To warm up, do some aerobics and stretching, and perform one set of 6 to 10 repetitions with a light to moderate load. This minimizes the chances of a muscle strain or pull during the subsequent training period.

3. After the warmup, find a starting load that is difficult to lift 6 times. This may take some experimenting on your first day. Once you have identified that load, that's what you will use until it becomes too easy.

Complete one set of 6 repetitions for each exercise listed in the routine you've chosen. Perform the positive phase (also known as the concentric or lifting phase) of each exercise as quickly as possible while maintaining proper form. Perform the negative (or eccentric or lowering) phase much more slowly, to a count of four.

4. After a few sessions, you will find that completing the 6 repetitions is easier. At that point, add repetitions, following proper form, up to 10 repetitions.

5. When you are able to perform 10 repetitions, make a note to add more weight at the next session.

6. With the added weight, drop back to 6 repetitions. Then repeat steps 3 to 5 until you have completed 12 weeks of the program. Then, if you still need to focus on leg workouts, you may move on to the intermediate level. Remember, we recommend that you do the balanced, full-body workouts rather than working on individual muscle groups.

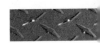

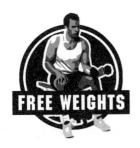

FREE WEIGHTS

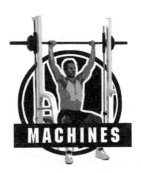

MACHINES

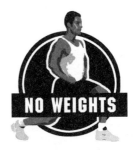

NO WEIGHTS

1. HEEL RAISE WITH DUMBBELLS (PAGE 215)
2. ANKLE FLEXION WITH WEIGHT PLATE (PAGE 216)
3. SEATED HEEL RAISE WITH BARBELL (PAGE 215)

1. TOE PRESS (PAGE 216)
2. ANKLE FLEXION WITH PULLEY (PAGE 217)
3. SEATED HEEL RAISE WITH BENCH-PRESS BAR (PAGE 217)

1. SINGLE-LEG HEEL RAISE (PAGE 218)
2. ANKLE FLEXION WITH BRIEFCASE (PAGE 219)
3. DONKEY CALF RAISE (PAGE 218)

POWERFUL LEGS
INTERMEDIATE WORKOUT

We recommend that you train with the balanced, full-body plan on page 52. But if you need to concentrate specifically on leg work, this program will produce quick gains. Choose one exercise routine to follow: free weights, machines, or no weights.

INSTRUCTIONS

1. Train 3 days a week. Allow enough recovery by waiting at least 48 hours between sessions.

2. Always warm up with some aerobics and stretching, plus one set of 6 to 10 repetitions with a light to moderate load. This minimizes the chances of a muscle strain or pull during the subsequent training period.

3. Your standard intermediate workout is three sets of 6 to 10 repetitions for each exercise listed in the routine you've chosen. The warmup set is your first set. The starting load for the second and third sets should be one that is difficult to lift 6 times. As your strength increases, increase the repetitions per set until you can do 10 repetitions while maintaining proper form. Then, for your next session, increase the load and drop back to 6 repetitions.

Perform the positive phase (also known as the concentric or lifting phase) of each exercise as quickly as possible while maintaining proper form. Perform the negative (or eccentric or lowering) phase much more slowly, to a count of four.

4. Vary your routines. Instead of some of the individual exercises, do combo lifts, or supersets, two exercises in succession (one rep of each) without a rest. You can do almost any two exercises this way. Combo lifts increase the intensity of your workout, create some variety, and can shorten your workout session.

Another variation is to use a lighter load than usual and do 15 to 20 repetitions, and/or to increase the load on successive sets and reduce the number of repetitions (this last variation is called pyramids). So, for example, in set 1, you might do 10 repetitions with 200 pounds; in set 2, you might do 7 repetitions with 250 pounds; and in set 3, you might do 4 repetitions with 300 pounds.

5. As you gain training experience, you might try experimenting with 1 or 2 partial repetitions at the end of each set, at the point where you can no longer complete a full repetition. This is called going to muscle failure, and it may enhance muscle development. *Note:* If you try this, you will need a partner to spot you, especially when you're using free weights.

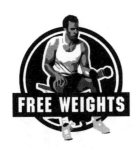

FREE WEIGHTS

1. HEEL RAISE WITH DUMBBELLS (PAGE 215)
2. ANKLE FLEXION WITH WEIGHT PLATE (PAGE 216)
3. SEATED HEEL RAISE WITH BARBELL (PAGE 215)

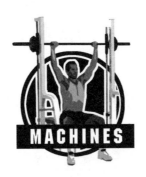

MACHINES

1. TOE PRESS (PAGE 216)
2. ANKLE FLEXION WITH PULLEY (PAGE 217)
3. SEATED HEEL RAISE WITH BENCH-PRESS BAR (PAGE 217)

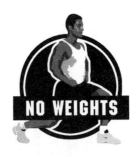

NO WEIGHTS

1. SINGLE-LEG HEEL RAISE (PAGE 218)
2. ANKLE FLEXION WITH BRIEFCASE (PAGE 219)
3. DONKEY CALF RAISE (PAGE 218)

POWERFUL LEGS
ADVANCED WORKOUT

We recommend that you train with the balanced, full-body plan on page 56. If you need to concentrate specifically on leg work, though, this program will produce quick gains. Choose one exercise routine to follow: free weights, machines, or no weights.

INSTRUCTIONS

1. Train 3 days a week. Allow sufficient recovery time by waiting at least 48 hours between sessions.

2. Your standard advanced workout is three sets of 6 to 10 repetitions for each exercise in the routine you've chosen. The first set, after your aerobics and stretching, is a warmup with a lighter-than-normal weight. The starting load for the second and third sets should be one that is difficult to lift 6 times. As your strength increases, increase the repetitions per set until you can do 10 repetitions. Then, for your next session, increase the load and drop back to 6 repetitions.

Perform the positive phase (also known as the concentric or lifting phase) of each exercise as quickly as possible while maintaining proper form. Perform the negative (or eccentric or lowering) phase much more slowly, to a count of four.

3. Vary your workouts as at the intermediate level, and try replacing some of the exercises with tri-sets and giant sets. Tri-sets are like combo lifts except that you add another exercise so that you're doing three in succession without rest. With giant sets, you do four exercises in succession without resting between them.

4. Do 1 or 2 partial repetitions at the end of each set when you reach the point where you can no longer complete a full repetition. This is called going to muscle failure, and it may enhance muscle development. *Note:* At the advanced level, you always need the assistance of a partner for safety when doing partial reps with free weights.

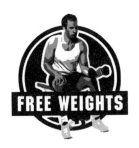

FREE WEIGHTS

1. HEEL RAISE WITH DUMBBELLS (PAGE 215)
2. ANKLE FLEXION WITH WEIGHT PLATE (PAGE 216)
3. SEATED HEEL RAISE WITH BARBELL (PAGE 215)

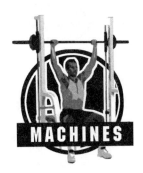

MACHINES

1. TOE PRESS (PAGE 216)
2. ANKLE FLEXION WITH PULLEY (PAGE 217)
3. SEATED HEEL RAISE WITH BENCH-PRESS BAR (PAGE 217)

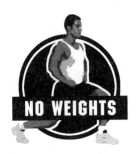

NO WEIGHTS

1. SINGLE-LEG HEEL RAISE (PAGE 218)
2. ANKLE FLEXION WITH BRIEFCASE (PAGE 219)
3. DONKEY CALF RAISE (PAGE 218)

EXERCISES THAT WORK MULTIPLE MUSCLE GROUPS
COMBO LIFTS

COMBO LIFTS, OR SUPERSETS, ARE FREE-WEIGHT EXERCISES THAT COMBINE TWO LIFTS: YOU FINISH ONE EXERCISE AND MOVE INTO A SECOND WITHOUT RESTING.

Combination lifting does two things. It provides a more intense workout, and it helps you complete your workout faster.

You choose how many combo lifts to include in a workout. Add more as you become stronger and more experienced at lifting. But if you are too fatigued or aren't seeing the muscle gains you expected, do fewer of them.

If you're really advanced, you can even try trisets and giant sets. That entails performing three and four exercises, respectively, without a break between them. "Once you get beyond three sets, it's very tough unless you're quite advanced," cautions our exercise coach, Peter Lemon, Ph.D.

INSTRUCTIONS

1. One way to do a superset is to combine two exercises that work the same muscle group but in slightly different ways. Example: the bench press and the incline or decline bench press. Each exercise works the pecs, but focuses on different parts.

2. Also try exercises that work opposing, or antagonistic, muscle groups. Example: dumbbell curls for the biceps, followed by dumbbell kickbacks for the triceps; or leg extensions for the quadriceps, followed by leg curls for the hamstrings. Combo lifts like this guarantee a balanced workout.

3. You can also do combo lifts that work completely separate muscle groups. Example: squats for the hamstrings and quads, followed by preacher curls for the biceps. Be aware, however, that if you train all the major muscle groups in 1 day, you have to wait 48 hours to resume working out because your muscles need to recover. There's nothing wrong with this, but if you like to lift weights 5 or 6 days a week rather than 3 or 4 days a week, don't do this type of combo lift.

4. Feel free to create your own supersets. This can add even more variety and challenge to your workout. Make sure that your program has balance and that you don't exclude any muscle groups.

ARMS

FOREARM EXTENSION AND CURL

[**A**] Sit on a bench with your legs a little farther than hip-width apart. Hold a dumbbell in your left hand, palm-down. Rest the meaty bottom part of your left forearm on your left thigh, with your wrist positioned just slightly over your knee for maximum mobility. Let your right hand rest on your right thigh. Keep your body upright, slightly leaning on your left leg for comfort. Let your left wrist bend naturally as the weight pulls it. This is the starting position.

[**B**] Using only your wrist and keeping the rest of your arm stationary, curl the dumbbell as high as you can. Hold for a second, then lower the dumbbell slowly, with control.

[**C**] Immediately roll your forearm over so that you're holding the dumbbell palm-up, with the top of your forearm against your thigh. Let your wrist bend back naturally as the weight pulls it down.

[**D**] Using only your wrist and keeping the rest of your arm stationary, curl the dumbbell as close to your body as you can. Hold for a second, then lower the dumbbell slowly, with control, and return to the starting position, rolling your forearm over to begin again.

Finish the set, then switch arms.

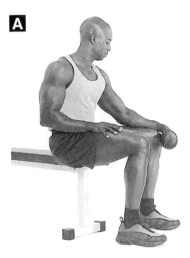

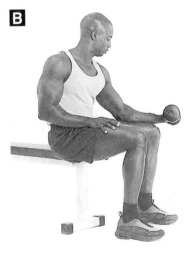

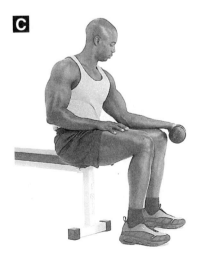

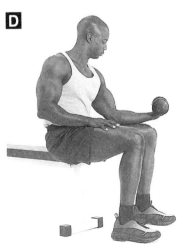

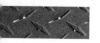

ARMS, CHEST, BACK, AND SHOULDERS

DUMBBELL CURL AND RAISE

[**A**] Stand straight with your feet shoulder-width apart and your knees slightly bent. Hold a dumbbell in each hand with your arms down at your sides and your palms facing in. This is the starting position.

[**B**] Slowly curl both dumbbells up toward your collarbone. As you do the curl, rotate your arms so that your palms face up. Pause for a second at the top of the lift.

[**C**] Slowly lower the weights until both arms are at your sides again.

[**D**] Slowly raise both weights as far as you can toward your armpits. Keep your elbows pointing out and the weights close to your body. Hold for a second, then slowly lower your arms to the starting position and begin the sequence again.

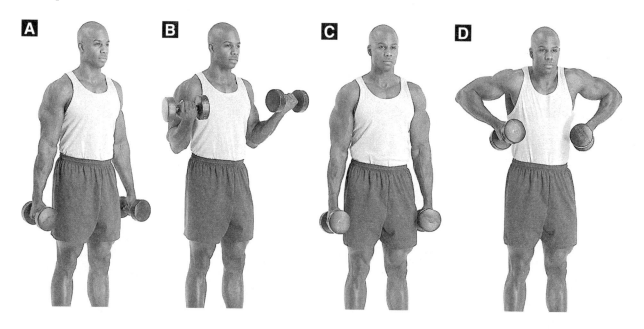

UPRIGHT ROW AND BEHIND-THE-NECK PRESS

Caution: *Begin with a light weight.*

[**A**] Stand with your feet shoulder-width apart and your knees slightly bent. Hold a barbell overhand with your arms fully extended and your hands shoulder-width or slightly farther apart. The bar should rest on your upper thighs. Lean forward slightly at the waist and let your shoulders droop forward just a bit, but keep your back straight. This is the starting position.

[**B**] Keeping the bar close to your body, slowly lift it until it's at shoulder level. Your elbows should point out.

[**C**] Carefully place the barbell so that it rests behind your neck, across the top of your shoulders. (Or keep the bar in front of your neck—an equally effective variation that some experts think is safer.) Your palms should face forward, and your elbows will point downward at this point. Keep your chest high.

[**D**] Slowly raise the barbell straight up, pulling your head slightly forward to allow space for the bar to move. Your elbows should point out again. Pause at the top of the movement.

Slowly lower the bar to your collarbone. Then lower the bar to your thighs and repeat the sequence.

A
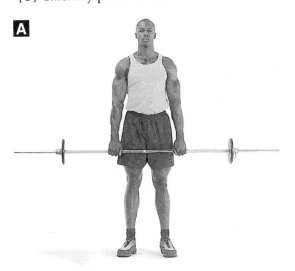

B
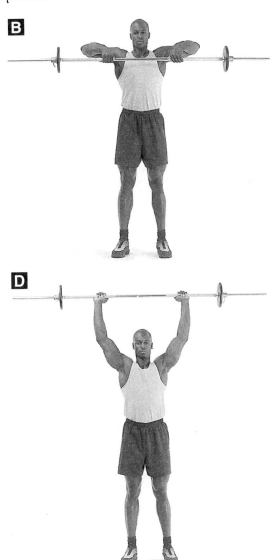

C
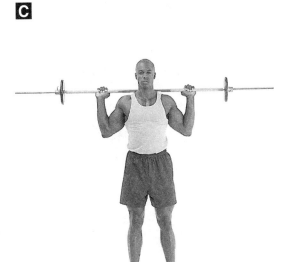

D

DUMBBELL FLY AND PRESS

It's a good idea to use a spotter for this move.

[**A**] Lie on your back on a bench with your legs parted and your feet firmly on the floor. Hold two dumbbells above you, your palms facing each other. The dumbbells should nearly touch each other above your chest. Your back should be straight and firm against the bench, and your elbows unlocked. This is the starting position.

[**B**] Slowly lower the dumbbells out and away from each other in a semicircular motion. Keep your wrists locked. Lower until the dumbbells are at chest level. Your elbows should be bent at roughly a 135-degree angle, while your back is straight. Hold for a second.

[**C**] Return to the starting position.

[**D**] Slowly lower the dumbbells both until they are even with your chest. Your elbows should be bent at 90 degrees. Hold for a second, then slowly raise back to the starting position and repeat the sequence.

A

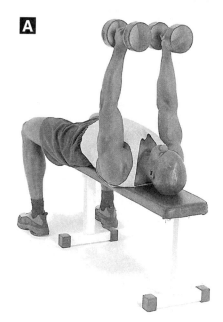

B

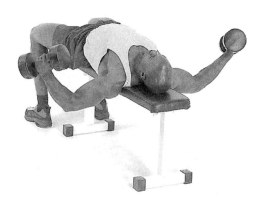

C

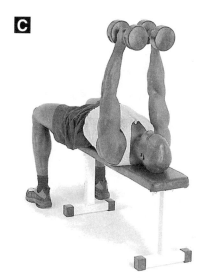

D

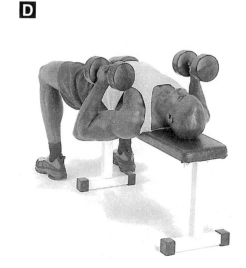

ABS, BACK, THIGHS, AND BUTT

DUMBBELL TRUNK TWIST AND STANDING TOE TOUCH

[**A**] Stand with your back straight, your chest out, and your head in line with your torso. Your feet should be flat and shoulder-width apart, and your knees should be unlocked. Hold a dumbbell in each hand, with your palms facing your body. Bend your arms and bring the weights close to your gut. This is the starting position.

[**B**] Slowly twist your torso to the left as far as you can comfortably go. Hold for a second, then slowly return to the starting position. Repeat to the right.

[**C**] When you have twisted to each side, face forward again as in the starting position.

[**D**] Slowly bending forward and to the right, touch the left dumbbell to your right foot. Bring yourself back to standing, then slowly bend and touch the right dumbbell to your left foot. Finally, bring the weights back to the starting position and repeat the whole sequence.

A
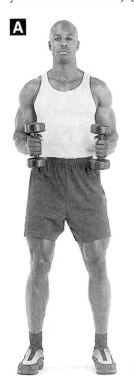

B
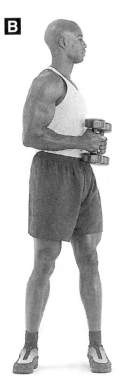

C
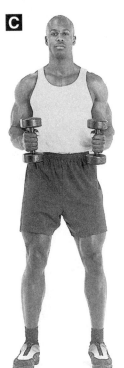

D
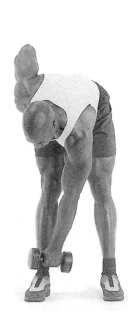

BACK, ARMS, AND SHOULDERS

DUMBBELL DEADLIFT AND MILITARY PRESS

Stand upright holding two light dumbbells in front of you, palms-down.

[**A**] Bend over at the waist, keeping your back straight. The dumbbells should be about shoulder-width apart measuring from the centers of the bars. Keep your legs stiff, but don't lock your knees. Let your arms hang down, but don't lock your elbows. This is the starting position.

[**B**] Lift the dumbbells by raising your torso to the upright position. Keep your back, arms, and legs straight, but don't let your knees or elbows lock. The dumbbells should be at about upper-thigh level when you're done raising your torso. Hold for a second.

[**C**] Lift the dumbbells to shoulder height, your palms facing in.

[**D**] Slowly raise both dumbbells overhead until they almost touch. Extend your arms fully, but don't let your elbows lock. Pause for a second, then slowly lower the dumbbells first to shoulder height, then to your thighs, and finally to the starting position.

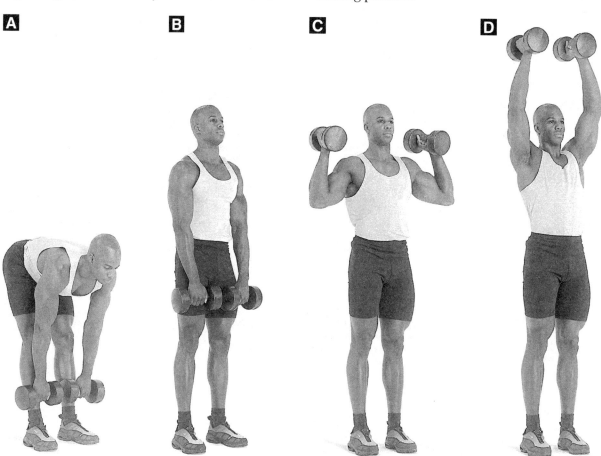

THIGHS, BACK, BUTT, SHOULDERS, AND ARMS

DUMBBELL SWING AND STANDING TRICEPS CURL

Hold on to a dumbbell with both hands. Stand with your feet about shoulder-width apart, your knees slightly bent, and your back straight.

[**A**] Bend at the waist while holding the dumbbell between your shins, arms fully extended. Keep the weight off the floor. This is the starting position.

[**B**] In an explosive movement, swing the dumbbell until it's over your head, simultaneously standing upright. Hold for a second.

[**C**] Keeping your upper arms close to your head, lower the dumbbell behind your head as far as it will go. [**D**] Hold for a second, then raise to the fully extended position. Then return to the starting position, the dumbbell between your shins.

A **B** **C** **D**

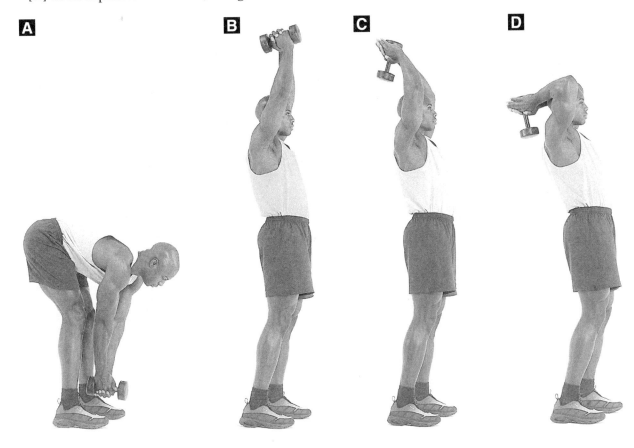

THIGHS, BUTT, SHOULDERS, AND BACK

DUMBBELL HACK SQUAT AND LATERAL RAISE

[**A**] With your feet hip-width apart, stand holding dumbbells at your sides, your arms fully extended and your palms facing in. Keep your head in line with your body. This is the starting position.

[**B**] Squat down until your thighs are close to parallel with the floor. Do not allow your knees to extend over your toes. Hold for a second.

[**C**] Rise, keeping your arms fully extended.

Your shoulders should be back, your back straight, and your knees slightly bent.

[**D**] With your elbows slightly bent, lean forward a little and slowly raise your arms up and out to your sides until the dumbbells reach shoulder level. Your palms should face the floor. Hold for a second, then slowly lower your arms to the starting position.

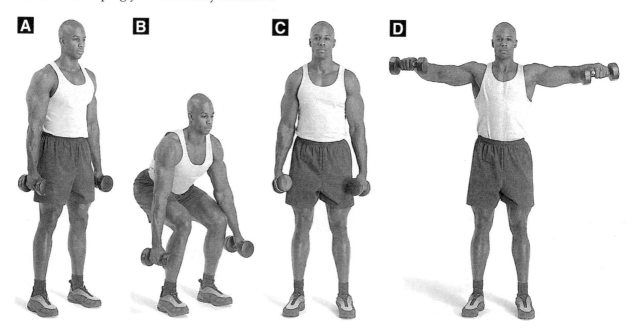

LEGS, SHOULDERS, CHEST, ARMS, AND BACK

SEATED DUMBBELL HEEL RAISE AND FRONT DELTOID RAISE

[**A**] Sit in the middle of a bench, near the edge. Rest the balls of your feet on a 6- to 8-inch platform in front of you, letting your heels stretch down as far as they will go. Your knees should be together and bent at a 45-degree angle. Hold a dumbbell in each hand, resting them both vertically on a folded towel on your thighs. This is the starting position.

[**B**] Push up as high on the balls of your feet as you can. Hold for a second, then return to the starting position.

[**C**] Let your arms hang at your sides, with your elbows slightly bent and your palms facing in. Lean forward slightly at the waist, keeping your elbows back, your chest out, and your lower back straight.

[**D**] Slowly raise both dumbbells in front of you until they're at shoulder height. Your palms should face down. Don't rock your hips or swing your arms for momentum. Hold for a second, then slowly lower the weights, returning them to the starting position.

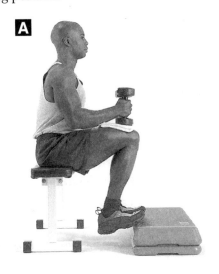

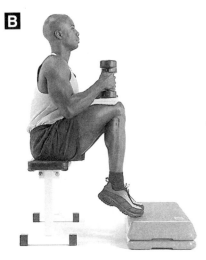

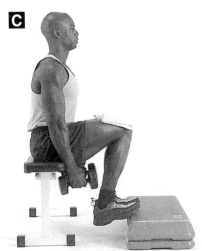

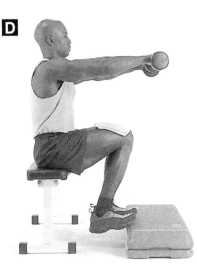

A Real Man's Guide to Heart/Lung Workouts
Cardio Routines

To burn serious fat and keep your heart and lungs healthy and strong means aerobic exercise. You don't have to dance, but you gotta move, baby, move.

Santa Claus has pumped iron and sweated out crunches for weeks, and his belly still jiggles like jelly. All he wanted for Christmas was that six-pack look for his abs, and instead he looks like he's been quaffing six-packs of egg nog. Why isn't he getting buff?

He has taken too many sleigh rides and spent too much time puttering around the toy shop when he should have been out running like the reindeer. It takes serious aerobic exercise to burn off serious fat.

Regular aerobic exercise does a lot more than help you look better. It strengthens your heart, lungs, and blood vessels; reduces risk factors for heart disease; improves strength and endurance; obliterates stress; and decreases anxiety and depression.

Aerobic exercise makes a man strong in ways that have nothing to do with muscles. And it's absolutely essential to an overall strength program. Work it into yours.

Aerobic Essentials

Aerobic exercise is defined as any sustained, rhythmic exertion involving large muscle groups (such as the legs, butt, and back) that raises your heart rate enough so that it works your cardiovascular system for a prolonged period of time. When you do it, you should breathe harder and deeper, but you shouldn't be panting. Proper aerobic exercise is intense but not so intense that you can't continue to carry on a conversation.

Lifting weights is not an aerobic exercise. Since you continually rest between sets, it is not sustained activity.

While aerobic exercise won't build big muscles, it will help you burn fat so that you can see the bulk you've added through weight training.

236

When you stop doing an aerobic exercise, your metabolism rate quickly returns to where it was before, says Peter Lemon, Ph.D., designer of the Hard-Body exercise program.

But when you lift weights, there is an increase in your base metabolism that continues 24 hours a day whether you exercise or not, Dr. Lemon says. He recommends doing aerobic exercise for an immediate energy burn, combined with weight training for a longer effect.

Sound like a hassle? It's not. There are so many activities that are aerobic that it's almost impossible *not* to find one or more that you enjoy. "The best exercises are the ones that you'll do on a regular basis," says Alan Mikesky, Ph.D., director of the human performance and biomechanics laboratory at Indiana University–Purdue University in Indianapolis.

It can be a kick-ass cardio routine such as kickboxing, or something comparatively sedate such as walking briskly on a treadmill or in your neighborhood. Or it can be a combination of activities. In the following pages, we describe 12 great cardio activities. They can be done alone or in a group. The list is by no means comprehensive.

HOW MUCH, HOW OFTEN

Most of us should do aerobic exercise at somewhere between 60 and 90 percent of our maximum heart rate. How low or how high you should go depends on what sort of condition you're in. If you're badly out of shape, you might even start at 50 percent of your maximum heart rate, Dr. Mikesky says.

You have two ways to figure out whether you are in this target range: You can guess, or you can actually measure yourself. Measuring is far better than guessing. But we'll still tell you how to guess: Observe your body. You should be breathing hard but still capable of conversation; your heart should be beating roughly double its usual rate, but it

shouldn't be pounding; and after a few minutes, you should be sweating lightly. If all of those things are happening, chances are that you're getting a good aerobic workout in your target range. A combination of two or more of the following signs indicates that you are going too hard: You are light-headed or dizzy; you are panting for air; you have an acute sense of your heart bamming away; you are dripping sweat; you can't speak a full sentence without gasping for air. Signs that you are going too light: When you stop, there is little noticeable adjustment by your body; you can't sense your heart beating; you can say the alphabet without breaking for breath; you're not sweating.

To actually measure your heart rate, you again have two choices: the low-tech way, which is to take your pulse every now and then, or the high-tech way, which is to wear a heart-rate monitor. Here are the details.

First, you need to determine your maximum heart rate. A way to approximate this is to subtract your age from 220. If you are 40 years old, it's 180—that is, 180 heartbeats per minute. To exercise at 60 percent of your maximum heart rate, multiply 180 times 0.6. That comes to 108. Ninety percent would be 180 times 0.9, or 162. If your reading falls between those numbers, you're working hard enough.

Once you've determined your healthy range, take your pulse periodically as you exercise and see where it falls in relation to these numbers. If your heart rate is too slow, pick up the pace of your workout. If it's too high, taper off a bit.

You can gauge your pulse by placing two fingers on your wrist or your neck and counting the beats for 15 seconds. It will probably be somewhere between 20 and 40 beats. Now, multiply the number by 4. Presto: your heartbeats per minute.

Or you might consider buying a heart monitor that straps around your chest and transmits your heart-rate readings to a special wristwatch. This way, you can keep constant track of whether you need to bump up or slow down your exertion without having to interrupt your workout to monkey around with finding your pulse, says Joe Ogilvie, a fitness instructor at spas in New York City and Lenox, Massachusetts.

Just as you can see the weight on that dumbbell you're curling, you can see what your heart's doing in the depths of your chest by looking at your wrist. Expect to shell out about $80 for one of these high-tech monitors.

Now you know how hard to do aerobic exercise, but how often should you do it? Novices ought to start out three to five times a week, 20 minutes at a time, Dr. Mikesky says. You can expand on this and burn more calories as you build more endurance.

With so many benefits to be had from aerobic exercise, it's little wonder that a new gimmick seems to come into vogue every week. You can find aerobics classes set to gospel music. Or how about capoeira? Capoeira was created by African slaves in Brazil approximately 400 years ago as a martial art. It is now a unique combination of dancing, singing, music, martial arts, acrobatics, and self-defense.

Or you can go through a firefighter's workout, complete with climbing ladders and hauling hoses. Stationary bikes and treadmills are even being equipped with slot machines so you can gamble while you ramble.

Sadly, sprinting to the buffet line and piling up your plate is not an aerobic activity.

You can, though, play speed golf.

SPEED GOLF

Golf as an aerobic exercise? That's as absurd as Keith Richards posing in a muscle magazine, or casting Rick Moranis as a bully. Unless you're talking about speed golf. The aim here is to zip around the course as if your plaid pants were on fire.

Speed golf was invented in 1979 by Steve Scott, an American record holder in the mile run. Then he went out and shot a 95—yes, in 18 holes—in 29.3 minutes.

Now there's an International Speed Golf Association governing the sport and tournaments. More important than all these stats, though, is the fact that speed golf is an aerobic exercise that's *fun*.

The Routine: The key to getting a good aerobic workout from speed golf is to not stand around studying your next shot like it's your financial portfolio. Remember, aerobic exercise is *sustained* physical activity.

• **Hit the ball and run.** That's right. After each shot, you run to where your ball lies.

• **Get a caddie.** Mercifully, you are not expected to carry your own clubs while you run from shot to shot. The caddie should be positioned down the fairway to spot your shot. As you run to the next shot, the caddie will be waiting with—you hope—the right club. An alternative is to ditch the caddy and run with two or three clubs in hand and a fanny pack containing extra balls so you don't waste time searching for errant shots.

• **Find the right footwear.** "Typically, the better players are all wearing running shoes," says Rob Duncanson of San Diego, who himself is one of the better players. "It's a bit uncomfortable to run in golf shoes for 18 holes." Besides, better golfers have balanced swings and less need to be concerned with the extra traction you might get in a golf shoe, he says.

• **Find a place to play.** This is the hardest part of speed golf. Golf courses have not yet begun setting aside specific hours or days for the game, with the exception of the occasional tournament. Call your local golf club ahead of time and explain that you'd like to zip through the course fast—while paying the full fee and being on the course before anybody else.

Duncanson has practiced by running 1 mile to a local park around 5:30 A.M., golf club in hand.

He finds an area where he won't damage the turf and hits shots 75 to 100 yards, runs to the ball and hits it back in the direction he came from. He does this for 30 minutes, then runs home. "You get the aerobic benefit of stopping and starting and swinging the golf club," he says.

The Warmup and Cooldown: Your warmup should get your heart rate up nearly as fast as it will be when you're running on the golf course, because you'll be off and running from the first tee, says Richard Cotton, chief exercise physiologist for the American Council on Exercise. Do the same stretches for your lower back, triceps, and shoulders that you'd do for a regular round of golf, followed by a few wind sprints.

You might also warm up by doing some interval running. Run 250 yards, then a shorter distance, and a still shorter distance after that. This mimics the progressively shorter running you'll do on the golf course as you drive, hit to the green, and putt.

Your cooldown should include gradually tapering off your activity and doing light stretching. "Don't ever just stop," Cotton advises.

WALKING

Chances are that walking hasn't been a big deal to you since you were about a year old and took your first, faltering steps. But for a painless way to burn off blubber and tone leg muscles, rambling along a road or tramping on a treadmill is tremendously efficient.

"The only thing walking won't give you that running will is injury," says Casey Meyers, author of *Walking: A Complete Guide to the Complete Exercise.* Now in his seventies, Meyers still walks 3 miles at a fast pace (13-minute miles) most mornings, and he does it with an artificial knee. We'll walk you through the routine. Follow these steps.

The Routine: In order to get your heart pumping, you're going to move at a brisker clip than when you saunter past the display window at Victoria's Secret.

• **Keep your heart rate up.** Go at a pace at which your heart rate is within your targeted heart range. Do this at least 3 days a week for at least 20 minutes.

That's the minimum. If you have time to walk every day, do, because there is no risk of injury, Meyers says. He recommends building up to 3 miles per walk. A brisk, calorie-burning speed would be to complete that 3-mile walk in 45 minutes—an average of 15 minutes per mile.

• **Try a treadmill.** If you walk uphill, your heart rate will rise quickly. But when you descend the hill on the other side, your heart rate drops just as fast. That's one advantage to walking on a treadmill: You can set it for hill hiking and never come down the other side. Don't set the degree of incline too high, though, or you will throw off your stride and posture. You can also walk faster on a treadmill than on a road, regardless of incline.

• **Bend your arms and swing them vigorously.** It helps you generate more speed when you walk for exercise, Meyers says. Try for somewhere between a 90-degree and 145-degree angle at the elbow. Lock your arm at the elbow so that the pivotal part of your swing is at your shoulder. Your forearm should not flop up and down.

• **Watch your form.** Look straight ahead and keep your chin up and parallel to the ground, with your head not tilted to either side. Each foot should track straight in your line of travel from heel plant to toe-off.

• **Choose the right shoes.** Wear shoes that have low, cushioned heels; good arch support; a flexible forefoot; and slip-resistant soles. Try on shoes at midday or after a walk when your feet have swelled, and when you do so, make sure that you're wearing the type of socks you'd normally walk in.

The Warmup and Cooldown: Meyers doesn't do his 3 miles all at one brisk, steady pace. He walks at a moderate pace the first ¼ mile, then picks up the tempo gradually, reaching full speed after ¾ mile. He tapers off a bit in the last ¼ mile, then does a few stretching exercises while his muscles are still warm.

Some experts suggest stretching your arms and legs in the warmup phase, after walking slowly for a few minutes and prior to your fast walk. The cooldown is important because it decreases the likelihood of light-headedness and prevents muscles from becoming stiff.

STAIRCLIMBER/ ELLIPTICAL TRAINER

When you hop on one of these devices at the gym, you signal to the rest of the crowd that you're climbing a solitary path to fitness. It's just man and machine; you don't need an aerobics class or any distracting chitchat. Or an elevator, for that matter.

Many guys like stairclimbers (as well as their newer cousins, elliptical trainers) because they can work away at their own pace while looking at a magazine or mulling over work matters, says Selene Yeager, a Lehigh Valley, Pennsylvania, personal trainer. And you can pop on a pair of headphones as a way to put out your "Do not disturb" sign.

These machines are a great way to burn calories, pump up your heart rate, and work the quads and hamstrings in your thighs as well as your butt muscles. It's also an activity you're likely to be able to enjoy even if your knees are tender from too much pounding while running.

The machines generally feature an interactive display that shows you how long you've been stepping, how many calories you've expended, and what level of intensity it's throwing your way. Stairclimbers will send your feet marching up and down, just as their name implies. You also step on an elliptical trainer, but your feet move more in the pattern of a flattened-out circle.

The Routine: Here's how to get more out of your stepping or climbing workout.

• **Start slowly.** It's best to step or climb for 30 minutes and work up from there. If the gym has posted a sign asking you to limit your time to, say, 30 minutes, be sure to hop off after your allotted time if others are waiting.

• **Position your feet well.** Users may feel their toes become numb and tingly before the end of the session. If you're getting weird messages from your southernmost reaches, you're probably putting too much pressure on the balls of your feet, pinching off blood circulation to your toes.

Move your feet forward or back on the foot pads until you find a position that lets them feel normal. Also, wiggle your toes periodically, Yeager suggests, as you tend to hold them more motionless while stepping than you would while running. That should help ward off the tingles.

• **Please step away from the armrest, sir.** You'll get more work out of your workout when you don't lean heavily on the armrest. For starters, you'll be bearing and moving around more of your own weight, and burning more calories as a result. Second, when you stand up straight, you give your abs a better workout because they have to support you during the exercise, Yeager says. To burn more calories, add your arms to the action, pumping them as you would during a run.

The Warmup and Cooldown: Be sure to ease into your workout to allow your muscles to warm up, and slow down at the end of the session to cool down. You'll probably find that your machine has warmups and cooldowns built into its workouts.

STUDIO CYCLING

When you picture a Hard-Body guy immersed in a group aerobics class at the gym, what image first comes to mind?

Perhaps something like this: Sweating profusely in a sea of spandex, he's trying to step through a group of intricately choreographed moves. Everyone else is facing one way. He's facing another, much to his embarrassment.

Well, here's another image to consider: studio cycling. You may have heard it called Spinning—that's one trademarked style of this exercise. Studio cyclists ride special stationary bikes together, but each person is the master of his own bike's resistance lever, so the workout can be as hard or easy as he needs.

After warming up the group, the leader may direct them to imagine that they're riding up a hill, pedaling across flatland, or zooming down a slope. Each cyclist shifts his weight on the seat and adjusts the bike's resistance to match the scenario. (Unlike in real life, you don't have to worry about cars zooming by just as you approach a curve.)

The bikes have a weighted wheel that builds momentum, mimicking the feel of a real bicycle, with handlebars that allow you to switch your grip and posture. Most classes will run about 45 minutes to an hour.

Because each person takes charge of how difficult his or her workout will be, no one has to worry about being left in the dust, says Yeager, who is a certified studio cycling instructor through the Reebok system.

So even if your last cycling experience was sometime in the sixth grade astride a Huffy with an electronic siren on the handlebars, you won't feel out of place among hard-core cyclists who shave their legs to cut down on wind resistance.

"Guys especially like it because it's not dancy and you don't have to follow choreography. It's kind of macho," Yeager says. "If you want to really challenge yourself, you can, and if you want to ease up on it, you can."

Because you're sometimes sitting and sometimes standing during a ride, you'll bring muscles throughout your lower body into the workout—particularly your butt, hamstrings, and quads. And

you can leave about 500 to 600 calories behind in a 40-minute class as you pedal away.

The Routine: Here are a few ways to make your studio cycling workout more comfortable.

• **Boost your cushion for comfortable pushin'.** You'll find that an investment of padded bicycling shorts or underwear can make your cycling session friendlier to your backside and neighboring regions. Look for the shorts in a bicycle shop or cycling catalog.

• **Drink hard.** Hydration is a must when studio cycling, because you'll sweat buckets. Keep a water bottle handy to sip as you pedal.

• **Use the delicate cycle if you need it.** Pace yourself so that you don't blow a gasket before your class is up. The other guys—and gals—in the class won't be watching to see how hard you've set your bike's resistance, so don't worry about impressing them.

• **Wipe properly.** Since you'll probably be sweating like a lawn sprinkler, bring a towel and keep it handy so you can dry off as needed.

• **Shop around.** Some instructors will give you simple drills to set the tone of the class, while others will try to simulate the experience you'd have while actually riding a bike out in the countryside. If you don't like how one class feels, give another teacher a try.

JUMPING ROPE

Think you're tough, fella? Are you ready for any exercise challenge you can find as you run, lift, and pump your way toward fitness?

Well, a group of schoolgirls out skipping rope at recess can teach you a lesson that you might not have pondered: Jumping rope gives you one intense workout you wouldn't want to, er, skip.

You'll torch calories like grease in a furnace—a 175-pound man will burn up about 225 calories in just 15 minutes—and you can get your heart rate briskly pounding. And, as you swing the rope and jump over it, you'll bring your legs, butt, forearms, upper arms, and shoulders into the action.

Plus, you can do it in your own home without having to beat the streets or head to the gym, and the only piece of equipment you need other than shoes (hint: it looks like a clothesline with handles) will set you back just $10 or so.

And if the thought of schoolyard kiddies reciting rhymes while they skip prevents you from considering this a manly exercise, think of all those boxers who furiously whirl the rope to get themselves ready to head into the ring.

The Routine: Here's how not to get tied in a knot on your first try behind the rope.

- **Soften the blows to your toes.** Wear shoes with plenty of cushioning on the ball of the foot. Cross-training shoes are a good choice.
- **Turn it up.** Put on some music with a quick beat to accompany your workout and boost the excitement.

- **Buy the right rope.** Find a lightweight rope with foam grips you can still clutch when your hands become sweaty. If you can step one foot on the center of a rope and pull the handles up to your chest level, congratulations: You've found the right length.
- **Watch your form.** As you swing the rope in a smooth arc, keep your shoulders relaxed. The motion that powers the rope should come from your wrists. Also, keep your back straight and resist hunching over.
- **Look before you leap.** Jump just about 1 inch in the air—enough to clear the rope—then land lightly on the balls of your feet with your knees slightly bent. You're not trying to stick your head through the ceiling or crash through the floor.
- **Take a break if you need it.** If you need a breather without interrupting your workout, stop jumping and just twirl the rope at your side.

The Warmup and Cooldown: Warm up before your session and cool down after with light exercise.

JUMP ROPE

This garden-variety jump requires minimal coordination.

Holding a handle in each hand, stand just in front of the center of the rope, which should be hanging down behind you. [**A**] Swing the rope over your head, using your wrists to propel it. [**B**] Jump as it approaches your toes. You should hop up only about 1 inch.

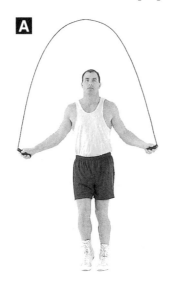

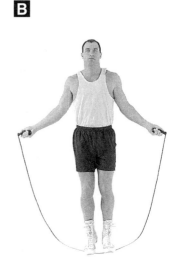

FRONT CROSS

This simple variation on the basic jump involves your arms more fully.

[**A**] Swing the rope normally until it is at its high point over your head. [**B**] As the rope swings down in front of you, cross the rope handles horizontally in front of you. Your arms should cross at roughly hip level. Leap over the rope as it hits the ground. [**C**] Keep your arms crossed as you continue to swing the rope up over your back until it reaches the high point over your head agian. [**D**] Uncross your arms on the downswing and jump the rope again as it hits the ground.

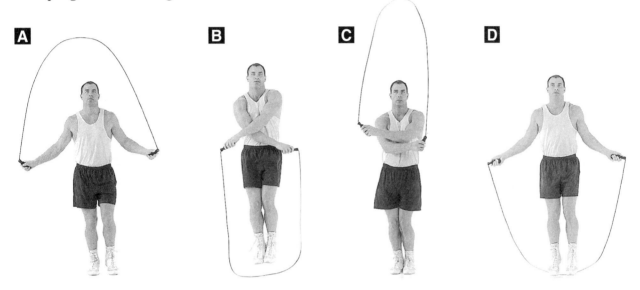

SKIER ROPE JUMP

The motion of this jump resembles the back-and-forth movement of your feet in downhill skiing.

Assume a usual jump-rope starting position. Instead of placing your feet back in the same spot as you clear the rope, land with your feet together but alternating about 6 inches from side [**A**] to side [**B**].

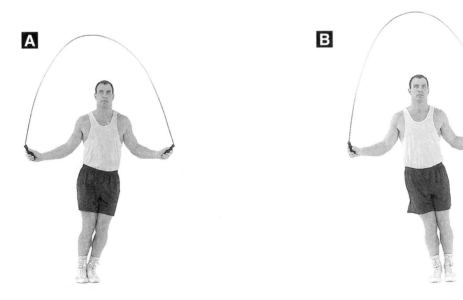

AEROBIC KICKBOXING

For decades, TV and movie screens have shown heroes from Bruce Lee to Chuck Norris to Jackie Chan using martial arts to teach bad guys a lesson at the school of hard knocks.

These days, though, people are looking to a hybrid of martial arts and aerobics as a way to kick their *own* butts too. Aerobic kickboxing combines punches and kicks culled from boxing and karate with a healthy dose of other heart-pounding action like jogging and rope-jumping.

You may know it as Tae-Bo, an exercise system available on videotapes that puts tae kwon do moves to music. Or you may see it billed as Cardio Karate, Aerobic Karate, or a similar moniker at your local gym or martial arts school.

The content of each class will differ depending partly on the instructor and partly on in what proportion the class draws from dance-type aerobics, boxing, and martial arts, says Mercy Van Aken, the aerobics director at Gold's Gym in Allentown, Pennsylvania, who has a background in aikido and karate.

Generally, the classes at Van Aken's gym run from about an hour to 90 minutes. Wearing aerobics or cross-training shoes, the students begin with several minutes of warmups and stretching.

The class then features a quick-moving series of drills involving punches and kicks; pushups,

KICKBOXING

All techniques originate from a body stance with one foot forward and one back, about shoulder-width apart, with all your toes pointed forward. For our purposes, we'll describe these as if you have your left foot forward. Both hands are held in fists in front of you; your right fist will be held just in front of your midsection, and your left fist will be further out and about level with your chin.

Punches

[A] **Jab:** Punch straight in front of you with your left fist, aiming for either midsection or face level.

[B] **Cross:** Give a straight punch with your right hand, also at midsection or face level.

[C] **Uppercut:** With either hand, throw a punch that starts in front of your midsection and angles up and away from you, ending about even with your upper chest. Your knuckles and the heel of your palm should be facing up.

[D] **Hook:** With either hand, punch with your arm bent as if you were trying to punch the side of a target at about head level. Imagine tightly hugging a heavy punching bag at about shoulder level to get an idea of how your arms will curve around.

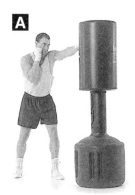 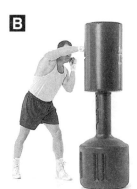 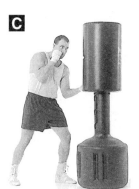 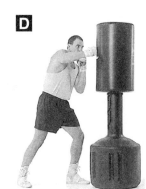

situps, and lunges; and more drills on heavy bags. Classes end with a cooldown featuring additional stretching.

The Routine: Here are a few tips to keep in mind when starting a kickboxing program.

• **Try a sample.** See if you can take at least one sample lesson to find out whether the workout is something you'll enjoy for the long run. Ask your teacher what sort of martial arts background or fitness training he or she has.

• **Stay loose.** Don't lock your joints or hyperextend your limbs when throwing punches or executing kicks.

• **Aim low.** If you're a beginner, don't throw high kicks until you're familiar with them and have gained enough flexibility and balance.

• **Pace yourself.** Stay within your limits so that you don't overexert yourself before the class is finished. Don't worry about looking good compared with the others. Their fitness is theirs, and yours is yours, Grasshopper.

• **Watch the knuckle sandwich.** When you throw a punch, focus on making contact with your two largest knuckles.

RUNNING

Right now, you're holding the potential to travel thousands of miles free of charge. You don't need to purchase a plane ticket or a bus pass or buy a car or even a bike.

Kicks

[**E**] **Front:** Bring your right leg up in front of you until your thigh is parallel with the ground. Kick your foot out with a snapping motion, making contact using the ball of your foot.

[**F**] **Side:** Bring your right leg forward and your right knee up toward your left shoulder. Shoot your right foot out to your right side, making contact with your foot pointed horizontally and striking with your heel.

[**G**] **Roundhouse:** Bring your right leg in front of you until your thigh is parallel with the ground, and turn slightly to your left, pivoting on your left foot and kicking out with your right foot. Your toes will be pointed away from you, and you'll imagine making contact using your lower shin.

[**H**] **Back:** Look over your left shoulder. Bring your left knee up slightly in front of you. Shoot your left foot straight back behind you at about hip level.

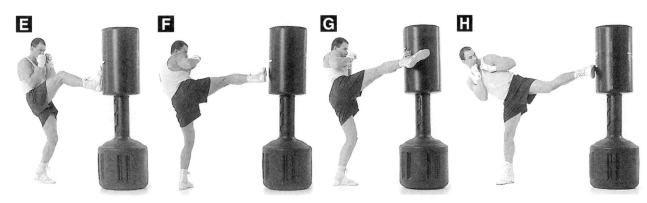

All you have to do is put on a pair of shoes and put one foot in front of the other. Do it relatively quickly and you're jogging. Pick up the pace and you're running. It's that simple.

You can run if you live near city streets or country roads. You can do it on the high school track or the gym treadmill. You can do it alone or with a group. You might even be able to set down this book and start enjoying it in a matter of moments.

While you're at it, you can enjoy the ever-changing sights, sounds, and smells of your surroundings throughout the year. The freshly cut grass gives way to colored piles of leaves, which soon disappear under expanses of unbroken snow. Instead of watching it rush past the car window, you'll be a part of it.

The Routine: If you've never run before, or if you do it only rarely, you'll probably get more enjoyment out of the activity if you ease into it. Follow these guidelines as you put the miles behind you.

• **Start slow.** If you're new to this, begin by walking 20 minutes a day for 4 days, then walk 30 minutes daily for the next 4 days, suggests Budd Coates, health promotion manager for Rodale and a four-time Olympic Marathon Trials qualifier.

Then start interspersing 2 minutes of jogging with 4 minutes of walking, for a total of 30 minutes. Each week, jog a little more of those 30 minutes and walk a little less. After 10 weeks, you can start jogging the whole 30-minute spell.

• **If possible, run on a soft surface.** A well-maintained track or path in a park will do nicely. If you don't have access to these, running on the crunchy surface at the edge of a paved roadway will be easier on your body than pounding down a cement sidewalk. Be sure to wear bright clothing and run *against* oncoming traffic.

Also, when you're choosing roadways, pick ones that are flat rather than steeply sloped from the center to the edge. Your feet will thank you.

• **Wear well-fitting shoes.** Since shoes are basically the only equipment you need for this activity, make sure that they fit well and suit your purposes. Visit a shop that specializes in running shoes, where you can discuss your personal running needs—such as how much you run, where you do it, and how your feet are shaped.

Also, shop in the late afternoon when your feet are at their largest, and wear the socks you'll be wearing while running. If the store will let you, take the shoes out for a brief run around the block to check their fit (be sure to avoid the mud puddles and dog droppings).

When you've logged 400 to 500 miles, reward yourself with a new pair of shoes. That's about how long you can use them.

• **Devise a weekly workout.** Once you've got the running habit down, try the following setup to schedule a week's worth of workouts, Coates suggests. Take a long run of about 8 miles; a medium one of 5 to 6 miles in which you run both quick- and slower-paced intervals, do some track work, or include hills; two or three runs of 2 to 4 miles; and 2 or 3 days of rest mixed in.

• **Stretch later.** Throughout much of this book, we advise you to stretch both before and after a workout, but Coates sees it differently for running. Although you should ease gently into each running workout to warm up, save your stretching for *after,* Coates suggests—unless you notice an overly tight muscle early in your run that needs some stretching attention.

CROSS-COUNTRY SKIING

There's a reason that most of us rarely see a guy cross-country skiing his way to work in the mornings.

CROSS-COUNTRY SKIING DIAGONAL STRIDE

[**A**] With your feet parallel, your torso leaning forward, and your knees slightly bent, begin pushing straight—not back—through your left boot into the ski as you initiate the kick.

[**B**] As you kick your left leg back, your weight will automatically shift to your right leg, which is driven forward for the glide. Your opposite arm will naturally follow, so plant your left-hand pole into the snow.

[**C**] With your left elbow bent, push the left pole. At the same time, initiate the glide forward with your left leg, repeating the sequence on the opposite side.

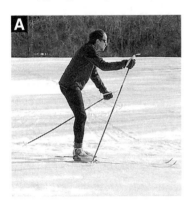
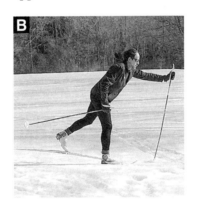
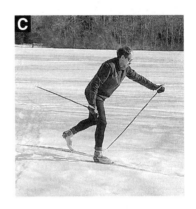

Well, there are several reasons, actually. The activity requires a layer of snow, for starters, which isn't an everyday occurrence for most of us. But more to the point of our discussion on fitness, cross-country skiing is a tough workout.

In fact, as aerobic activities go, it's often regarded as one of the top calorie-burning exercises. A 175-pound man will get a full-body workout while burning through about 820 calories in an hour. That may not be an appealing selling point for the average Joe, but it's a good reason to try it in your quest to be a Hard-Body Man.

If you live in an area with ample snow and enjoy crisp winter air, you can take up this activity, which has been traced back to the Norwegians of 5000 B.C. Or, if you have no snow or desire to be in it, you can hop on an indoor cross-country skiing machine to simulate the exercise.

For the Great Outdoors: Here's some advice if you're willing to brave the cold.

• **Try before you buy.** Before you commit to a set of cross-country equipment, rent several different types of gear from a ski shop and take it out on a real-world test.

• **Shop around.** When you buy, try to find a shop that specializes in cross-country skis, with a knowledgeable staff. Salespeople should take the time to answer your questions and ensure that the equipment you buy will work well for the kind of skiing you like to do and the kind of snow you'll likely encounter.

• **Do a systems check.** Make sure that your skis are compatible with your boots and the system that binds them together.

• **Ease into it.** Be sure to warm yourself up and, if you like, do light stretching before you barge into a skiing session.

For the Great Indoors: Here's some advice for you machineheads out there.

• **Try 'em out.** If you're unaccustomed to skiing, you might find that the motions of using an indoor ski machine don't come as second nature. If you're going to buy one, first try several models to find a style that lets you get into a groove.

• **Add an aural element.** Since you won't be reveling in nature's wonders when you use an indoor ski machine, you may want to listen to music, books on tape, or a "sounds of nature" recording while you're burning the calories.

CROSS-TRAINING

Wouldn't it be great if the only healthy food on the Hard-Body Plan were iceberg lettuce? Mmm, day after day, bowl after bowl, you could eat all the crunchy, white iceberg lettuce that you could stomach.

On second thought, maybe that wouldn't be so great. Who wants one thing all the time, even if it's something you happen to like? The same goes for exercise. After a while, you might find that the same aerobic routine week after week grows tiring.

That's why the variety of cross-training becomes so important. You become engaged in different activities that give your mind novel situations and actions to think about, plus you give more areas of your body a chance to join the fun. Also, if you have an injury, cross-training may let you give the sore part a rest. Or, better yet, it might help you avoid overuse damage in the first place.

The Routine: Here are some options to consider when choosing cross-training ingredients.

• **Switch between high and low.** If you normally run or cycle, incorporate activities that work your upper body—say, rowing, swimming, or tennis.

• **Alternate hard and soft.** If you frequently jog or play racquetball, choose an activity to add to the mix that's gentler on your joints, such as biking or swimming.

• **Combine fast and slow.** You can also do some low-exertion exercise, such as a session on the stationary cycle, interspersed with a few minutes of a harder workout, such as jumping rope.

• **Mix up the machine work.** Turn a workout session into a cross-training experience by splitting your time up on the different aerobics machines at the gym. Jog on the treadmill, hop on the stationary cycle, and then follow it up with a session on the elliptical trainer.

Another choice, if the weather permits, will also save you a little gas money: Jog to the local pool, swim for a while, and jog back home.

MOUNTAIN BIKING

The sport of mountain biking has a colorful phrase that you want to avoid: doing an "endo" (or even worse, a "gnarly endo").

Short for "end over end," it's the mishap you secretly hoped to see Evel Knievel do but dread yourself—flying over the handlebars with the grace of a sack of doorknobs.

Though the endo represents an experience you *don't* want from mountain biking, the hobby offers plenty of good stuff too.

For starters, your thighs, hips, and butt get a workout from pedaling the bike, and your forearms and upper arms work to put on the brakes and steer.

You'll also hone your balance and agility and, depending on your surroundings, get to enjoy natural surroundings as you pedal away down the trail.

The Routine: Here are some ways to get more of a Hard Body (and less of a bruised body) from mountain biking.

• **Wear a helmet while riding.** Choose one that cradles the lower back part of your head, suggests elite cross-country racer Ned Overend in his book *Mountain Bike Like a Champion*. (His name, interestingly enough, is an anagram for "end over end.")

MOUNTAIN BIKE DESCENT

To keep your face from meeting the ground in front of you while going down a steep descent, push your butt back and lean over the seat.

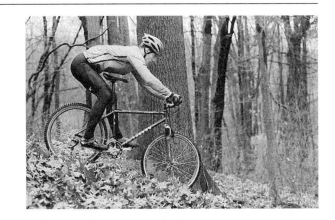

BUNNY HOP

Pick up some momentum and position yourself in the attack position when approaching an obstacle. [**A**] Stop pedaling when your front tire is about 1 foot away from the obstacle, and press down on the handlebar and pedals like you are loading a spring. [**B**] Spring up for your liftoff by pulling up the front wheel with your arms. [**C**] Once your front wheel is over the object, push the front wheel forward and suck up your legs to lift the rear wheel over.

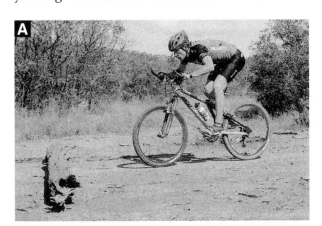

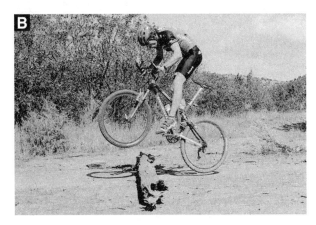

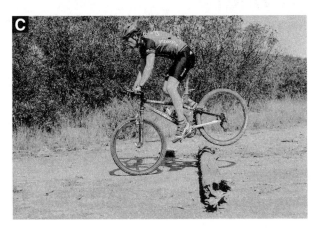

MOUNTAIN BIKE JUMP: TAKE-OFF AND LANDING

[**A**] Keep your cranks (the bars the pedals are attached to) horizontal. Ease your backside off the seat and shift your weight back a bit. [**B**] Pull up and back on the handlebar while going over the obstacle. [**C**] Upon landing, try to hit the ground rear wheel first or both wheels together with your front wheel pointed straight. Keep your weight back and stay loose to absorb the impact by keeping your knees and elbows bent.

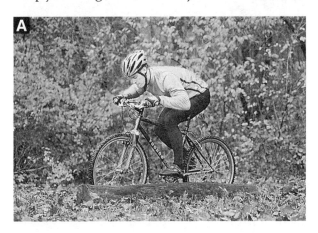

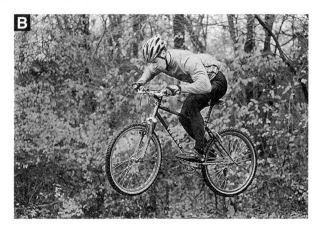

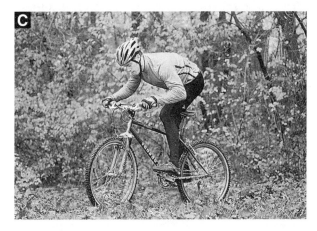

Make sure that it's snugly attached—if it budges more than an inch, tighten the strap—so it won't fly off your head if you fly off your bike.

• **Don't let your bike write a check your body can't cash.** In other words, know your own limits. If you see a challenging piece of trail you're not ready for, get off and push your bike. Similarly, be careful on unfamiliar trails.

• **Watch out for others on the trail.** Also allow plenty of room between you and the rider ahead.

• **Ride relaxed.** Keep your elbows and knees bent, not locked.

ROWING

Hard-Body Men of the Viking age got some of their aerobic exercise by rowing. Of course, they weren't seeking the fitness benefits when they tugged on the oars; their goal was simply to zoom their ship up as quickly as possible to a village and then loot it.

Nowadays, rowing, whether in a boat in the water or on a machine at the gym, is still a fine way to give your muscles and cardiovascular system a serious workout. Just keep your war cries to yourself,

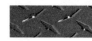

Olaf, or you might attract unwanted attention. (And remember, looting will get you 5 to 10 in the pen.)

If you don't have access to one of those nifty, streamlined rowing shells (which would put you in plenty of company), don't worry—it's easier to get a good workout on a rowing machine, or "erg," in the gym than out in the water, says James Stratton, the coach for the Johns Hopkins University novice crew team.

These devices look like a long, low track with a seat that slides up and down its length. You sit on the seat facing a covered flywheel at one end of the track. You grip a handle, push your feet against two foot plates, and pull back on the cable connected to the flywheel.

The erg in the gym is more stable than its equivalent watercraft, Stratton says, so you can focus on your workout without rocking back and forth trying to keep your balance over the water.

What you *are* doing is sailing along your imaginary river powered by your quads, hamstrings, lats, and lower back. And you're toning your shoulders and forearms, he says.

The Routine: Here's the proper form to use while working out on the rowing machine so that everyone in the gym will think you're a natural. (Using the word *erg* liberally will help too.)

Step 1: Start in the "finish" position. Your legs are straightened out but not locked, you've pushed the seat back as far as you can take it, and you've pulled the handle back against your upper abdomen.

Step 2: Slide forward into the recovery position. Begin by extending your arms, then bend at the hips, and finally bend your knees and allow the slide to roll toward your heels. Keep your back erect and your shoulders squared while you're bending forward. When your body is close enough to the flywheel that your shins are vertical or nearly so, you're ready to begin your slide back.

Step 3: Press with your legs to begin your backward slide. Your back is still straight, you're leaning forward at the hips, and your arms are extended. Right now, all your power is coming from your legs.

Step 4: As your legs become nearly straight, lean back, putting power into your stroke from your lower back. When your legs are straight and you're leaning back slightly, *then* bring the handle in to your upper abdomen. The arms will be the weakest part of the stroke, and you save them for the end.

Step 5: Start the cycle back at step 1.

Your slide forward (as if you were pushing the oars forward) should be slow, taking about three times as long as your slide back (where you would be digging the oars into the water and pulling back on the handles), Stratton says.

INLINE SKATING

Let's watch a guy have a very bad inline skating experience, one that he probably could have avoided if he had approached the hobby differently.

Without strapping on a helmet or other protective equipment, he takes off across town, skating hesitantly down streets, across broken sidewalks, and over curbs. With no training and little practice, he falls down frequently.

Approaching a steep hill, he picks up speed on wobbly feet (he hasn't gotten the hang of braking, either). In one fell swoop, he somersaults over, hitting his head on the pavement and scattering nasty road rash around his body. Fortunately, he's not badly injured, and he sells his skates to a used-sporting-goods store without ever wearing them again.

That's how *not* to do it. On the other hand, when it's done right, inline skating can be a terrific—and very cardiovascular—sport, as about 29 million Americans are discovering. In addition, you'll pump up muscles in your ankles, calves, knees, inner thighs, and hips.

The Routine: Before you strap on the skates and zoom off, make sure that you're ready.

• **Wear safety gear or you'll feel more than the burn.** A number of studies have found that the body parts most commonly injured while skating are the wrists and lower arms. So be sure to wear wrist protectors. Hard Body or not, you're not going to impress your lady if she has to cut your steak for you.

And while you're slapping on protective gear, continue with a helmet and elbow and knee pads. Someday you'll thank us for this wisdom.

• **Rent first.** Rent a pair of skates and equipment before you buy so that you can get the feel for the hobby. Your skates should fit snugly but shouldn't cause any uncomfortable pressure. Move around on them a little in the store to make sure they fit.

Expect to pay at least $100 for a pair of skates when you're ready to buy. Plenty of styles retail for $250 and above.

• **Start smooth.** Begin your inline skating endeavors on a flat, smooth surface away from cars, obstacles, and, of course, angry dogs. A parking lot is a good choice.

• **Learn to stop.** You may remember, way back when, that your driver's-ed instructor made sure right away to teach you the importance of that horizontal pedal just to the left of the gas. Inline skating is no different. Study the instructions with your skates, and practice using your brake.

• **Learn to go.** Position yourself so that your knees are slightly bent and your feet are parallel. Lean forward slightly. Turn your right foot to a 45-degree angle and push out to the side with it. As you push yourself, put your weight on your left foot and lean in the direction you're moving. Once you've pushed off, bring your right foot up and parallel with your left, and do the whole thing over with your left foot.

• **Seek help.** Ask at your local skate shop about upcoming lessons and clinics in your area. The International Inline Skating Association certifies instructors; seek out one of them.

STRENGTH TRAINING FOR 32 SPORTS AND ACTIVITIES

FUNCTIONAL FITNESS

The serious Hard-Body Man using the Hard-Body Plan will find that this program helps him excel in all the sports and games he plays. And particular exercises will particularly help with particular sports. What follows are 32 athletic events along with the exercises from the Hard-Body Plan that will best work the muscles for each. If you don't have machines handy, you can replace those exercises with the equivalent free- or no-weight exercise.

Why 32? Well, great athletes such as Jim Brown, Sandy Koufax, and Magic Johnson wore that number. More important, that's all we could come up with.

ARCHERY

Any quivers should be limited to the case holding your arrows, not the shaking that occurs if you have insufficient strength in your arms, shoulders, and upper back.

Hard-Body Plan exercises to do:
- **Alternating dumbbell curl** and **cable pulldown** for upper-arm strength
- **Wrist roller** to develop strong wrists

- **Lying side deltoid raise** to strengthen upper-back and shoulder muscles

ARM WRESTLING

You mostly need upper-body strength in the biceps, forearms, chest, and shoulders before you can slam your opponent's wrist to the table.

Hard-Body Plan exercises to do:
- **Bench press** to help you develop your pectoral muscles
- **Parallel dip with weight plate** for your triceps
- **Barbell curl** for building biceps
- **Forearm curl** to help strengthen your wrists and forearms

Throw in some mirror work too—practice making scary grimaces to spook and distract your opponent.

BADMINTON

Even for a backyard game like this, you need strong forearm muscles and legs powerful enough to enable you to make quick stops and starts.

Hard-Body Plan exercises to do:
- **Dumbbell fly** for chest muscles
- **Forearm curl** to strengthen your forearms and wrists
- **Leg curl** to develop your hamstrings
- **Leg extension** for building your quadriceps
- **Seated twist** to work your abdominals

BASKETBALL

You need strong leg muscles for running and jumping, plus powerful arms to wrest rebounds away from opponents.

Hard-Body Plan exercises to do:
- **Squat** for leg and hip thrust
- **Leg curl with ankle weights** to strengthen hamstrings and protect them from injury
- **Bench press**, with a narrow grip, to strengthen your chest for upper-body thrust
- **Romanian deadlift** for back extension
- **Lying triceps extension** to help strengthen your triceps

BICYCLING

As you would expect, you need strong leg muscles for bicycling, and you need some upper-body power to stabilize your body in the saddle.

Hard-Body Plan exercises to do:
- **Seated heel raise** and **leg curl** to strengthen calf and hamstring muscles for more pedal power
- **Deadlift** to keep your lower back from hurting
- **Wrist raise** to give you the upper-body strength to stay as steady as a cowboy in the saddle

BOWLING

Overall strength can improve your lane prowess. Powerful arms and shoulders are especially important.

Hard-Body Plan exercises to do:
- **Alternating dumbbell curl** and **wrist roller** for more power throughout your arms
- **Dumbbell military press** to strengthen your shoulders
- **Lat pulldown** to develop your upper back and provide balanced strength

BOXING

Powerful punches come from having strong pectorals, deltoids, and triceps. You also need strong calves to stay on your toes round after round.

Hard-Body Plan exercises to do:
- **Barbell curl** for big biceps
- **Desk dip** for strengthening triceps
- **Bench press** for developing pectoral power
- **Lying side deltoid raise** for stronger shoulders
- **Seated heel raise** to strengthen calves

CANOEING AND KAYAKING

A strong back, strong shoulders, and strong arms will get you rolling down the river.

Hard-Body Plan exercises to do:
- **Bent-arm pullover** to work the lower pectoral muscles in your chest and the latissimus dorsi in your mid- and lower back
- **Dumbbell military press** for strengthening shoulders

- **Lying triceps extension** to work triceps and, with the other exercises, give you more paddling power
- **Curl-up** for more abdominal development

CLIMBING

This sport requires good overall body strength. You have to be able to pull, push, twist, shove off with your legs, brace yourself, and maintain balance.

Hard-Body Plan exercises to do:
- **Parallel dip with weight plate** for building triceps strength
- **Barbell curl** to bolster biceps
- **Seated row** to strengthen the back
- **Leg extension** to work the quadriceps
- **Leg curl** to build the hamstrings and provide good overall strength
- **Dumbbell trunk twist** to strengthen obliques, making twisting easier

DIVING

Overall body strength will help you make a splash in this sport, but especially important are the deltoids, abdominals, and calves.

Hard-Body Plan exercises to do:
- **Seated heel raise** to strengthen calves
- **Crunch** (do a variety) for stronger abdominals
- **Seated twist** for the oblique abdominal muscles, which run along your sides
- **Side deltoid raise** to strengthen deltoids

FENCING

Sturdy legs and strong pushing muscles are essential. You thought we were going to say arms, didn't you? Arms are important, too, bud. But without legs, you'll fall right over.

Hard-Body Plan exercises to do:
- **Parallel dip with weight plate** to work your triceps
- **Incline bench press** to build your pectorals and shoulders
- **Leg curl** for your hamstrings
- **Squat** for your quadriceps and hamstrings

FOOTBALL

The emphasis on muscles can vary depending on what position you play, but football requires good overall strength, especially in your legs and back and the muscles that you use to push.

Hard-Body Plan exercises to do:
- **Leg extension** to work your quadriceps
- **Leg curl** for your hamstrings
- **Toe press** to develop calf muscles
- **Bent-arm pullover** to build chest muscles
- **Incline dumbbell bench press** for chest muscles
- **Parallel dip with weight plate** for triceps development
- **Deadlift** to strengthen your back

GOLF

Powerful legs and shoulders improve your swing, well-developed obliques help you twist your trunk and support your back, and strong forearms and wrists give you greater club control and more accurate shots.

Hard-Body Plan exercises to do:
- **Stationary lunge with dumbbells** for hip and leg thrust

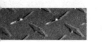

- **Oblique trunk rotation** for strong torso rotation
- **Upright row** to help you drive the ball farther
- **Crunch** (a variety) for a stronger abdomen
- **Forearm curl** for strong forearms
- **Wrist roller** for strong wrists

HIKING

Your legs and upper back are most apt to tire if you're carrying a backpack.

Hard-Body Plan exercises to do:
- **Wide-grip row** to work your back muscles, your shoulders' rear deltoids, and your hamstring and gluteal muscles
- **Leg extension** to develop your quadriceps
- **Leg curl** to develop your hamstrings

THE PLAYER

At only 5 feet 7 inches, PGA great Gary Player is a believer that strength training can improve your game. Early in his career, he ran up and down the dusty gold-mine hills of his native South Africa to develop his legs, he says in his book *Fit for Golf*.

Then Player began doing 70 fingertip pushups spread throughout the day, to build up his arms and fingers. Eventually, he retained a professional bodybuilder to start him on a series of exercises using weights.

"By training the correct muscles, you can easily increase the strength and coordination you need for a powerful golf swing," Player says in his book.

HOCKEY

Well-developed leg muscles, abdominals, and shoulders are vital for success on the rink.

Hard-Body Plan exercises to do:
- **Stationary lunge with dumbbells** for hip and leg thrust
- **Curl-up** for strong abs and better balance
- **Oblique trunk rotation** for strong abs
- **Shrug** for powerful shoulders that help you hit the puck with power

INLINE SKATING

Strong abs and legs are the key to spending more time on your feet than on your butt.

Hard Body Plan exercises to do:
- **Curl-up** for your abdominals
- **Seated twist** for the obliques
- **Oblique trunk rotation** for the obliques
- **Leg extension** to build your quadriceps
- **Squat** to strengthen your butt, quadriceps, and hamstrings

JUDO

Powerful legs and the ability to grasp and pull are needed.

Hard-Body Plan exercises to do:
- **Bent-arm pullover** to build the lower pecs in your chest and the lats in your mid- and lower back
- **Parallel dip with weight plate** for developing your triceps
- **Barbell curl** for beefing up your biceps
- **Leg extension** for more powerful quadriceps

KARATE

This martial art requires a combination of upper- and lower-body strength. The pushing muscles of your upper body are particularly important.

Hard-Body Plan exercises to do:
- **Leg extension** for more powerful quadriceps
- **Leg raise** to tighten abdominal muscles
- **Parallel dip with weight plate** to strengthen your triceps
- **Barbell curl** to build your biceps

RACQUETBALL AND SQUASH

For these two similar sports, you must have strong legs to start and stop quickly, in addition to upper-body strength and great wrists.

Hard-Body Plan exercises to do:
- **Squat** to build your hamstrings, quads, and butt
- **Stationary lunge with dumbbells** for your thighs and butt
- **Leg extension** also for your hamstrings, quads, and butt
- **Seated heel raise** to strengthen calves

- **Wrist roller** to develop your wrists
- **Seated twist** to work your obliques
- **Barbell curl** to work your biceps

RUGBY

Forget the joke about leather balls: What this rough-and-tumble sport *really* takes are strong legs, a strong back, and strong pushing muscles.

Hard-Body Plan exercises to do:
- **Leg extension** for stronger quadriceps
- **Leg curl** to develop your hamstrings
- **Seated row** to work your entire back but especially your upper middle back
- **Alternating dumbbell curl** or **hammer curl** to build your biceps
- **Seated overhead triceps extension** for stronger triceps

RUNNING

If you're running any distance, you need leg muscles that can contract repeatedly over pro-

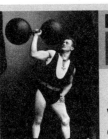

HARD-BODY FACT

Distance runners take note: Lifting lighter weights at a high number of repetitions will work your slow-twitch muscle fibers and may boost your strength and endurance during the kick at the end of a race. Weight training is probably most useful during preseason training. It should never be used as a substitute for running in your training regimen. If you run, be careful not to use weight training to obtain too much additional muscle mass, though; it may be counterproductive since you have to carry this weight.

longed periods. You also need arms, shoulders, and an upper back that won't tire or cramp before you finish.

Hard-Body Plan exercises to do:
- **Lat pulldown** to strengthen your upper back
- **Deadlift** for your lower back
- **Bench press** to work your chest and triceps
- **Barbell curl** to develop your biceps
- **Curl-up** to strengthen your abs

SCUBA DIVING

You need strong legs and pulling strength in order to swim under water.

Hard-Body Plan exercises to do:
- **Bent-arm pullover** to develop the lower pectoral muscles in your chest and the latissimus dorsi muscles in your back
- **Parallel dip with weight plate** to strengthen your triceps muscles
- **Leg extension** to work your quadriceps muscles
- **Leg curl** to work your hamstrings
- **Seated heel raise** to strengthen calves

SEX

You're more apt to be a star performer in this favorite indoor activity if you have strong chest, arm, and abdominal muscles.

Hard Body Plan exercises to do:
- **Bench press** for chest power that enables you to support your arms and shoulder muscles, especially important in the missionary position
- **Pushup** for the same reason as the bench press

- **Crunch** (do a variety) to work the abdominals and obliques

SKIING

You may be forced to spend more time recovering in bed than gliding over slopes or trails unless you have strong shoulders, quadriceps, hamstrings, abs, and lower-back muscles.

Hard-Body Plan exercises to do:
- **Shrug** for shoulder development
- **Upright row** to build shoulders
- **Stationary lunge with dumbbells** to strengthen quadriceps and hamstrings
- **Leg curl** for quads and hamstrings
- **Seated heel raise** to build calf strength, especially important for cross-country skiing
- **Curl-up** to develop firmer abdominals
- **Cable row** to fortify your lower back

SOCCER

Obviously, you need tremendous leg muscles to excel at soccer, but you also need some upper-body strength, too, for accurate throw-ins.

Hard-Body Plan exercises to do:
- **Squat** for leg and hip thrust
- **Leg curl with ankle weights** to prevent hamstring injury
- **Romanian deadlift** for back extension
- **Dumbbell military press** to improve upper-body thrust
- **Seated overhead triceps extension** for triceps power

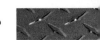

SOFTBALL AND BASEBALL

Even a leisurely game of softball requires strong legs for running and powerful forearms and shoulders so you can slam like a slugger.

Hard-Body Plan exercises to do:
- **Bent-over lateral raise** or **side deltoid raise** to strengthen shoulders
- **Forearm curl** for stronger forearms
- **Seated heel raise** to build up calves

SWIMMING

Gotta work your fins if you want to swim like the fishies. It takes overall body strength in addition to proper technique in order to excel as a swimmer.

Hard-Body Plan exercises to do:
- **Incline bench press** for your chest
- **Upright row** to build your shoulders
- **Crunch** (various forms) to hit all your abdominal muscles
- **Seated heel raise** to strengthen your calves

TENNIS

Strong legs for sudden starts and stops while changing direction are essential if you want to be an ace on the tennis court. You'll also need upper-body strength, especially in your shoulders and forearms.

Hard-Body Plan exercises to do:
- **Squat, stationary lunge, leg extension,** and **leg curl** to strengthen your quadriceps, hamstrings, and butt

- **Barbell curl** to build biceps
- **Forearm curl** to work your wrists and forearms
- **Side deltoid raise** and **bent-over lateral raise** to strengthen your deltoids

VOLLEYBALL

You need strong legs for leaping and upper-body strength for spiking the ball in order to be a whiz on the volleyball court.

Hard-Body Plan exercises to do:
- **Vertical leg press** to build your quadriceps and hamstrings
- **Seated heel raise** for stronger calves
- **Side deltoid raise** to strengthen shoulders
- **Seated twist** to work the obliques

WATER POLO

To be adept at water polo, develop the muscles that you use in swimming and throwing.

Hard-Body Plan exercises to do:
- **Bent-arm pullover** for a more powerful chest
- **Cable pulldown** to strengthen your triceps
- **Crunch** (do a variety) to work the abdominals
- **Leg curl** for stronger hamstrings
- **Vertical leg press** for your quadriceps and hamstrings
- **Seated heel raise** to develop your calves

WATERSKIING

To stay upright in this activity, you need strong thigh and upper-body muscles.

Hard-Body Plan exercises to do:
- **Vertical leg press** to strengthen your quadriceps and hamstrings
- **Seated row** for stronger back and shoulder muscles
- **Forearm curl** to work your forearms and wrists

WRESTLING

You need overall body strength to compete in wrestling, with emphasis on the muscles used in gripping and pulling your opponents.

Hard-Body Plan exercises to do:
- **Parallel dip with weight plate** to develop your triceps
- **Bent-arm pullover** to develop chest and back muscles
- **Barbell curl** to build your biceps
- **Squat** to strengthen quadriceps, hamstrings, and butt
- **Curl-up** for strengthening your abdominals
- **Seated twist** for abs
- **Wrist roller** to develop your wrists

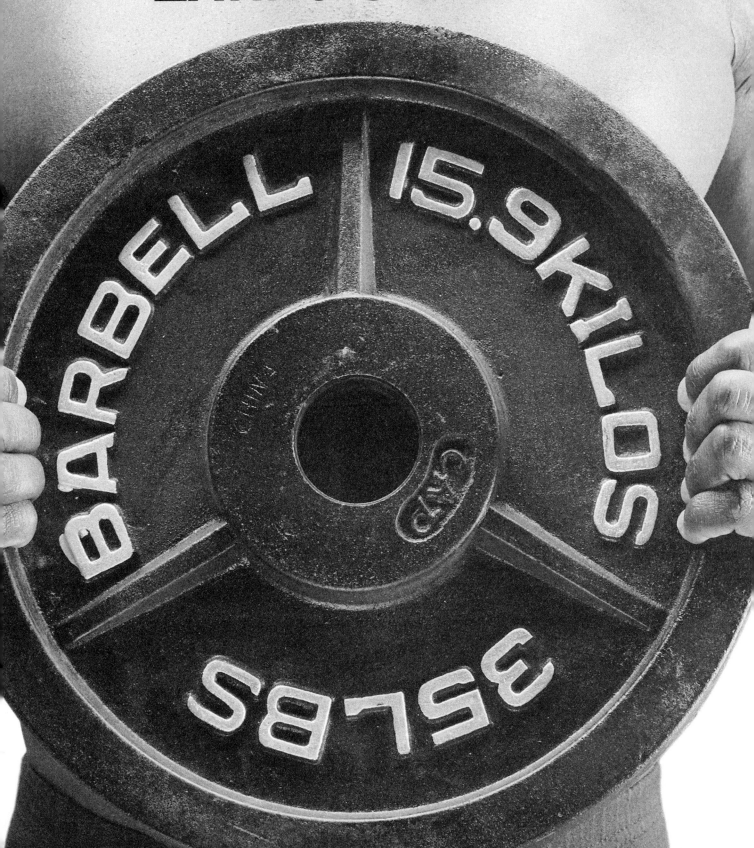

PART 3

EATING SMART

HERE'S THE PLAN
STRATEGIC EATING

EXERCISE MAKES MUSCLES STRONGER AND CONSEQUENTLY BIGGER. THE RIGHT FOODS FUEL THE PROCESS. THE HARD-BODY MAN FUELS UP WITH LOW-FAT, HIGH-CARBOHYDRATE ENERGY FOODS. HE EATS AMPLY, REGULARLY, AND OFTEN.

You have to eat if you want to lose fat and build muscle, and you have to eat right. Although the food you put into your body doesn't build the muscle, it does fuel your muscle-building workouts and help speed recovery.

Take it from Gail Butterfield, R.D., Ph.D. "What you put in your mouth determines whether you'll be able to do the kind of training day after day that you need to do to bulk up," says the sports nutritionist, researcher, and registered dietitian.

How you eat also affects aesthetics, helping you achieve the true Hard-Body look.

You don't get that lean, cut, bulging-muscle appearance if those hard-won muscles are hiding beneath a layer of fat. So a key part of Hard-Body eating is reducing and holding down body fat, says Thomas Incledon, M.S., R.D., a sports nutrition specialist in Plantation, Florida, and designer of the Hard-Body Diet.

We're not suggesting that you drop to just 3 or 4 percent body fat, as some extreme body-builders do to show off their ripples. It's not healthy. But with the Hard-Body Plan, you do lose the jelly and highlight the cuts. You do that by eating *lower*-fat foods and by burning more calories than you take in.

You need to develop and stick to a sensible eating plan that is easy to live with and easy to follow wherever you are.

The plan that we offer works. It works if you wield garlic presses and whisks with the dexterity and aplomb of a chef on cable TV. It works if your idea of home cooking is canned spaghetti for breakfast and slapping cold cuts and cheese onto white bread for the more formal meals. What you have in your hands is a top sports-nutritionist-approved, man-made plan for men. Really. We tell you how to eat well at the 24-Hour Quick Mart and at Joe's Drive-Thru Burger Joint or Mickey D's.

A TYPICAL DAY IN THE LIFE OF THE HARD-BODY MAN

6:45 A.M. Hard-Body Man empties his bladder, then starts the coffeemaker. He drinks a glass of water.

7:08 A.M. He enjoys a cup of coffee while shaving.

7:22 A.M. Hard-Body Man downs a banana, a cup of low-fat yogurt, and a bagel with peanut butter—a workable combination of protein, carbs, and fat—and heads out the door. He doesn't have to, but he often eats the same thing for breakfast. Yesterday, though, he had a bowl of cornflakes instead of the bagel.

7:46 A.M. While gassing up at Ourtown Quick-Stop, he grabs a 10-ounce bottle of orange juice for the road.

9:03 A.M. At work, he goes into the break room and pours another cup of coffee and a large mug of ice water.

10:30 A.M. Morning snack. Hard-Body Man is lifting at noon, so he makes this a preworkout snack. He eats an apple and three graham crackers and drinks a glass of fat-free milk—foods high in carbs and easy to digest.

11:06 A.M. He pours a 16-ounce glass of ice water, which he gradually drinks over the next hour.

12:07 P.M. At the gym, he lifts for 45 minutes. In between sets, he occasionally hits the water fountain—before he is actually thirsty.

1:01 P.M. On the drive back to the office, he eats a high-glycemic cereal bar and drinks a pint of sports drink to replace lost fluid and electrolytes.

1:15 P.M. Hard-Body Man drops into the company cafeteria and orders a small, tossed salad, a plate of spaghetti with meat sauce, and a breadstick. He eats at his desk and washes it down with another 16-ounce glass of water.

1:30 P.M. He refills the ice water for the afternoon. He always keeps water at his desk. He prefers water because it contains no calories. Juices, lemonade, and soft drinks without caffeine all replace fluids just as well.

2:30 P.M. Feeling a siesta beckoning, Hard-Body Man wards it off. He heads downstairs and slips outside for a quick, vigorous 5-minute walk—a Not-a-Smoke Break.

3:30 P.M. He's wide awake and a little hungry. He snacks on an apple, crackers, and a bit of string cheese.

6:33 P.M. Now home, Hard-Body Man places two skewers of fresh-sliced vegetables and a marinated chicken breast on the backyard grill. He brushes the food with herbs and olive oil and enjoys a glass of red table wine. In the kitchen, a potato bakes in the microwave.

6:58 P.M. After a small salad with light dressing, he eats the grilled fare and the potato, garnished with salsa and fat-free sour cream. He drinks heartily from a pitcher of lemonade. Although he cooked tonight, yesterday he ordered out a plain pizza and topped it with his own fat-free mozzarella cheese and fresh vegetables. For dessert, he had fruit. His formula for dinner is simple: Go easy on the meat and dressings and load up on vegetables, potatoes, bread, and rice. He limits himself to two glasses of wine or beer.

8:30 P.M. He guzzles a half-glass of apple juice and then sips ice water while reading a magazine.

10:00 P.M. Sitting down to watch his favorite TV show, Hard-Body Man snacks on a bowl of air-popped popcorn sprinkled with a bit of salt and light butter. Some nights, he eats low-fat chips or a couple of fig bars.

11:06 P.M. He swallows a final glass of water and hits the sack.

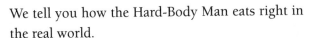

We tell you how the Hard-Body Man eats right in the real world.

This is not about denial. This is not about starving yourself. No leaf-of-lettuce-and-half-ounce-of-tuna Cindy Crawford lunches here. You eat real food, and plenty of it. "You're working hard. You've got to feed the machine," says Jackie Berning, R.D., Ph.D., a sports nutritionist in Colorado Springs, Colorado.

You'll personalize and adapt this plan to your body size and weight and to your workout program objectives. It's not hard to do, and we'll tell you exactly how. Maybe you want to lose weight. Maybe you want to gain weight. To help illustrate concepts, this plan uses a reference man—a 175-pound, 5-foot-10, medium-build guy who'd like to bulk up a little. We show you how to adjust the plan based on your goals and how much you vary from that reference man. You will adjust things, but the keys are the same for all guys.

Don't stuff. Don't starve. Eat small, frequent meals. Do this to keep your energy level stable and your calorie intake more even. You get the calories you need and not a lot of excess. This encourages your body to use them as muscle fuel rather than to store them as fat.

The Hard-Body Plan calls for six or seven meals each day. These are not all-you-can-eat gorgefests. You don't pack away a chicken at every sitting. Actually, you don't have to think of them all as meals. Think meals and hearty snacks. The point is, with six or seven meals a day, you get all the fork action you need, says Incledon.

Because you eat more frequently, you take in smaller meals—enough to curb your hunger, but not enough to leave you feeling fat and overly full.

This is simply basic, sound eating and common sense. You need to eat—and eat often.

"I always tell athletes that if they're hungry, they should eat. The body is very good at adjusting appetite levels to activity levels," Dr. Butterfield says.

Learn to listen to your body. Your *body*—not your lusty imagination when it's dreaming of cream-filled pies, greasy fries, or other sweets or junk foods. You'll find that your body always tells you when it needs fuel. And you'll find that it never, ever says "Stuff me and make me hurt and feel sluggish." Listen to your body. It's an amazing and smart machine.

Eating small, frequent meals spreads your calorie intake over the entire day during the time when you tend to be more active and burning calories. See how that differs from forcing down your biggest meal at the end of the day when you're ready to kick back and flip through the channels?

The active man who works out and feeds his body the way it wants to be fed will probably burn calories at the same rate he consumes them. That's a *good* thing. It prevents the calories from turning into ugly fat.

Eating frequently also keeps insulin levels fairly stable. Insulin regulates your muscles' uptake of nutrients and calories. Steady levels of insulin mean that calories are more easily converted to the glycogen that fuels muscle activity.

Think of calories as units of energy or gallons of gas. Put in too much and it weighs down your machine. Put in too little and your machine coughs and sputters to a stop and has to be pushed to the station.

All foods provide calories. The amount of calories in a serving of food is listed on the nutrition label on the can or package. Make it a habit to eyeball those figures for a while to get the hang of Hard-Body eating.

Carbs are more important than protein. You don't need more protein. Carbohydrates fuel your workouts and provide you with ready energy.

We have a formula for proper fuel mixing. It's basic and easy to follow once you grasp which foods fall into which categories. And to make it even easier, we provide literally dozens of sample Hard-Body meals later in the book. The formula: *Each day—no matter what foods you eat—you should take in roughly 15 to 20 percent protein, 20 to 25 percent fat, and the rest carbohydrates, says Incledon. That means that well over half of everything you eat is a high-carbohydrate food.*

"But what about protein?" you ask. "Those muscleheads down at the gym with the scary grimaces and forearms with veins like garden hoses are always talking 'Protein, protein, protein.'"

We're talking back. We're saying "Nonsense." Nonsense. Want to hear it again? Yes, protein is the key nutrient for repairing and growing muscle. But chances are that you already are getting *too much* protein. You don't need more. Don't buy protein powders and don't go on the latest Liver, Steak, and Eggs for Breakfast diet.

"If you eat more protein than the body requires, it either flushes it out of the system or uses it as fuel. Eating more doesn't help at all," Dr. Berning says. "In fact, it hurts your energy levels."

No food or nutrient endows you with bigger muscle. What builds muscle is training and hard workouts.

Eat foods that fuel high-intensity weight training and allow you to work out day after day. Carbs are your best high-test fuel because they're much more easily converted to energy by your body than protein is, says Incledon.

Also, when your body burns carbs for energy, it doesn't have to burn up as much protein for fuel. More protein then does what it *should* be doing: repairing tissues and helping the muscles grow as you progress in the Hard-Body program.

It might seem that fats (and their liquid version, oils) would be the perfect food for energy. Fats contain more energy per gram than carbs or protein. But you don't want to start eating fat for energy. Fats are easily converted to fat. So instead of bulging muscles, you just end up with bulges.

Fat isn't all bad, though. You need it to make hormones that are used for muscle building. You need fat for some important metabolic processes. And you need fat to give flavor to your food. You just don't need *too much* fat.

Shoot for a fat intake of 20 percent if you need to trim off some flab. Otherwise, up to 25 percent is optimum for achieving and maintaining the Hard-Body lifestyle, says Incledon.

One of your six or seven daily feedings is actually split in two and served on either side of your workout. The first prepares your body for the exertion, and the second helps patch it up afterward.

About an hour to 90 minutes before your workout, you'll eat a snack that's high in carbs with a bit of protein. This floods your body with glucose for your muscles to burn off during the exercise and lessens the normal damage done to your muscles during lifting. You can make a half-portion of one of the snacks on our menu pages, or pick up an energy or nutrition bar that meets the criteria.

Within 15 to 60 minutes *after* your workout, you'll eat another high-carb snack—but this time

EATING OUT

Eating out is when guys tend to fall off the wagon of good Hard-Body eating. Maybe it happens to you because you order a meal not understanding how the food is prepared or how much fat it contains.

Here are some hints to help you know whether you are eating the right stuff.

Avoid menu items that say "fried," "crispy," "breaded," "scampi-style," "creamed," "au gratin," or "gravy." These all suggest lots of fat.

Better choices are food descriptions that say "steamed," "broiled," "charbroiled," "poached," "marinara," "tomato sauce," or "prepared in its own juices."

Make sure that there is something green on your plate, Dr. Berning says, and take care to eat a wide variety of foods each day.

More than 40 nutrients essential to health and growing muscles are found in foods, she points out. Eating a balanced variety of foods ensures that you're taking in enough vitamins, minerals, and fiber.

How it all adds up at the end of the day is what counts, not the ratio of carbs, protein, and fat at any given meal—except for that postworkout snack, which needs to be heavy in high-glycemic carbs.

Whether you get most of your protein by eating a turkey burrito with scrambled eggs for breakfast or by having a grilled chicken sandwich at dinnertime is completely up to you. You can be flexible with this. To keep it simple, in part 4, we've made every breakfast, lunch, dinner, and snack selection relatively balanced. This makes it easy to follow the plan perfectly, and you may want to do just that. But you don't have to be that precise.

With the exception of pre- and postworkout snacks, most of the time, we aren't running on the fuel that we just fed ourselves. Instead, we're drawing fuel from our reserve tanks. Hard-Body eating is a process of replenishing the reserves—keeping the tanks topped off.

"The body has pools of nutrients that it keeps on hand and taps when needed. You should eat to maintain those pools," Dr. Berning explains.

In the chapters that follow, we'll focus on each essential aspect of the plan, and we'll show you how they all add up to equal your new Hard Body.

you need to make sure that it's a high-glycemic carb, which goes to work quickly in restocking your muscles with fuel and helping muscle fibers repair themselves. More on that in "Boosting Glycogen" in the next chapter.

Your pre- and postworkout eating is a key part of the plan's timing, which we will explore in more detail in the next chapter. The total calorie count of the pre- and postworkout snacks needs to roughly equal the calorie count of one of your regular snacks.

Day in and day out, you need a varied diet of vegetables, fruits, meats, and grain to obtain the minerals, vitamins, nutrients, and fiber necessary for building your Hard Body.

WHEN YOU EAT IS AS IMPORTANT AS WHAT YOU EAT
PERFECT TIMING

BUILDING MUSCLE REQUIRES A STEADY FLOW OF NUTRIENTS AND CALORIES. TO MAINTAIN THAT FLOW, EAT SMALL, FREQUENT MEALS. TIME THOSE MEALS AROUND YOUR WORKOUTS AND EAT A COMBINATION OF CARBOHYDRATE AND PROTEIN TO ENHANCE THE HORMONE AND ENZYME ACTIVITY THAT BUILDS MUSCLE.

Here's a familiar scenario for a working stiff: You eat a big breakfast at 7:00, but by 10:00 you're already prowling the break room looking for a doughnut and coffee. When lunch rolls around, you're hungry—big-time hungry.

You buy a wiener from a street vendor, walk down to the food court for a couple of slices, and come back with a monster soda to wash it all down. By 3:00, you're feeding quarters to the vending machine for a Coke and a packet of salty peanuts. You put off dinner so you can go to the gym to lift. When you finally meet your main squeeze for surf and turf, it's 7:30. In the next hour, you devour two appetizers, a couple of beers, and the all-you-can-eat crab leg entrée.

But that's okay. Right? After all, you need the calories, and besides, you worked out today.

Wrong, buddy. All wrong. Not only are you eating the wrong stuff but you're also eating it out of sync with your body. Three big squares a day and snacking on junk food in between to hold off hunger has nothing in common with the body's biological requirements. It just isn't natural.

We real men, hunters and gatherers, were made to graze. Unfortunately, true grazing isn't practical in the modern world. That's why we've created the Hard-Body Plan. It assumes that you're going to eat about every 2½ hours a day and that you'll time those meals to your workouts and your body's needs.

Not only will you eat better, you'll enhance

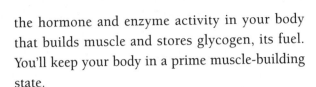

the hormone and enzyme activity in your body that builds muscle and stores glycogen, its fuel. You'll keep your body in a prime muscle-building state.

Meal timing is at the cutting edge of sports nutrition. Several studies show that consuming a combination of carbs and protein before and right after your workout can have wondrous effects on muscle building, says Susan Kleiner, R.D., Ph.D., a sports nutrition researcher and consultant in Mercer Island, Washington, who has written two books, *High-Performance Nutrition* and *Power Eating*.

"It's something we suspected for some time, but now we have more evidence to confirm it," she says. "Smaller, more frequent meals eaten at the right time can be the difference between seeing results and not seeing results in muscle growth."

Frequent meals keep your body fueled, provide nutrients as needed, and help your body maintain a muscle-building state.

Eating about every 2½ hours—rather than every 5 or 6 hours as in Typical Joe's three-meal-a-day plan—is a more efficient way for your body to take in nutrition, says sports nutritionist Thomas Incledon, M.S., R.D., designer of the Hard-Body Diet.

Frequent meals give your body food as needed in the amount that it can handle effectively, rather than overloading it every few hours, says Ann Grandjean, Ed.D., a nutrition researcher in Omaha, Nebraska.

When you go to a buffet and stuff yourself like a Christmas turkey, your body simply can't efficiently absorb all those calories and nutrients, so it uses what nutrients it can and packs away excess calories as fat. Because the digestive tract can only pick up a certain amount of nutrients such as cal-

cium or protein, any extra just passes through and is flushed out of the body unused.

Hard-Body eating is efficient. Compare it to the industrial concept known as just-in-time delivery, where tractor trailers loaded with auto parts arrive at an assembly plant just as workers need the parts to build an automobile.

With Hard-Body eating, it's no different in your body. You deliver the raw materials just when your muscles need amino acids and carbohydrates to repair tissues and recharge glycogen for muscle fuel.

To keep this delivery fleet rolling, eat on a frequent schedule. Never wait until you feel hungry, Dr. Kleiner says.

Hunger is a sign that your body is already on the hunt for raw materials. Unless the trucks pull up soon, your body starts scavenging internally and making what it needs by breaking down tissue, an effect known as catabolism.

You don't want to become catabolic. You want to stay in an anabolic state, which is the state of actively building and maintaining tissue, Dr. Kleiner says.

Frequent feedings also raise your metabolism because your body has to burn calories to digest the food. That's a good thing. "Keep that metabolism revved up if you're trying to burn body fat," says Claudia Wilson, R.D., a sports nutritionist in Salt Lake City.

By eating several times a day, you accentuate this effect, especially if you take in high-carb and low-fat foods. Why these foods? Because it takes more energy to process and store carbs than it does fat, Wilson says.

To build more muscle mass, most guys have to increase their calorie intake. Eating more frequently—about every 3 hours—is a convenient way to add more calories to your diet.

(continued on page 272)

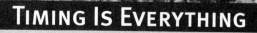

TIMING IS EVERYTHING

Your schedule of snacks and meals will vary depending on when you like to work out. Let's say that you like to lift at noon. You might eat a good breakfast, have a light meal at 9:00 A.M., have a preworkout snack at 11:00 A.M., lift at noon, have a postworkout snack or go out for lunch immediately after leaving the gym, eat a snack at 3:00 P.M., grill up a dinner at 6:00, and have another light snack before bed.

Morning Workout

5:00	5:00 Preworkout Snack
6:00	6:00–7:00 Workout
7:00	7:15 Postworkout Snack or Breakfast
8:00	
9:00	9:30 Snack
10:00	
11:00	
Noon	Noon Lunch
1:00	
2:00	
3:00	3:00 Snack
4:00	
5:00	
6:00	6:00 Dinner
7:00	
8:00	
9:00	9:00 Snack
10:00	
11:00	

Midmorning Workout

5:00	
6:00	
7:00	7:00 Breakfast
8:00	
9:00	9:30 Preworkout Snack
10:00	10:30–11:30 Workout
11:00	
Noon	
1:00	1:00 Postworkout Snack or Lunch
2:00	
3:00	
4:00	4:00 Snack
5:00	
6:00	6:00 Dinner
7:00	
8:00	
9:00	9:00 Snack
10:00	
11:00	

Lunch Workout

5:00	
6:00	
7:00	7:00 Breakfast
8:00	
9:00	9:00 Snack
10:00	
11:00	11:00 Preworkout Snack
Noon	Noon–1:00 Workout
1:00	1:15 Postworkout Snack or Lunch
2:00	
3:00	3:00 Snack
4:00	
5:00	
6:00	6:00 Dinner
7:00	
8:00	
9:00	9:00 Snack
10:00	
11:00	

But if you lift in the early evening, you'll have to adjust your dinner schedule to incorporate a preworkout and postworkout meal. You can either drink your meal as a sports drink or eat food, suggests Claudia Wilson, R.D., a sports nutritionist in Salt Lake City.

Check out these timelines to get some ideas on how to schedule your eating and workout needs into your day.

Midafternoon Workout

5:00	
6:00	
7:00	7:00 Breakfast
8:00	
9:00	9:30 Snack
10:00	
11:00	
Noon	Noon Lunch
1:00	
2:00	2:00 Preworkout Snack
3:00	3:00–4:00 Workout
4:00	4:15 Postworkout Snack
5:00	
6:00	6:00 Dinner
7:00	
8:00	
9:00	9:00 Snack
10:00	
11:00	

After-Work Workout

5:00	
6:00	
7:00	7:00 Breakfast
8:00	
9:00	9:30 Snack
10:00	
11:00	
Noon	Noon Lunch
1:00	
2:00	
3:00	3:00 Snack
4:00	
5:00	5:00 Preworkout Snack
6:00	6:00–7:00 Workout
7:00	7:15 Postworkout Snack
8:00	8:00 Dinner
9:00	
10:00	
11:00	

Evening Workout

5:00	
6:00	
7:00	7:00 Breakfast
8:00	
9:00	9:30 Snack
10:00	
11:00	
Noon	Noon Lunch
1:00	
2:00	
3:00	3:00 Snack
4:00	
5:00	
6:00	6:00 Dinner
7:00	7:45 Preworkout Snack
8:00	8:30–9:30 Workout
9:00	9:45 Postworkout Snack
10:00	
11:00	

Calories essentially are energy units. It takes extra energy to build extra muscle. It seems like a paradox, but meal timing can help you bulk up as well as lose body fat.

If you're just beginning to work out and build muscle mass, you likely need more calories than you're currently taking in. Muscle building requires a lot of calories: Your body needs about 2,700 calories of energy to build 1 pound of lean muscle. A weight lifter will build that muscle over a period of a week or so, and likewise he must take in and burn a steady supply of calories during that period. The only way to ensure a steady supply of calories is to eat more often.

If you're only eating three meals a day now, it's easy to make the change to the Hard-Body eating plan. Just add some tasty snacks that meet your muscle-building needs, Dr. Grandjean says. She suggests eating snacks of peanut butter and crackers, or an apple and trail mix, or dried fruit with slices of cheese. If you're looking to increase your protein intake at the same time, you could supplement your snack with a can of salmon, tuna, or chicken.

"You don't need to stuff yourself at each eating, but you've got to be consistent about having several meals a day," Dr. Grandjean says. "Even if you eat just 100 calories each day above your normal intake, you will eventually gain weight."

If you're lifting regularly, don't worry. That gain will be in the form of muscle.

If you're putting on muscle, expect to gain between ½ pound and 1 pound a week. Monitor your weight gain to make sure that you're not putting on extra fat too. Body-mass measuring devices that also serve as bathroom-type scales have become quite affordable and are available for home use. A Hard-Body Man might want to make an investment in one of these high-tech scales, as they offer a precise way of monitoring body fat.

Before lifting, eat an easily digested, high-carb, low-protein snack. This way you'll have some extra glucose floating about in your bloodstream for energy, and you may reduce muscle tissue damage from lifting.

Research suggests that eating a combination of carbohydrate and protein before intense exercise decreases the tissue breakdown of training.

Dr. Kleiner says that researchers aren't sure why, but apparently the combination of the nutrients limits the injurious chemical reactions that take place after you make microscopic tears in muscle fibers.

Tearing is one of the natural results of stressing muscles during weight training. If you lessen the injurious chemical reactions through scientific eating, however, you may also shorten the buildup and recovery period afterward, Dr. Kleiner says.

The bottom line: bigger muscle in a shorter time. That's the Hard-Body Plan.

"We're finding that this can be extremely significant. You'll have less soreness after lifting and quicker recovery," she says.

Protein has another important effect when mixed with carbohydrates in the way we recommend. It slows down the digestive process and regulates the conversion of carbs into glycogen.

Without the protein, carbs move quickly into the bloodstream and spike insulin levels. Insulin, in turn, hastens the conversion of glucose into glycogen. After a workout, when you're trying to recharge glycogen, that's exactly what you want. But just before and during your workout, it's better to have more glucose floating around as available energy.

"You don't want everything you just ate to go into storage," Dr. Kleiner says. "This way, the body can use the glucose in the bloodstream first, and later go to its glycogen stores."

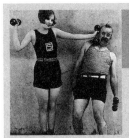

THAT'S DUMB

Guys who lift in the morning before breakfast shortchange themselves energywise, says Dan Benardot, R.D., Ph.D, author of *Nutrition for Serious Athletes* and a sports nutritionist and researcher in Atlanta.

You're essentially fasting when you're asleep. After 8 hours in the Land of Nod, the levels of glycogen in your liver and glucose in your blood plummet. First thing in the morning, there's little carbohydrate energy available for weight lifting. It isn't long into your workout before your body starts breaking down muscle to power up those weights, says Dr. Benardot.

"Not eating is really a classic error of early risers," he says. "You should at least get in a couple of hundred calories before you go the gym."

The best choices are easily digested carbs such as fruit, yogurt, or a slice of toast, or a sports drink with a high carb content.

Incledon recommends a nutrient ratio of about 2 parts carbohydrate to 1 part protein for your pre- and postworkout snacks. Many energy bars and popular sports drinks have roughly this ratio; eating or drinking one of them will do the trick. Incledon points out, however, that scientific research is continuing and that the carb-to-protein ratio is not at all firmly established. In fact, he says, anything between 2:1 and 4:1 should be okay. If you're using energy bars for your workout snacks, do check the ratio: Some are way, way off the Hard-Body recommendation. One bar we found was 10 parts protein to 1 part carbohydrate.

Of course, you'll also find ample sources of carbs and protein in *real* foods too. We'll talk more about those in detail in the next two chapters.

In total, you should take in between 100 and 200 calories about 60 to 90 minutes before you lift, Dr. Kleiner says.

A great way to maximize muscle building during your workout is to halve one of the tasty snacks we list in part 4. Eat half of it an hour to 90 minutes before your workout, and eat the other half 15 to 60 minutes following your workout. Or have a designer energy bar both times. Or have one of those jam-filled cereal bars and ½ cup of fat-free milk (to add the needed protein).

Also, you might read food labels for the first week or so. That way, you'll get the hang of calorie counting, and you won't have to give it much conscious thought. Here's another recommendation from Dr. Kleiner.

After you put down the last barbell of your workout, you need to pick up a postworkout snack within 15 to 60 minutes and then eat a regular meal within 2 hours. It's important that the postworkout-snack carbs are of the high-glycemic kind (but not simple sugars). This jump-starts your muscles' repair and recovery process.

BOOSTING GLYCOGEN

When choosing which foods to eat after a workout, look for carb-rich munchies with a high glycemic index.

The glycemic index measures how quickly a particular food causes blood sugar to rise. A high glycemic rating means that the body turns the food into sugar very quickly. Boosting blood sugars enables your muscles to more quickly convert glucose into glycogen.

Although candy has a very high glycemic index, it causes insulin to quickly spike and then fall. The result is a sugar rush and crash.

Instead, for your postworkout snack, choose foods such as wheat bread, bananas, cornflakes, instant rice, crackers, watermelon, fruit juices, and potatoes. They'll do the job, suggests Dan Benardot, R.D., Ph.D., author of *Nutrition for Serious Athletes* and a sports nutritionist and researcher in Atlanta.

And include some protein in your postworkout meal to help replenish glycogen faster, suggests Thomas Incledon, M.S., R.D., designer of the Hard-Body Diet.

High-glycemic foods are those that your body quickly converts to energy by breaking them down into sugars. Don't confuse these with sugary junk foods, though: The best high-glycemic foods are items such as pastas, some fruits and juices, cereals, and breads.

A banana would do nicely. Or grab a low-fat, low-fiber, jam-filled cereal bar at a convenience store and down it with ½ cup of fat-free milk. Or have a bagel. Because these high-glycemic foods are rapidly digested and absorbed, they quickly elevate insulin levels—a process that, strategically timed, speeds the uptake of nutrients to your muscles.

And timing is key to recharging your muscles after a workout.

Short-burst, anaerobic activity such as weight lifting is fueled almost entirely by muscle glycogen. An hour or so of lifting dramatically depletes your muscles' glycogen stores. After your workout, the enzymes that convert carbs to glycogen are in a highly excited state, geared up to begin glycogen synthesis—essentially, to refill the glass just emptied. Also, your muscles are pumped with blood and your metabolism is in overdrive, ready to deliver the goods.

"Everything is in place, raring to go," Wilson says. "If you feed those enzymes right after exercise, you accelerate glycogen synthesis."

Usually, your body needs up to 48 hours to completely recharge its glycogen stores. But eat a postworkout snack and you can cut that time in half or better, she says, giving you "a window of opportunity you don't want to miss." It's also essential that you move on to one of your regular meals within 60 to 90 minutes after this snack. That keeps the process going, says Incledon.

Don't forget the protein in the postworkout snack, though. It also seems to boost the rate of glycogen replenishment and enhances the muscle-building effects of the growth hormone you release during exercise.

In addition, your body starts assembling more protein after exercise, as muscles start repairing and rebuilding damaged fibers. That's another reason to have some protein coming in, Wilson says.

"That way, you know that there are amino acids readily available for the body to synthesize new muscle protein," says Wilson.

ENERGY FUEL
HOT CARBS

OF THE THREE MAJOR NUTRIENTS—PROTEIN, FAT, AND CARBOHYDRATES—CARBS ARE MOST EASILY CONVERTED TO GLYCOGEN, YOUR MAIN SOURCE OF MUSCLE FUEL FOR STRENGTH TRAINING. CARBS POWER WORKOUTS, PROVIDE EXTRA CALORIES FOR MUSCLE GROWTH, AND SPARE THE PROTEIN IN YOUR BODY FOR MUSCLE REPAIR AND BUILDING. CARBOHYDRATE-RICH FOODS MAKE UP THE CORE OF THE HARD-BODY EATING PLAN.

When most weight lifters hear the word *carbohydrates,* they picture a scrawny runner seated in front of a colander of spaghetti, spooning in gobs of pasta to load up for the half-marathon on Saturday.

It's less likely that they associate carbs with intense weight training sessions, major muscle growth, and fast recovery from workouts.

They should. Carbohydrates are your best source of fuel whether you're pounding up hills in a 10-K or doing hammer curls in front of a mirror, says Dan Benardot, R.D., Ph.D., a sports nutritionist and researcher in Atlanta.

In other words, carbs *are* Hard-Body food. You want to build muscle? Think carbohydrates.

"Much of the initial research on carbs and en-

WHY IT MATTERS

A Hard Body is an efficient system that uses the food it takes in and takes in no more food than it can use. Eating foods that are rich in carbohydrates is the best way to give your muscles a fast-acting supply of fuel to burn when they need it.

As your hardworking muscles fire up carbs as fuel, they burn them fast and clean, with no waste to ship off and no leftovers to store away. And since you're feeding them what they need, your muscles spend less time leaching nutrients from your body and more time doing what they're supposed to: getting bigger.

ergy involved distance runners, so there's this lingering myth among strength trainers that carbs are only for endurance athletes. Instead, bodybuilders have overemphasized protein because muscle is made of protein," he explains.

But, he says, think of the rippling muscles on a thoroughbred racehorse. Horses don't eat meat. A racehorse builds all those powerful muscles by exercising and eating oats and hay. We don't want to shovel hay onto our plates with a pitchfork, but the point is that hay is full of carbohydrates. And muscles need carbs.

You don't have to munch your lawn, talk like Mr. Ed, or "carbo-load" like a wiry marathoner, but according to Dr. Benardot, a guy who regularly lifts weights should get at least 60 percent of his calories each day from carbohydrate-rich foods—cereals, pastas, vegetables, fruits, rice, even the sugars in sports drinks.

Carbohydrate is the body's primary fuel for exercise because it's directly converted into muscle glycogen. Carbs pump up your energy levels, fuel workouts, and provide the calories needed for muscle building, which burns energy. "If you're expending lots of energy, you need to be taking in lots of energy," says Dr. Benardot. Just remember this simple formula: carbs = fuel. Here's why.

Carbs break down in the body to form glucose and glycogen, sugars that provide energy. Insulin, a hormone, enables the muscle cells to convert glucose into glycogen and store it until it is needed.

Carbs provide quick energy because they're easily digested. Mashed potatoes, breads, and candy bars—all high-carb foods—break down significantly with just saliva. To borrow the old slogan from M&M's candies, carbs melt in your mouth. By the time they get to your stomach, they're already well on the way to powering your next workout.

"Carbs really move into your bloodstream quite fast. A banana, a cracker, or fat-free milk does not stay in the stomach very long before the body starts converting it into glucose and glycogen," explains Leslie Bonci, R.D., a registered dietitian and nutrition consultant for the Pittsburgh Steelers and all athletic teams at the University of Pittsburgh.

What's required for glycogen storage is the hormone insulin. Every time you eat, the levels of insulin in your bloodstream increase. The insulin coaxes receptors in your muscle cells to open up and allow glucose to enter. Once in the cells, glucose is either metabolized quickly to supply energy or converted to glycogen by special enzymes.

"If you eat some carbs an hour or so before a workout, you'll have more glucose floating around in your bloodstream," says Bonci. "That's why a high-carb meal before lifting can give you a little added boost of energy."

Make carbohydrates the central food of each meal and snack and you'll have more energy, staying power, and intensity in your workouts. Eat carbs throughout the day to keep your glycogen stores—your energy reserves—at peak readiness.

When a basketball player sprints up the court on a fast break or a lifter hoists a hunk of iron on the weight bench, he is drawing energy primarily from muscle glycogen.

Such short-burst activities are referred to as anaerobic because they're fueled by chemical reactions occurring in the *absence* of oxygen. Aerobic exercise works just the opposite: Longer, less in-

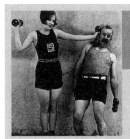

THAT'S DUMB

You may have heard that carbs make you fat. At least that was the hype—and the controversy—over the Zone Diet a couple of years ago.

But let's take a closer look.

Sure, carbs can make you fat. But so can protein and fat if you eat enough of them. To gain weight, all you have to do is eat more calories than you burn.

Now, if you're a guy who eats loads of spaghetti and pizza and does little more than watch hours of obscure sports like the Canadian national curling championships on cable TV, yes, you're probably going to get fat eating carbs.

But if you're a Hard-Body Man, you've got nothing to worry about. You eat small, frequent meals, lift weights three or four times a week, do some aerobics, and burn carbs like crazy—both when you're exercising and on your recovery days when your body is building muscle. You're getting bigger, but you're packing on muscle, not fat.

tense activities such as jogging or swimming drive oxygen *into* the muscles. The presence of oxygen in muscles enables runners to burn fat as well as muscle glycogen for energy. That's why runners are so lean.

Strength trainers, however, burn almost no fat because their lifts and sets last only a minute or so. Consequently, a Hard-Body Man really depends on his glycogen stores.

A 175-pound, physically active guy can store about 2,100 calories of glycogen in his body, with the vast majority—approximately 1,600 calories' worth—residing in his muscles. The remaining glycogen is in his liver and in his bloodstream in the form of glucose.

Once those reserves are used up, the body simply can't mobilize enough fat to keep going, and fatigue sets in.

"Your glycogen storage is really quite small. An hour or so of lifting is going to deplete it. After that, you need to refuel," says Bonci.

As we've said, your best sources of fuel are car-

bohydrate-rich foods because your body prefers to run on carbs rather than protein or fat. If you're athletic and you work out hard every day or every other day, your body will become superefficient, and carbs will flow directly into your muscles as glycogen.

"When you're exercising regularly, your muscles are in a continual state of utilizing glucose. They can always use more fuel," says Bonci.

The amount of glycogen you can store increases with training. A trained muscle holds more glycogen than an untrained muscle. As you get stronger and your muscle mass grows, you'll need to eat more carbs and calories to load those muscles with glycogen.

Muscles depleted of glycogen by exercise need time to recharge. You can speed up that process by consuming carbohydrate-rich foods immediately after lifting, says Bonci.

Your muscles need at least 24 hours—and up to 48 hours—to recharge with glycogen. They also need energy and recovery time to mobilize amino acids (contained in protein) and repair microtears from lifting.

You should eat about 200 calories of carbohydrates within 15 to 60 minutes after lifting. The sooner the better, says Bonci, and a fast-acting carb will hit the spot. Bananas, pizza, pasta, a cereal bar with some fat-free milk, or a sports drink will do for an after-workout meal. And then you can go right on to a regular Hard-Body meal within an hour or two after that.

Another way to stay charged up is to make sure that you're consuming plenty of carbs in every meal and snack, so that you're always refueling. Never let the tank get low, counsels Bonci.

"Don't shortchange your body with a lack of carbohydrates. It will catch up with you," she says. When you don't eat enough carbs, your energy levels gradually decline. You'll find yourself lifting less weight, doing fewer sets, and even having to skip workouts. You'll simply need more recovery time.

To build more muscle, you may have to increase your calorie intake. When you're eating more to gain muscle mass, carbohydrates are your best source of additional calories.

Many physically active men barely take in enough calories to support the muscles they already have, let alone grow more, says Dr. Benardot.

A clue that this is happening? You lift and lift and lift and lift, and you don't see any gains in mass. It's time to lift more carbs from your plate to your mouth.

When you don't take in enough calories and

carbs, bad things happen. As your body starts craving fuel, it siphons off protein (amino acids) in your bloodstream for energy. It may even break down your muscles to get at the protein. What could be worse? You go to the gym to build muscle, but your body has to rob your muscles in order to support your gym work. Your gains and losses equal zero.

The solution? You guessed it: Give your body the carbohydrate fuel it needs, so that the protein in your diet is available for muscle building, says Dr. Benardot.

Don't reach for that hot fudge sundae just yet, though. This "eat more carbs, eat more carbs" plea doesn't mean that you should automatically start eating more food altogether. And it doesn't mean that you should eat foods full of refined sugars, such as candies and ice cream and cakes.

If you're carrying too much flab, you may actually need to cut calories. Even then, you'll probably want to cut the calories by cutting fats and protein, not by chopping carbs.

Most of your carbohydrate intake should be in the form of complex carbohydrates, which are found in brown rice, whole grains, pastas, whole-grain breads, and vegetables. Complex carbs, with some exceptions, break down more slowly and provide a steady source of energy. Eat only a small amount of simple carbs and sugars.

Carbohydrates come in two varieties: complex and simple. Simple carbs are found in things like white table sugar, honey, the fructose in and from fruits, and highly refined white flours. Simple carbs pack lots of calories but few nutrients. That's why

FIGURE YOUR PERSONAL CARB NEEDS

Hard-Body Men need to chew on plenty of carbohydrates each day because 95 percent of their energy for weight lifting comes from muscle glycogen, which is simply stored carbs.

To figure out how many carbohydrates you need each day, you calculate from your percentage of daily calories. We're recommending that the Hard-Body Man get 60 to 65 percent of his calories from carbs.

If you know how many calories you currently eat each day, you can use the following formula to determine your approximate carbohydrate needs. As an example, we'll use a 175-pound guy who eats 3,300 calories per day because he wants to bulk up a little.

The formula?

Daily calories × recommended carbohydrate intake (60 percent) = calories from carbs per day

How does that work with our reference man?

3,300 calories × 0.60 = 1,980 calories from carbohydrates

Now, to determine how many grams of carbohydrate are needed each day, take the number of carb calories and divide by 4. That's because 4 is the number of calories in each gram of carbohydrate. So, in this example,

1,980 ÷ 4 = 495 grams per day.

nutritionists refer to candy bars and sweets as empty calories and advise us to avoid them.

Simple carbs tend to quickly raise blood sugar levels and turn on insulin. The effect, however, is short-lived, and blood sugar levels usually soon fall below where they were before they encountered that candy bar.

It's like flooring the gas pedal to take advantage of a gap in bumper-to-bumper freeway traffic. You might move up a little, but you really don't get anywhere in the long run. Soon you're back in the pack, crawling along with the traffic. You are much better off eating complex carbohydrates, also known as starches.

Complex carbs are neither simple nor empty. Unrefined or unprocessed foods containing complex carbs also contain plenty of calories, vitamins and minerals, nutrients, and fiber. And unlike simple carbohydrates, they tend to be absorbed gradually, so the flow of sugars into your bloodstream is slow and continuous. You lessen the spikes in insulin and energy.

Eating complex carbohydrates is like being plugged into a steady power source instead of being given a jolt every few hours.

You'll find complex carbs in bulky, dense, moderate-calorie foods such as cereals, pasta, vegetables, and grains. And because they don't carry as many calories per gram as fat does, it can actually be a challenge to eat enough of them during the day to support muscle building. So the good news is that you won't starve on the Hard-Body Plan. You'll eat well and you'll eat plenty. You'll just adjust your eating toward more complex-carb foods.

To meet your body's needs, eat carbohydrate-rich foods at every feeding, says Bonci. Eat cereal

CARBOHYDRATE CONTENT OF COMMON FOODS

	Size	Carbs (g)	Calories	Protein (g)	Fat (g)
Apple	3¼-in. diameter	32	125	0	1
Bagel, plain mini	3½-in. diameter	38	195	7	1
Banana	1 medium	28	109	1	1
Chef Boyardee Beef Ravioli	1 cup	37	229	8	5
Chili beans in sauce	½ cup	21	117	7	0.4
Corn on the cob	5-in. piece	19	83	3	1
Cranberry sauce	½ cup	54	209	1	0.2
Fig Newtons, fat-free	4 pieces	44	180	2	0
Gatorade	8 oz	14	50	0	0
Hummus with pita bread	¼ cup hummus, 1 piece pita	42	269	10	7
Hunt's Snack Pack Chocolate Pudding	1 pudding cup	22	140	2	5
Kellogg's Corn Flakes	1 cup	24	102	2	0
KFC extra-crispy thigh	1 piece	18	370	19	25
Kidney beans, canned	1 cup	40	218	13	1
Lean Cuisine French bread sausage pizza	1 pizza	41	420	19	4
Minute Instant Brown Whole Grain rice	⅔ cup cooked	34	170	4	1.5
Old El Paso refried beans	½ cup	17	100	6	0.5
Peanut butter and jelly sandwich on whole wheat	1 sandwich	43	370	13	16
Pizza Hut hand-tossed cheese pizza	2 pieces	86	618	28	18
Potato, boiled	2½-in. diameter	27	118	2	0
PowerBar, apple-cinnamon	1 bar	45	230	10	2.5
Quaker Maple and Brown Sugar Instant Oatmeal	1 packet	33	160	4	2
Subway 6-in. turkey sub on wheat bread	1 sub	45	282	17	4
Taco Bell bean burrito with red sauce	1 burrito	54	370	13	12
Thin spaghetti with Ragu Chunky Gardenstyle tomato, garlic, and onion sauce	2 oz pasta (uncooked weight), ½ cup sauce	60	320	9	4.5
Twinkie	1 piece	27	157	1	5
Whole-wheat bread	1 slice	13	69	3	1

for breakfast; fruits and crackers for munchies; rice, pasta, or potatoes for dinner; and always lots of vegetables. You can't go wrong with vegetables because nearly every food in a vegetarian diet contains carbohydrates.

And be sure to eat a wide variety of carbs each day. Different carb-heavy foods interact with your blood sugar in different ways. The measurement of this interaction is called a food's glycemic index. This isn't always easy to determine: A baked potato has a high glycemic index, meaning that it quickly sends your blood glucose soaring, but an apple has a low glycemic index. A single food type can also behave differently depending on how it has been processed.

For your postworkout snack, a high-glycemic food is fine. Simple carbohydrates are often high-glycemic, so a sugary treat is okay here—but we're not talking candy bars. A jam-filled cereal bar is fine, though, as long as it is paired with a bit of protein, such as that found in a half-cup of fat-free milk. The rest of the time, eat plenty of carbohydrates from many sources, along with a bit of protein to slow their digestion, to mix up the glycemic indexes and thus keep your blood sugar more stable.

Bonci says that if you're a guy who likes precision and will read food labels, you should try to eat 3 grams of carbohydrate per pound of body weight every day. By this formula, a 175-pound guy should be eating in the neighborhood of 525 grams of carbs daily.

Because most athletes she counsels are not willing to count grams of anything, Bonci recommends that they cover at least two-thirds of their lunch or dinner plates with complex-carb-rich foods. Now there's a plan that's easy to follow. Another simple strategy is to build every meal around a carbohydrate rather than a meat.

"You can also do simple things like always eating bread with a meal or a snack," she says. "Pizza works very well for this. So do tortillas, pita, and crackers."

If you're as human as most of us, of course you're going to have a candy bar once in a while. And that's okay, as long as your definition of *once in a while* isn't "daily." Candy, jams, juices, fruits, and syrups should make up a small (read that as "SMALL!") part of your carb intake. We all know that we're supposed to be eating several servings of fruit each day, but, while training, that just isn't in the cards. You'll have *some* fruit, as you'll see in the meal plans in part 4.

The meal plans in this book take much of the guesswork out of eating. Follow the Hard-Body guidelines and meal suggestions and you'll get all the carbs you need.

No matter how you operate—counting grams, following recipes, or just using common sense—remember that a Hard-Body Man cannot eat the average Joe's high-fat, nutrient-poor diet.

Hard-Body Man really does eat like a racehorse and like those wiry distance runners. He just looks better. Lots better.

GROWTH FUEL
THE TRUTH ABOUT PROTEIN

THE BODY USES PROTEIN TO REPAIR AND GROW MUSCLE. ALTHOUGH PROTEIN IS THE KEY MUSCLE-BUILDING NUTRIENT, THERE IS NO BENEFIT—AND THERE ARE SEVERAL DRAWBACKS—TO INGESTING TOO MUCH. MOST MEN SIMPLY DON'T NEED PROTEIN SUPPLEMENTS OR A HIGH-PROTEIN DIET. CONSUMING A NORMAL, VARIED DIET OF PLANT AND ANIMAL PROTEIN WILL DO THE JOB.

By the 6th century A.D., Olympic athletes began hiring coaches to teach them how to eat and train. Milo of Kroton, a champion wrestler from southern Italy, followed a robust meat diet that was advocated by the leading nutritional authorities of the day.

According to legend, Milo would devour 30 pounds of beef and bread at one sitting and then wash it down with 2 gallons of wine. For training and sheer spectacle, he routinely carried a cow across the length of the Olympic stadium.

His carnivorous diet and choice of exercise equipment spoke a clear message: Strong guys get strong by eating meat.

Zip forward to today and you'll hear brawny guys down at the weight room extolling the potency of skinless chicken breasts, soy burgers, and amino acid supplements.

WHY IT MATTERS

As you settle into a weight lifting routine, the workouts create tiny tears in your muscles that your body repairs with protein to make the muscles bigger and stronger. But you don't want to overload your body with protein any more than you'd glob handfuls of mortar into the spaces between bricks in a wall. It's wasteful and messy: The excess protein is either excreted or tucked into unnecessary storage.

Get just the amount of protein that your muscles need from a spectrum of animal and plant foods, from lean chicken breasts and 1% milk to tofu and beans.

It might seem a stretch from Milo to these guys, but their message is the same. Be it flank steaks or hummus, strong guys eat lots of protein.

Well . . . maybe.

Protein is absolutely essential to producing bigger muscle. It's the one nutrient directly channeled to the repair and growth of muscle fibers. Men who pump iron need to eat more protein than sedentary, lie-around-the-house, watch-ESPN-all-day wannabe weight lifters do.

But that doesn't mean that you need to eat tons of the stuff. The *Men's Health* Hard-Body eating plan recommends that you get about 15 percent of your daily calories from protein-rich foods such as fish, poultry, red meat, tofu, beans, and dairy products.

If you're the size of our 175-pound, 5-foot-10-inch reference man, you'll need to scarf about 143 grams of protein a day. That's roughly the equivalent of two chicken breasts, a cup of low-fat cottage cheese, and ½ cup of black beans—and it's much easier to swallow than Milo's 30-pound steak sandwiches.

That may not seem like enough, but it's plenty if you channel every bit of this protein into muscle building, says Thomas Incledon, M.S., R.D., the sports nutritionist who created the Hard-Body Diet.

"What determines your protein needs is how much you exercise. You only want enough protein to synthesize more muscle," Incledon says. "There is a limit to how much protein your body can use. More isn't necessarily better."

If you're a guy who likes burritos from quick-serve gas stations and who eats dinner at drive-thru burger joints with talking signs, you're probably already overloading on protein.

If that sounds like you, then, as you begin training, you may need to cut protein consumption, or at least change what you're eating to make sure that your protein isn't laden with wads of fat and cholesterol.

We know, we know: High-protein diets are the craze. They are touted as beneficial for maintaining optimum insulin levels. The Hard-Body Plan does that without unnecessary food restrictions and boring meals. Frankly, the foods in the Hard-Body Plan are much tastier. Yes, you can have all the hamburger you want on one of the high-protein fad diets. But you can't have the bun. You can't have the mustard. You can't have the pickle. Do you really want just lots and lots of hamburger, day in and day out?

Eating lots of protein by itself will not help you grow muscle or speed muscle building. You can't have steak and eggs for breakfast and extra-cheese pizza slices on the ride home from work and expect to develop terrific triceps. That takes intensive strength training and probably less protein than you're currently eating.

Growing muscle is a recurring process of damage and repair, damage and repair. Every time you lift weights, you stress muscle fibers and create tiny tears in them. That's the source of the soreness you feel the next day.

Your body, using protein as a raw material, rebuilds the fibers and, as a form of protection, coaxes them to grow. Protein is your repair and construction kit.

The biochemistry of how protein works in the body is complicated, but here's the simple version. Protein consists of different types of amino acids, which are strands of oxygen, carbon, hydrogen, and nitrogen atoms wound together in various combinations.

When you eat dietary protein—the type found

THAT'S DUMB

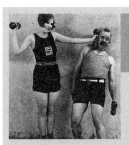

A Denver Broncos football lineman was downing 45 chicken breasts a day. That is serious protein loading and, as we now know, protein loading hurts rather than helps.

"Can you imagine anyone eating 45 chicken breasts?" asks Jackie Berning, R.D., Ph.D., who serves as a consulting sports nutritionist for the Denver Broncos.

The lineman was a huge guy, but when he came to Dr. Berning seeking her advice, he was essentially a 280-pound weakling. He hardly had enough energy to make it through his workouts and weight training sessions.

Dr. Berning told him that he was eating too much chicken—way too much chicken.

"He wasn't getting enough carbohydrates, and his body was absolutely overloaded with protein. It had no choice but to use protein as fuel," she explains.

The take-home lesson: Protein is a poor fuel.

in food—the body breaks it down into its individual amino acids. It then rearranges those acids in different combinations to create new proteins for maintaining tissues. Besides building muscle, protein also helps you grow hair, manufacture hormones and red blood cells, transport nutrients through your body, and support your immune system.

The Hard-Body Man should eat about double the protein per day that the Recommended Dietary Allowance (RDA) calls for. But cool it there: Eating protein beyond your needs will actually *hinder* muscle building by lowering your energy reserves.

You don't need to buy enough prime rib each week to make your butcher's Cadillac payment. If you've been getting that impression from amateur weight-room nutritionists, understand that these guys are misinterpreting the biology of protein and muscle building.

Once your muscles incorporate the protein required for repair and growth, the body diverts any excess to other pathways. Protein gets burned as energy, converted into carbohydrate, packed away as fat, or flushed from the body via urine. Since none of these other pathways builds muscle, excess protein is really wasted protein, Incledon says.

What's actually more important than protein intake is total calorie intake. To build hard muscle, you need to work out hard and consistently. That requires lots of energy, and your best source of energy is carbohydrates, not protein, says Incledon.

Protein isn't a very efficient fuel. Before it can power your workouts, you have to convert it to carbohydrate and then to glycogen (muscle fuel) in the muscle. Or it can be turned into fat and stored for later use. Did you hear that? *Turned into fat!* That's not the goal here.

If you eat enough carbs, your body will rarely have to call upon its pools of protein to fuel your workouts. Your protein will be spared and used for muscle growth and repair.

Consider this: After a hard workout, your muscles may need nearly 2 days to completely recharge with glycogen—and that's after you've given them complete rest and eaten a high-carbohydrate diet. If you're working out intensely day after day and eating a high-protein, low-carbohydrate diet, your glycogen stores will gradually diminish, like an aging battery losing its charge, says Jackie Berning, R.D., Ph.D., a sports nutritionist in Colorado Springs, Colorado.

You'll have less energy to lift and you'll fatigue faster in your workout. You'll be able to do fewer repetitions, you'll have to lighten your weight loads, and you'll require more time to recover. Ultimately, you'll grow less muscle.

And you may actually hurt yourself. Eating too much protein over an extended time may be tough on your kidneys. That's because the kidneys process the waste left by protein metabolism, and too much protein prevents them from getting rid of these wastes properly, says Susan Kleiner, R.D., Ph.D., a sports nutrition researcher, in her book *Power Eating*.

Nutrients—including protein—are better absorbed through food than any type of supplement.

CALCULATE *YOUR* PROTEIN REQUIREMENTS

How much protein should you be eating each day?

The RDA (Recommended Dietary Allowance) for protein is 0.8 gram per kilogram of body weight, but that's for a sedentary, lie-around-the-house type of guy. A Hard-Body Man definitely needs more.

Sports nutritionists, coaches, and athletes disagree on exactly how much daily protein is enough for strength training, but it's likely to fall somewhere between 1.4 and 1.8 grams per kilogram of body weight, according to an often-quoted 1995 study done by Hard-Body Plan architect Peter Lemon, Ph.D. He did the work at the Applied Physiology Research Lab at Kent State University in Ohio.

You can determine your approximate protein requirements with the following formula. Divide your body weight by 2.2 (the number of pounds in a kilogram) and then multiply by the number of suggested grams of protein.

If you're 175 pounds, it would go like this:

175 pounds ÷ 2.2 pounds per kilogram = 79.5 kilograms

Low end of protein needs: 79.5 kg × 1.4 g/kg = 111.3 g

High end of protein needs: 79.5 kg × 1.8 g/kg = 143.1 g

You don't have to do this calculation, though. We've worked it all out for you in the "Daily Quotas" chart on page 326.

Maybe at this point you're staring at that $60 gallon of "Instant Biceps in 10 Days!" protein supplement you just received from an advertiser in one of the muscle magazines. Don't pour the stuff down the sink just yet. You can still use it.

A supplement is a convenient way to ensure that you're taking in enough protein each day. Use the supplement on days when all you've found to munch is rabbit food and the nearest steakhouse is just too far away (or if you're a vegetarian and eat *only* rabbit food).

Normally, though, you'll get all your protein from the food you eat. Certainly, you will when you follow the Hard-Body Plan. We like to eat and we think you do too. So we're steering you toward whole foods, not dry, nasty powders. Drink milk, graze the veggie trays at office parties and buffets, and grill chicken and an occasional steak in the backyard. That's the *Men's Health* protein secret.

Research shows that protein is best assimilated by the body when it is consumed in a diet of whole foods rather than with a diet of hybrid food supplements like designer powders and gels. It seems that whole foods contain substances that help your body absorb nutrients. Scientists call them food factors. These food factors aren't necessarily found in nutritional protein supplements.

Although many manufacturers of protein powders and amino acid supplements say that their products are more rapidly absorbed than the protein in food, research does not back up these claims. Nor is there any evidence that rapid absorption of protein and amino acids would have any effect on muscle building, Dr. Berning explains.

A lot of weight lifters drink protein shakes right after exercise. Don't. Instead, consider guzzling a sports drink that contains a ratio of carbohydrates to protein that falls somewhere between 2:1 and 4:1 carbs to protein, says Incledon. That will help you recover and build muscle. We tell you why in Thirst Quenchers beginning on page 295.

Your body needs several hours to synthesize muscle proteins after intense exercise. As long as you're eating some protein-rich foods daily, you'll have plenty of amino acids in your system readily available for muscle repairs after workouts, says Dr. Berning. The Hard-Body Plan gives you the optimum amount of protein at all times throughout your workout day and recovery periods.

Besides being largely unnecessary, protein supplements and many amino acid supplements also tend to be expensive. You'd be just as well-off— and quite a few bucks richer—if you ate a 50-cent can of tuna.

Remember: Good meals and hard training are what you need to build muscle, not protein supplements or amino acid pills and potions, Dr. Berning says. No matter what the power boys are telling you, if they're true muscleheads, they spend a lot of time in the gym pumping iron. And *that's* how they got the massive muscles.

Getting your protein from an animal source ensures that you take in all the essential amino acids—building blocks—you need for growing muscle. If you're a strict vegetarian, you'll need to eat a combination of several foods or take a protein supplement.

Your body cannot manufacture amino acids on its own, so it must get them through food. Food contains two types of protein: complete and incomplete.

Complete protein, or animal protein, contains all the essential amino acids in sufficient quanti-

PROTEIN: HOW SOME COMMON FOODS STACK UP

	Size	Protein (g)	Calories	Carbs (g)	Fat (g)
All-Bran cereal	1 cup	8	160	46	2
Black beans, cooked	½ cup	8	114	20	0
Cheddar cheese	1 oz	7	113	0	9
Chicken breast, roasted, skinless	6 oz	53	284	0	6
Chickpeas	1 cup	14	269	45	4
Clams, steamed	10 clams	24	141	5	2
Cottage cheese, small-curd, 1% fat	1 cup	28	164	6	2
Egg, hard-cooked	1 egg	6	77	1	5
Fat-free milk	1 cup	8	85	12	0
Flounder, baked	4 oz	27	132	0	2
Hamburger patty, extra-lean	4 oz	32	299	0	18
Morningstar Farms spicy black bean burger	1 burger	11	113	15	1
Peanut butter and jelly sandwich on whole wheat	1 sandwich	13	370	43	16
Pumpkin kernels	1 oz	7	151	5	13
Shrimp, boiled	16 shrimp	18	87	0	1
Sirloin steak, lean	4 oz	34	228	0	9
Starkist tuna in springwater	6-oz can	36	180	0	3
Sunflower seeds	¼ cup	8	205	7	18
Swanson Premium Chunk chicken breast in water	1 can	27.5	150	2.5	2.5
Tofu, regular	½ cup	8	76	2	5
Turkey breast fat-free lunchmeat	2 pieces	8	44	2	0
Ultra Slim Fast Chocolate Royale	1 ready-to-drink can	10	220	38	3
Venison, roasted	4 oz	34	179	0	4
Wheat germ, toasted	½ cup	16.5	216	28	6

ties. Consider it one-stop eating for protein. If you eat eggs, meat, cheese, fish, or milk or other dairy products, your protein needs are easily met.

Plant proteins—beans, pastas, lentils, and nuts—are known as incomplete proteins. No single food from this group contains adequate quantities of all the amino acids required for metabolism and muscle building.

If you are a vegan (pronounced VEE-gun)—someone who doesn't consume any type of animal product, including milk and eggs—you'll have to eat a calculated combination of plant foods to get all your amino acids. But if you're a guy whose vegetarian diet excludes only meat, you can get what you need by eating eggs, fish, and cheese and other dairy products along with your plant proteins. We cover all this in easy-to-follow detail in Beef Up without Meat on page 317.

If you eat low-fat dairy products, lean cuts of meat, and plenty of plant protein, you'll get all the protein you need and still keep down the fat and cholesterol content—and that's the goal.

A diet high in animal protein is probably a diet high in fat and cholesterol, which is not good. It probably doesn't have much fiber, either, and fiber is important for good digestion and elimination.

It's not that meat is necessarily bad for you. You just need to be selective about what cuts you eat and how it's prepared. Choice, lean cuts of beef, lamb, and pork are good low-fat sources of protein.

Skinless chicken breast is a favorite of body-builders.

You can also cut down on the grease content of your meat by cooking it properly. Grill or broil the critter to allow some of the fat to melt and drip away, says Incledon.

Another way to balance the bad effects of animal protein is to eat more meatless meals. If you like dairy products, you can get high-quality protein from reduced-fat cheese, low-fat yogurt, and fat-free milk, says Incledon. Eggs are fine if eaten in moderation. Tofu, beans, peas, lentils, and vegetables contain large amounts of protein. Eating more plant protein is also easier on your wallet.

"Whether you're a vegetarian or a meat eater, your best strategy is to eat a wide variety of foods," Incledon says. "Not only will that help with muscle building; it will also raise your overall nutritional status."

That's a cool thing, nutritional status. If you have high nutritional status, lowly carrots will stand up and bow down to you as you pass the produce bins.

Chubster Fuel
Fat to Burn

KEEP YOUR FAT INTAKE LOW, BUT DON'T BE FAT-PHOBIC. TREAT IT LIKE ANY OTHER IMPORTANT NUTRIENT. IN MODERATION, FAT IS A GOOD SOURCE OF CALORIES, AN AID TO VITAMIN ABSORPTION, AND A NUTRITIONAL BUILDING BLOCK FOR GROWING MUSCLES. THE MAJORITY OF YOUR FATS SHOULD COME FROM PLANT SOURCES RATHER THAN MEATS.

If you were a Hard-Body guy 400 years ago in Nebraska, part of your job would have been finding ways to turn a 2,000-pound buffalo into a meal. Needless to say, the animals weren't too cooperative about the idea, so you'd have to be resourceful to bag one.

Killing a buffalo fed your band for a while, but what really supersized your meal was an opportunity for serious slaughter: an isolated herd grazing in a narrow draw that funneled downhill and emptied over a steep cliff. Then, with half your hungry tribe screaming and waving hides on each side, you chased the beasts off the edge, where they piled up like so many steaks in a freezer.

For days after, everyone butchered and ate like gluttons, devouring all the fresh meat and fat they could stomach and pounding the rest into pem-

WHY IT MATTERS

As a Hard-Body Man, you'll treat dietary fat like a good friend who leads you into trouble too easily. You'll allow it into your life, but only in measured doses and certain situations.

While it's true that too much fat can give you just the kind of soft physique that you're bench-pressing yourself away from, when you get plenty of exercise and keep the fat in your diet moderate and of the right sort, you won't have to worry about it heading to your belly.

It will, however, help support your body's vital functions and stock it with a slow-acting supply of calories to help keep you going.

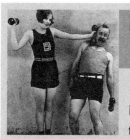

THAT'S DUMB

You may have heard about high-fat diets and fat supplements that supposedly increase your body's ability to burn fat as fuel. There is a certain amount of truth in those claims for runners, but for a strength trainer it's a case of the cure being worse than the disease.

You'd best stay clear of high-fat diets, for this reason: When you eat a high-fat diet, you decrease both your carb intake and the amount of glycogen you store in your muscles. When your body gets low on glycogen, it will turn to fat for energy, but that does not make fat a good fuel for you. Fat cannot power high-intensity training such as weight lifting.

Studies show that people exercising vigorously on a high-fat diet soon run out of steam. They simply can't mobilize enough fat to continue exercising when glycogen stores get low.

mican, a mixture of berries, meat, and fat. When winter came and buffalo were scarce, you lived off the pemmican and the body fat you accumulated during the summer hunt.

Fat was fuel. Fat was life itself for a Plains native in the 1600s.

Much has changed. Few of us ever experience a feast-or-famine situation, some supermarkets carry farm-raised bison, the only guys running toward cliffs are strapped to hang gliders, and fat is now the great big bogeyman of nutrition. Listening to the alarmist hype—"Don't eat fat. Eat low-fat. Buy no-fat. Fat begets fat."—you'd think that fat is poison rather than one of the body's key nutrients.

Fat is crucial to metabolism, muscle building, and the production of enzymes and hormones. You can't have a healthy Hard Body without literally chewing the fat. The trick is to match your fat intake to your body's needs.

Our Native American friend did. He walked hundreds of miles a year, lived outdoors, and took down beasts as a big as your SUV using only a stick. His lifestyle required an enormous amount of calories. Chowing down on fat made perfect sense.

"Fat can still be your friend. It doesn't have to be your nutritional enemy," says Ann Grandjean, Ed.D., director of a nutrition center in Omaha, Nebraska. "Most men who are athletic and live an active life probably have nothing at all to fear from fat."

The problem arises if you are genetically predisposed to heart disease, Dr. Grandjean says. If you have high cholesterol, if your father had a heart attack at 42, and if half of your aunts and uncles have had bypasses, you should be vigilant about your fat intake no matter how much you exercise.

The rest of us who exercise and are health-conscious are probably doing pretty well fatwise, Dr. Grandjean says. It's even possible that we've taken the no-fat message to the extreme and don't consume enough of it.

"You need to look at fat as you would any other nutrient. Too little fat isn't good, and too much isn't either," she says.

Eating less than 20 percent of your daily calories in fat can tamper with your efforts to build muscle.

Fat is everywhere in our bodies. It fills the outer membrane of each cell. It dissolves, transports, and aids in the absorption of vitamins D, K, E, and A. It supplies the body with essential fatty acids needed for the growth and reproduction of tissues, including muscle. Fat cushions our inner organs and acts as a storehouse of energy.

We obtain fat from both animal and plant sources. Saturated fats, which are solid at room temperature, come from animal products such as meats, butter, cheese, and egg yolks, along with plant sources such as coconut and palm oil. Unsaturated fats (liquid at room temperature) are found in vegetable oils and some plants, nuts, and seeds.

The American Heart Association recommends that you eat 30 percent or fewer of your daily calories in fat, mostly in the form of two types of unsaturated fats: polyunsaturated and monounsaturated. The recommendations are for average guys, but as you've heard us say before, a Hard-Body guy isn't average.

You should shoot for 20 to 25 percent of your daily calories in fat. Keep it closer to 20 percent if you're fighting flab, but don't go overboard in an attempt to look more ripped, says Claudia Wilson, R.D., a sports nutritionist in Salt Lake City.

Extremely low fat diets deny you necessary calories, are low in nutrients, may lessen the effectiveness of workouts, and can even harm your immune system. Also, they're hard to maintain, says Dr. Grandjean.

Unless you're a bodybuilder longing to have people gawk at every vein and fiber in your musculature, there's simply no point to it. Stick to our recommendations and your muscles will be plenty well-defined and impressive, guaranteed to turn admiring heads on the beach next summer.

Keeping your fat intake around 20 to 25 percent also leaves room for the carbs you have to eat to fuel exercise and muscle building, Wilson says. Although fat can be used as a fuel (most of us pack enough body fat to fuel a 500- to 1,000-mile walk), it runs a poor second to carbs when it comes to weight lifting.

Strength trainers burn almost entirely muscle glycogen during workouts. To burn fat, you must either diet or do low-intensity exercise such as walking or jogging. That's why fat was a good fuel for a Hard-Body guy wandering the Great Plains, but not for you, a guy who drives to work every day and tosses around weights four times a week.

Except for the meals or snacks surrounding workouts, it's a good idea to include a bit of fat in every meal. Fat makes food taste good and slows digestion. You'll feel fuller longer and be less likely to overeat between meals.

Strangely enough, fat may help you eat less and get leaner.

Unlike carbohydrates, fats empty more gradually from the digestive tract. Including fat in a meal increases its *satiety value*, a measure of fullness and satisfaction.

Remember on your Caribbean cruise when you ate two lobsters dipped in melted butter (two because your girlfriend thought her steamed crustacean still looked too alive)? Afterward, you pushed back from the table and realized that you were stuffed. And you stayed stuffed for hours.

It wasn't the volume that you ate and drank but rather the fat in the meal that made the lobster seem to hang in your belly for hours and hours. You were satiated.

Now, let's say that every morning you eat a plain bagel (300 calories) for breakfast. (Actually, the Hard-Body Plan calls for 400 calories for the typical guy.) The bagel, being almost entirely carbohydrates, takes just 2 hours to break down and move into your bloodstream. That's what makes bagels great energy food. The problem is that you barely get to work before you're hungry again.

The alternative is to eat only half of the bagel, but this time spread on some cream cheese. The fatty cream cheese slows digestion and holds off hunger for 3 to 4 hours.

"By adding a little fat, you eat less and still maintain the same 300-calorie count," Wilson explains.

Fat also has psychological value because it adds texture and makes food taste good. Perhaps you've tried some no-fat cookies and potato chips and found them as pleasurable as munching on bits of plywood. Maybe you tried to compensate by eating several more, thinking that it was okay because, after all, they're fat-free.

Watch out, Wilson warns. Many manufacturers try to offset the lack of taste by dumping in loads of sugars. Hence, a low-fat food may not necessarily be a low-calorie food.

"In this case, it's better to eat two full-fat cookies rather than six or seven no-fat cookies," she says. "You'll be more satisfied and, in total, take in less calories."

If you're eating an extremely low fat diet (less than 20 percent of your daily calories from fat) and you are unable to add muscle, eating more fat can supply the extra calories you need to bulk up and support muscle building.

Fat, of course, is feared for its capacity to make you flabby. That's because it packs a potent caloric punch. It has more than twice as much energy per gram (9 calories) as does carbohydrate (4 calories).

For a thin guy looking to bulk up or a football lineman trying to more closely resemble a large building, eating more fat can be a good thing, Dr. Grandjean says.

Elite athletes who burn calories like a furnace frequently eat diets containing as much as 35 percent fat.

CALCULATING HOW MUCH FAT TO CONSUME

If you like to be precise and don't mind counting calories and grams, here's a formula to determine approximately how much fat you should be eating each day, according to sports nutritionist Susan Kleiner, R.D., Ph.D., in her book *Power Eating*. First, you'll have to determine roughly how many calories you eat each day. A good way to get an accurate count is to tally up your intake for several days in a row and then divide by the number of days to get your daily average.

Let's say that you're eating an average of 3,300 calories each day and want to hit a target of 20 percent of calories from fat. Use the following formulas:

Daily calories × recommended fat intake (20 percent) = calories from fat per day

3,300 × 0.20 = 660

Calories from fat per day ÷ number of calories in a gram of fat = grams of fat per day

660 ÷ 9 = about 73 grams per day

"Nutritionists frequently say that dietary fat is too easily packed away as body fat. That's true for someone who is overweight, not exercising, and eating excess calories," Dr. Grandjean says. "But it isn't as accurate for people who are active and working out regularly. They may need more calories from fat." Maybe you are finding it impossible to consume enough carbs and protein to support muscle building. Maybe you've lifted and lifted for months but haven't gotten bigger. A little fat might fix you right up.

But don't take that as a license to start eating containers of ice cream, whole milk, and fast food, Wilson says.

Saturated fats in animal products contain high amounts of cholesterol and can cause plaque buildup in your arteries. That's the stuff that heart disease is made of. Eat saturated fats sparingly, and opt instead for unsaturated fats from plant foods such as olive oil and peanut butter. Also, avoid hydrogenated fats whenever you can.

Even if you can afford extra calories in your diet from fat, you still need to be choosy about which kind of fat to eat, Wilson says. A good rule of thumb is to get most of your fat calories from polyunsaturated and monounsaturated fats.

If you like to eat meat, though, go ahead and have a steak or a chop. Meat eaten in moderation is good muscle food. Simply look for leaner cuts, slice away the visible fat, and cook your meat on a grill to let some of the imbedded fat drip away.

Grilling, along with baking, broiling, and steaming, is a lower-fat way to prepare not only meat but also other foods. Frying is the opposite extreme. Fry as little as possible, but when you do,

use olive or canola oil: Both are rich sources of monounsaturated fat.

Pick or prepare foods that have no more than 3 grams of fat per 100 calories, and keep a close eye out for hydrogenated oils on labels. Manufacturers may put the fats in their food products through a process called hydrogenation, which makes the food creamier and gives it a more pleasing texture. The hydrogenation process, however, makes the food unhealthier for several reasons. First, it shifts the fat from polyunsaturated (good) toward a more saturated form (bad). Second, it creates trans fatty acids, which tend to raise the harmful type of cholesterol in your blood and lower the beneficial kind. So try to eat a minimum of processed foods containing hydrogenated oils.

If you're a guy who's resourceful in the kitchen, you can take steps while cooking to lower the fat content of your meals. You can use margarine instead of butter, fat-free yogurt instead of sour cream, and egg whites instead of whole eggs.

To minimize hydrogenated oils when buying margarine, pick one that has liquid vegetable oil, such as canola, olive, or safflower, as the first ingredient and that contains no more than about 2 grams of saturated fat per tablespoon.

Many men find that their weak spot centers around cheese. Learning to like low-fat cheese is mostly a matter of retraining your palate, Wilson says. If you've made the transition to fat-free milk, you'll remember those days when fat-free milk seemed watery and tasteless. But once you made the move from whole milk to 2% and eventually to fat-free milk, you found that fat-free milk really does taste like milk.

"One strategy is to eat lowered-fat cheese with strong flavors, like sharp Cheddar, Parmesan, and feta," Wilson says. "Let flavor overcome the lack of fat."

The Veggie brand makes soy-based cheeses that are very close in flavor and texture to tradi-

FAT CONTENT OF SELECTED FOODS

	Size	Fat (g)	Saturated Fat (g)	Calories	% Calories from Fat	Carbs (g)	Protein (g)
Ben and Jerry's Chocolate Chip Cookie Dough ice cream	½ cup	16	10	300	48	34	5
Brazil nuts	6 to 8 nuts	19	4.6	186	92	3.6	4
Campbell's Chunky New England Clam Chowder	1 cup	15	5	240	56	21	7
Dinty Moore Beef Stew	1 cup	8	3.5	180	40	18	10
Doritos Nacho Cheesier	11 chips	7	1	140	45	17	2
Dunkin' Donuts BlueberryCake Donut	1 doughnut	16	3.5	290	50	35	3
Dunkin' Donuts Coffee Coolatta with Cream	16 oz	22	14	410	48	51	3
Jif Extra Crunchy peanut butter	2 Tbsp	16	3	190	76	7	8
Kraft Monterey Jack Cheese with jalapeño peppers	1 oz	9	6	110	74	0	7
Little Debbie Nutty Bars	2 bars	18	3	310	52	32	5
McDonald's Quarter Pounder with cheese and large fries	1 burger	52	17	980	48	95	34
Planters cocktail peanuts	1 oz	14	2	170	74	6	7

tional cheeses, and much, much lower in fat, notes Thomas Incledon, M.S., R.D., designer of the Hard-Body eating plan.

Sometimes, the difference in taste and texture is unacceptable. If you can't imagine eating a bagel without butter, then go ahead and use a dab, but use fat-free milk rather than cream in your coffee.

If diet salad dressing tastes awful to you, then use the real thing, but eat your dinner roll plain.

"Food should be fun to eat. Sometimes you need to just enjoy eating and not worry about every fat gram," Wilson says. "You can do that by making choices: full-fat here, low-fat there. As long as your overall diet is balanced, it's okay."

WATER, SPORTS DRINKS, AND OTHER COOL REPASTS
THIRST QUENCHERS

DRINKING LOTS OF WATERY DRINKS IS ESSENTIAL TO SPORTS
NUTRITION. A HARD-BODY MAN CANNOT TRAIN AT HIS BEST
UNLESS HE PUMPS UP HIS BODY, ESPECIALLY HIS MUSCLES,
WITH FLUID. FOR EVERYDAY ACTIVITIES, DRINK LARGE AMOUNTS
OF WATER AND OTHER SUITABLE BEVERAGES. DURING EXERCISE
AND BEFORE AND AFTER, CONSUME SPORTS DRINKS, WHICH
AID REHYDRATION, FLOOD YOUR BLOODSTREAM WITH
CARBOHYDRATES, AND SHORTEN RECOVERY TIMES. UNLESS YOU
ARE TRYING TO LOSE WEIGHT: THEN STICK TO WATER.

Maybe you witnessed something like this in 1973, or even years later when high school coaches were supposed to be more enlightened.

It's late August, 93°F, an hour into the afternoon session of preseason football camp. You slam your shoulder guard into the blocking sled ridden by the defensive coach, a hefty guy nicknamed Bucky. He screams: "You call that a hit, boy? Do it again. Again! Move this sled!" Among his many wisdoms, the coach has a hydration theory, one he

picked up from his drill sergeant back in boot camp long ago: In hot weather, once a man starts drinking, he won't be able to stop. Thirst toughens the troops.

Bucky wants you to be tough too. So he's put the water keg off-limits. No drinking until the end of practice. And there it sits: over on the bench, guarded by the wimpy manager. Water beads on its insulated surfaces; the silver cup dangles empty on its string.

Jimmy DeAngelo, a lineman, has been staring at that keg for a long time. Finally, he rips off his helmet, stumbles to the sidelines, and drinks and drinks—not from the forbidden keg but from a mud puddle along the track. "Hey, boy!" Bucky yells. "Just what in tarnation are you doing?"

Okay. So it didn't happen. But it'd make a good movie, huh? And it gets us to the point: No matter what archaic belief systems you've been asked to swallow, you do need to gulp down fluids if you want your workouts to pay off. Nobody should avoid fluids while exercising. Hydration is essential to peak performance. You need good hydration to:

- store the muscle fuel glycogen
- turn protein into new muscle
- and cool the body during exercise.

Whether he's working out or recovering on rest days, a Hard-Body guy should always be well-hydrated, drinking from the time he gets up in the morning until he goes to bed at night.

Muscle is three-quarters water. Loss of fluid significantly affects athletic performance. When you're dehydrated, you'll lift less, fatigue more quickly, and take longer to recover.

When you consider that up to 65 percent of a man's weight is water, it's no surprise that water is one of your body's primary nutrients.

Water pumps up blood volume and transports nutrients and oxygen. It fills the spaces between cells and acts as a medium for biochemical reactions. It contains electrolytes, the dissolved chemicals that carry electrical messages between nerves and muscles. It lubricates joints.

Unless muscle stays well-hydrated, it shrinks in size like a dried-up sponge. Nerve signals scramble, nutrients reach their destinations more slowly, muscle contractions weaken, and athletic performance declines dramatically, says Julie Burns, R.D., a registered dietitian and nutrition consultant in Western Springs, Illinois. Her professional clients include the Chicago Bears, the Chicago Blackhawks, and the Chicago Bulls. Being well-hydrated can make the difference between good and bad workouts, Burns says. Some studies show that just a 1- or 2-percent drop in body weight due to dehydration can have a significant negative effect on athletic performance.

"The number one reason for early fatigue is dehydration, not a lack of fuel," Burns says. "Just drinking lots of fluids is a simple way to keep a muscle working at its peak."

Water is also critical to glycogen storage and to the process of replenishing spent glycogen stores. For every one part of glycogen tucked away, the muscle requires three or four parts water, says Susan Kleiner, R.D., Ph.D., a sports nutrition author and owner of High Performance Nutrition in Mercer Island, Washington.

"Unless you're well-hydrated, you won't recover quickly from your workout," she says.

Many men walk around in a continual state of mild dehydration, not taking in enough fluids to meet even their everyday needs. The fluid needs of a Hard-Body Man tend to be even greater than those of less active, less muscled guys.

Fluid requirements are based on metabolism and increase with temperature, physical activity, and altitude.

An average, sedentary guy who eats 2,500 calories per day, lives at sea level, and spends his days

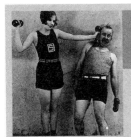

THAT'S DUMB

As far back as 1947, good research showed the dangers of denying liquids to men involved in strenuous physical activities, especially when they were exercising in warm conditions.

But it wasn't until the 1970s that guidelines on fluid intake during physical activity found their way into textbooks and onto the practice field.

In the meantime, dozens of athletes and military recruits died from exertional heat stroke complicated by dehydration.

reclining in a moderate-temperature, low-humidity, air-conditioned house *requires* about 12 8-ounce cups of fluid per day—and more wouldn't hurt, Dr. Kleiner estimates.

But a Hard-Body Man *isn't* average. He eats more, exercises harder, builds muscle on recovery days, and lives an active life. His fluid needs are much higher—probably about a gallon a day, and even more on workout days when he's really sweating.

"Men will say that that much fluid makes them run to the bathroom all the time. Well, they're right. And that's okay. It's good to urinate often and get rid of those toxins being filtered out by the kidneys," says Dr. Kleiner.

Urine is an indicator of good hydration, notes Dr. Kleiner. Assuming you haven't just loaded up on B vitamins, which your body pees off quickly and colorfully, your urine should be nearly colorless and odorless. If your urine is darker than the color of straw, or smelly, it's loaded with nasty things that your kidneys needed to flush but couldn't for a lack of fluids.

More subtle signs of mild dehydration include dry eyes and mouth, weakness, fatigue, and headaches.

Water should make up at least half your daily fluid intake, Dr. Kleiner says. Create a plan or schedule that reminds you to drink throughout the day.

Don't wait until you're thirsty to drink. By then, you're already slightly dehydrated. To avoid that, put together a hydration plan—essentially a schedule and several visual cues to remind you to drink frequently. (If you want to call it a drinking plan, that's fine, but it has nothing to with Saturday night on the town.)

Here are Dr. Kleiner's suggestions for how a Hard-Body Man can pour more water into his life:

• Drink a couple glassfuls of water when you first get up in the morning and before you go to bed, even though a late-night drink might wake you up to urinate.

• Have water with every meal and snack.

• Keep a pitcher of cold water in the fridge and drink it dry every day. Put another pitcher on your desk, so you're not tempted to drink just soda, tea, or coffee.

• Take water to the gym.

If you don't like the taste of the water coming from the tap, you have options. You might add a twist of lemon or lime, stir in a splash of fruit juice, or freshen it with a little seltzer. A home water filtration system can remove chlorine and contaminants like lead and improve taste. Or you can buy bottled, filtered water, anything from a pint-size bottle at the convenience store to one of those big, blue water cooler bottles delivered weekly. Most of the bottled stuff tastes pretty good.

Water isn't your only choice for meeting your daily fluid requirements. While you're not exercising, you can help to meet your fluid needs with fat-free, soy, or rice milk; diluted fruit juices; seltzer water; soups; organic, noncaffeinated herbal teas; sports drinks; and even the moisture present in food (especially juicy, water-laden fruits and vegetables).

Sorry, but you have to back off the coffee and alcohol. These things actually *hurt* hydration.

Anything with caffeine or alcohol—that includes coffee, tea, beer, wine, and mixed drinks—is a diuretic. Diuretics are liquids that actually accelerate fluid loss.

You know all about diuretics. You belly up to the bar for a draft beer and 20 minutes later in the bathroom most of it seems to be swirling down the drain. And then 15 or 20 minutes later, déjà vu. Drink beer all evening and the headache you feel the next morning will be due in large part to dehydration.

Coffee, tea, and soda aren't much better than beer. "I wouldn't even count a caffeinated beverage. Caffeine's a negative in my book. If you drink a cup of coffee or a can of caffeinated soda, you owe yourself an equal amount of water," Burns says.

By the way, decaffeinated black tea and decaf coffee are okay and are exceptions to this rule.

Drink all you want and count them toward your total daily minimum intake of fluid.

Sports drinks are not beverages for everyday thirst, but they are especially well-suited for workouts. Choose one that's tasty, that contains an adequate number of carbs, and that replaces lost electrolytes, advises Burns.

Water and other fluids suffice for sedentary activities, she says, but when it comes to exercise, consider a sports drink—unless your goal is to lose flab. If that's the case, stick to water. Sports drinks are most appropriate before, during, and after exercise. They speed up hydration, unleash a shot of easily and quickly digested carbohydrates, and replace electrolytes lost during serious sweating.

You'll find a dizzying array of these products on the store shelf, but be forewarned: They aren't all created equal, Burns says. She recommends that you buy only products that meet the following guidelines. They should be noncarbonated, and they should have the following nutrients per 8-ounce serving:

- 14 to 17 grams of carbs
- about 100 milligrams of sodium
- and at least 30 milligrams of potassium.

Sports drinks also should tantalize your taste buds. Some taste much better than others. Studies show that people are more inclined to drink flavored and sweetened beverages than plain water after exercise.

Many manufacturers of sports drinks like to ballyhoo the vitamin content of their products. And though the vitamins probably don't hurt, they aren't really necessary in a sports drink, Burns says. You don't need to spend extra bucks on specially vitamin-fortified drinks because you get sufficient vitamins with the Hard-Body Diet.

And avoid carbonated sports drinks, Burns adds, because carbonation slows digestion and causes stomach distress.

Also beware of caffeine in these beverages. Some "energy drinks" are chock-full of caffeine. Instead, look for ones with extra helpings of carbs and a bit of protein, recommends Dr. Kleiner. That way, if you don't like eating food before exercise, you can drink your preworkout meal. Watch the calories, though, warns Thomas Incledon, M.S., R.D., designer of the Hard-Body Diet. Make sure that if you're guzzling sports drinks, you aren't exceeding your total recommended calorie intake. (You determine your personal quotas using the "Daily Quotas" chart on page 326.)

And remember: If you're trying to burn flab, you don't need the extra calories you'll get from a sports drink; so stick to water and low-calorie fluids, says Incledon.

While sports drinks hydrate you, they also raise glucose levels in your bloodstream and supply a bit of extra energy to burn during exercise, says Dr. Kleiner.

Before you work out, start by having a drink. Dr. Kleiner's prescription: Drink 2 cups of fluid 2 hours before. That way, it's fully absorbed before you start pumping the muscles. Then, immediately before lifting, take in another 4 to 8 ounces.

This is when a carb-rich sports drink is better than water. The simple sugars raise insulin levels and load your bloodstream with glucose. Your body will mix that glucose into its burners and thus burn less muscle glycogen, leaving muscle glycogen to carry you through your workout and provide those last bursts of energy before exhaustion.

The American College of Sports Medicine recommends that exercisers who are working out for longer than an hour or who are sweating heavily because of intensity or heat should drink at regular intervals—between 4 and 8 ounces every 15 to 20 minutes.

During the first 30 to 60 minutes of an average-intensity workout (brisk walk, moderate cardio workout), you can get by just fine on water. After that, or if you are doing more intense exercise such as playing in a soccer game, you may want the more readily absorbed fluid, extra carbs, and extra calories of a sports drink.

If you can't stomach the idea of drinking anything during a workout because it makes you feel

WEIGHING YOUR WATER LOSS

When training hard, you lose a lot of fluids through respiration and perspiration. A simple way to know whether you're replacing all your fluids is to weigh yourself before and after exercise. For every pound of body weight lost during exercise, you should drink 20 to 24 ounces of fluid, says Julie Burns, R.D., a sports nutritionist in Western Springs, Illinois.

Many men are surprised how much weight they lose during exercise, says Burns. When Burns first started working with the Chicago Blackhawks, she found that some hockey players lost 8 to 10 pounds of weight during a single game.

"Replacing fluids is something you need to think about every time you work out," Burns says. Weighing yourself is a great reminder to drink. And it will help you learn just how quickly you sweat off liquid.

bloated, here's Dr. Kleiner's advice: Start slow, with just a bit of fluid, and work your way up over several weeks—especially if you're in a warm, sweaty gym.

A sports drink *after* a workout is superior to water. It replaces lost electrolytes, speeds rehydration, and boosts the replacement of muscle glycogen.

The perfect combo after a workout is a sports drink and high-glycemic foods, such as bread, pasta, rice, or a cereal bar. You also need a bit of protein, notes Incledon. The food and drink flush carbohydrates into your bloodstream, raise your insulin levels, and encourage your muscles to soak up glycogen. (Check the label on your sports drink, though: Incledon warns that some sports drinks get most of their carbs from fructose. Those drinks won't help.)

Sports drinks also help you rehydrate more quickly than water alone. Sodium and glucose assist with absorption by pushing more water molecules into the cells. Sodium (salt), of course, also makes you thirsty and virtually drives you to drink—which is a good thing when you need to rehydrate, says Dr. Kleiner.

And finally, sports drinks replace those lost electrolytes, one of the sources of all those killer muscle cramps you remember from that first week of preseason way back when, explains Dr. Kleiner.

If only Bucky, your coach, had understood the physiological benefits of hydration. It would have been better for you, better for the team, and certainly better for Jim DeAngelo, who at every class reunion still has to endure hearing someone tell that mud puddle story.

BARHOPPING
A GUIDE TO ENERGY BARS

SOME HANDY DESIGNER BARS OFFER QUICK ENERGY FOR WORKING OUT AND THE NUTRITION NEEDED AFTERWARD. SOME EVEN TASTE GOOD.

It takes fuel and powerful workouts to burn fat and build muscle.

Nutritional bars hold out the promise of a high-octane, designer fuel—and some actually deliver. They provide your needed calories, carbohydrates, and protein in one compact and easy-to-consume package. And they don't fill you up and weigh you down while you're working out.

Some of these bars, though, are junk food. And some are overpriced and unnecessarily loaded with vitamins and herbs. And some don't come close to meeting the carb-protein-fat ratios of the Hard-Body Plan.

Downing a good bar is a convenient way to take in your needed calories for a workout, says Laura Spanbauer, R.D., a registered dietitian and sports nutrition counselor based in Albany, New York.

In a perfect world, we would find the perfect bar. Such a bar would have about 200 calories and two to four times more carbohydrates than protein. It wouldn't go overboard on added vitamins, minerals, and herbs. And it wouldn't boast simple sugars such as sucrose and fructose and high-fructose corn syrup among the first items on the ingredients list.

Also, in a perfect world, you would actually have *two* bars that fit the profile: a preworkout bar with a low glycemic index to keep your motor running, and another with a higher glycemic index to help you with your postworkout recovery.

"You want something with a higher glycemic index after your workout to replenish your glycogen stores," notes Alan R. Stockard, D.O., medical director of sports medicine at the Osteopathic Medical Center of Texas at Fort Worth.

Furthermore, in a perfect world, the bar that you eat would taste like a Mrs. Field's cookie or a candy bar.

Dream on.

The world ain't perfect and neither are the energy bars. But some come closer than others.

Here's a quick reference guide to help you survey the bars you can find in nearby supermarkets, drugstores, convenience stores, and health food shops.

301

WHAT'S IN A NAME?

Don't worry too much about how the bar is classified. It might be called an energy bar. It might be referred to as a meal replacement bar. It might be a "nutritional bar." It may even be a simple "cereal bar." Whatever. There are plenty to choose from. On a recent trip to a convenience store we counted 38 different bars available.

"The idea behind most bars is to give you a quick and ready source of energy for your exercise activity," Dr. Stockard explains.

"You'll need to try a few out so that you can find out which bars taste good and which ones do not upset your stomach or make you feel bloated," says Gunnar Brolinson, D.O., who practices sports medicine and family medicine in Toledo, Ohio.

"Watch out, though, because some of the bars have more protein in them than carbohydrates," warns Richard B. Kreider, Ph.D., the assistant chairman of the department of human movement sciences at the University of Memphis. "You should minimally get at least 8 to 10 grams of protein in a bar. But the overall ratio of carbohydrates to protein should be between 4:1 and 5:1."

Thomas Incledon, M.S., R.D., designer of the Hard-Body Diet, is less convinced that weight lifters need a ratio that high, and he says that bars with as low as a 2:1 carb-to-protein ratio are fine for Hard-Body pre- and postworkout snacks.

If your bar meets those criteria, then how much carob, oats, and spinach it contains is the next matter of interest. That's because we're more concerned with the bar's glycemic index, and you won't find information about that, specifically, on the labels. Glycemic index is hard to determine unless you have a mobile lab or a highly trained nutritionist with you at the store. We can offer some rough guidelines, though.

If the first ingredients listed on the bar are recognizable, substantive food items—such as a grain

or, as we kidded, carob, oats, and spinach—then the bar probably won't give you just a sugar high. (We want to avoid a sugar high.) Avoid bars that have simple sugars at the top of the list. As we said earlier, they are just too high-glycemic.

Another key to glycemic index is the amount of fiber listed. A high-fiber bar is unlikely to be high-glycemic, and therefore it would not be as useful as an after-workout snack, but it might be perfect for the preworkout snack.

A typical jam-filled cereal bar, the kind you buy in grocery stores, is fine for the postworkout snack, says Incledon, provided that you down it with 4 ounces of fat-free milk to add a bit of protein.

A MATTER OF TASTE

Just because a bar seems to have a good glycemic index and the proper amount of carbs and protein means nothing if you can still taste the spinach through the carob. You have to be able to stomach the things. We thought maybe we could help. We gathered a tasty collection of the bars and, to review their palatability, we used a crackerjack team of . . . normal folks. The kind of people you work with, live with, and run around town with. Not one of them regularly consumes raw eggs and chalky protein shakes. We asked.

"Personal preference is really important with energy bars," Spanbauer stresses. "If you like the taste of the bar and it doesn't have anything particularly wrong with it nutritionally, it's probably a decent choice."

We did try to be as objective as possible by picking one general category for all of the bars we reviewed. We did this scientifically. We went "eeny, meeny, miny, *chocolate!*"

Unfortunately, we can't say that they all tasted like chocolate.

And we realized that it's probably best not to

name names here because manufacturers are constantly discontinuing flavors and issuing new ones and changing formulas as new research is published and for who knows what other reasons. What do the things taste like? Well, most of them don't taste really good. Okay? Need proof?

Here are a few of our reviewers' comments about various bars.

• "The bar somehow manages to be both too soft and too chunky, and the flavor is reminiscent of a stale peanut butter cup dipped in warm milk."

• "The texture is smooth, with just a hint of crunch in the cookie dough flavor and a thick nougatlike consistency in the chocolate-peanut flavor."

• "Although the bar has a slight 'chemical' flavor at first, it quickly smoothes out to taste like a soft brownie."

• "The flavor is not bad but is very faint and slightly bitter." One reviewer likened it to a "bar that was frozen and then was thawed." The texture is a bit like a grainy Tootsie Roll.

• "Good taffy-fudge texture and flavor." One reviewer complained that while this bar tasted fine, it felt heavy in the stomach 20 minutes later.

There you have a good sampling. Now go do your own taste test.

MIX AND MATCH

We found that many of the bars fall quite comfortably in a carb-to-protein ratio range of 2:1 to 4:1. Some are way off, though.

Most of the ones we looked at were close to the 200 calories you need, too.

But if you cannot find a single bar that meets all your needs, think about mixing them up. If one bar you like is too low in carbohydrates and another one is too low in protein, guess what?

You could be super-adventurous and eat half of each bar.

As long as the total calories and overall ratio of carbs to protein fits the Hard-Body parameters, you are okay in our book.

Or here's another idea, courtesy of Spanbauer: Combine a bar with an energy gel, which is a carb-rich packet of thick, flavored liquid. These gels are becoming more and more popular, particularly among runners and bicyclists. Lifters can use them too. There's no law about these things. And the gels provide another advantage.

"While bars are great for giving you carbohydrates for energy and replenishing glycogen, they don't provide H_2O," Spanbauer points out. "But gels—and power drinks for that matter—can give you hydration as well as carbohydrates."

The gels usually have no protein, they tend to be fairly low in sugar, and they have around half the calories of most bars. So if the bar you like best is both low in carbs and too high in sugar for your preworkout snack, eat half of the bar and drink down a packet of a low-sugar energy gel to round out your calories and carbs.

Play with other combinations too. Work with the bars you have handy and whatever else you like.

VITAMINS, MINERALS, AND HERBS THAT ENHANCE MUSCLE GROWTH
VITAMIN VITALITY

WE ALL NEED OUR VITAMINS AND MINERALS. BUT A HARD-BODY MAN WHO EATS WELL DOES NOT NEED TO POP PILLS TO SUPPORT HIS BASIC BODILY FUNCTIONS. A MULTIVITAMIN IS ALL THE INSURANCE YOU NEED.

If there's a shelf somewhere in your kitchen or pantry that has so many bottles of vitamin and mineral supplements on it that you could open your own little health food shop right now, then listen up:

It might be time for a good spring cleaning.

For one thing, the great balanced eating program we provide in the Hard-Body Plan gives you a well-rounded dose of vitamins and minerals. Sports nutritionist Thomas Incledon, M.S., R.D., who devised the program, saw to that.

If you eat a great, balanced mix of foods, you won't need to down a bunch of pills, capsules, liquids, and powders to meet your body's basic, minimal nutritional needs. So contend the American Dietetic Association and the National Research Council.

But, understand that many people—including a surprisingly large number of doctors—now look to vitamins and minerals not only as essential nutrients that protect against illness but also as medicinal healers in their own right. Why so? Researchers are finding that certain supplements, including vitamins such as C and E and minerals such as selenium, when taken in appropriately large doses, can have a medicinal effect on the body that goes far beyond their standard support function. If you've heard the term *nutraceutical,* that is what they're talking about—natural ingredients being used for medicinal purposes.

To the Hard-Body Man, supplements are a type of nutritional health insurance—additional nutrients that guarantee that he gets the building blocks that he needs to keep his body in top shape. Here are the basics of what your Hard Body needs, and why.

VITAMINS AND MINERALS: YOUR DAILY DOSES

Few things in the world of vitamins and minerals are more contentious than the words *recommended daily allowance*, which now have been superceded by the words *Daily Value*.

The National Research Council says that these levels are the bare minimum you need to prevent health problems. Other experts contend that you should shoot for getting upward of 200 percent (or even much, much more) of the Daily Value for most vitamins and minerals. "The DV's were never set up with an optimal nutrition status in mind. This is why they are critiqued, since lots of data indicate that some nutrients are required in greater dosages," adds Incledon.

Vitamins and minerals *do* play a role in muscle making. We'll explore that role vitamin by vitamin, mineral by mineral.

VITAMINS

Your body relies on 13 vitamins to maintain the delicate balance of your metabolism, keep you alert, fight off infection, initiate chemical reactions, and perform a host of other duties. You need every last one of them to remain healthy. You get all of them when you eat the Hard-Body Diet.

Here are a few that directly relate to building a Hard Body.

Folate: Daily Value, 400 micrograms. Also known as folic acid, this vitamin is used to metabolize protein and to convert many amino acids for cell growth.

If you are using a folate supplement, make sure to take vitamin B_{12} as well. This is important because folate masks the symptoms of a vitamin B_{12} deficiency, says Laura Spanbauer, R.D., a sports nutritionist in New York State.

Niacin: Daily Value, 20 milligrams. This vitamin is required to help break down the carbohydrates, fats, and proteins you consume.

Niacin is very powerful. It is sometimes prescribed by physicians to deal with high cholesterol. At those therapeutic dosages, side effects can include flushing, itching, nausea, and cramps. At very high doses, niacin can cause liver damage.

Niacinamide, typically used in multivitamins, lacks the therapeutic properties of niacin itself.

Pantothenic Acid: Daily Value, 10 milligrams. This vitamin helps to metabolize carbohydrates, protein, and fats for energy.

Pantothenic acid is very safe and has been taken at doses as high as 10 to 20 grams a day with no ill effects except for occasional diarrhea and water retention. But keep your dosages close to the Daily Value unless you want some really expensive urine.

Riboflavin: Daily Value, 1.7 milligrams. Also known as vitamin B_2, this nutrient helps convert glucose and fats into energy.

Riboflavin is one of the safest vitamins; it's water-soluble and excess amounts are quickly excreted from your system.

Vitamin B_6: Daily Value, 2 milligrams. It assists in metabolizing protein and amino acids.

"Some people have claimed that this vitamin helps to increase energy output during physical activity, but most studies have failed to prove that," says Spanbauer.

Avoid doses above 100 milligrams, except under medical supervision. Excess amounts can cause pain, numbness, and weakness in the limbs.

Vitamin C: Daily Value, 60 milligrams. This most popular of vitamins is essential to the formation of connective tissue (bone, teeth, cartilage, and skin), helps protect the body against oxidants, and helps the body make efficient use of other vitamins and minerals, among other functions.

Dosages as high as 5,000 milligrams per day are often used. Excess doses may cause diarrhea, which is easily solved by cutting back on the dosage or taking divided dosages throughout the day with meals.

MINERALS

Fifteen minerals are required by your body to regulate cell function and to provide the structure for those cells. Here are a few for the Hard-Body Man to keep a close eye on.

Calcium: Daily Value, 1,000 milligrams.

"If I had to suggest one mineral that a lot of people should consider supplementing, it would probably be calcium," Spanbauer says. "Bone strength is a very important component of optimal health and fitness."

Teenagers and men over age 50 need from 1,200 to 1,300 milligrams per day.

People who consume a lot of caffeine in their diets or who smoke should also consider bumping up their calcium intake a bit, says Spanbauer.

And don't forget to obtain your Daily Value of vitamin D (400 international units), which is needed for your body to absorb calcium.

Chromium: Daily Value, 120 micrograms.

One of chromium's functions is to assist in the process of converting fats and carbohydrates to energy. Studies, though, haven't shown that chromium supplementation increases muscle mass or fat loss.

If you wish to supplement, 200 micrograms daily is quite safe according to numerous research studies.

Magnesium: Daily Value, 400 milligrams. This mineral helps break down glucose, fatty acids, and amino acids; assists in metabolizing carbohydrates and protein; and helps transmit electrical impulses across nerves and muscles.

Manganese: Daily Value, 2 milligrams. Manganese is necessary to synthesize cholesterol and strengthen bones.

"Manganese also helps metabolize glucose, which is your primary source for energy and endurance," Spanbauer says.

Daily amounts of up to 10 milligrams seem to be safe, but there is really no need to go that high.

Phosphorus: Daily Value, 1,000 milligrams. Like calcium and manganese, this mineral plays a role in building strong bones. And it assists the body in processing carbohydrates, fats, and protein.

Because phosphorus can be found in so many different kinds of foods, supplements are unnecessary for the vast majority of people.

HERBS: THE GREEN TEAM

Wouldn't it be great if there were a plant substance you could ingest that would turn up your fat burners, speed up muscle growth, and give you endless energy? That's the promise of some herbal supplements that you've seen on health food store shelves and advertised in fitness magazines—and that some guys in the gym swear by.

We looked into them. We talked to one of the world's foremost herbalists, David Winston. We looked at studies. We looked at claims. We looked for, but didn't discover, any magic bullets. We found some herbs that might have some small, beneficial effect. We found a lot of misunderstandings about herbs.

Let's clear up the misunderstandings.

• You've been exposed to the concept that herbs are somehow safe, innocuous, always-healthy substances because they come from plants as opposed to big, bad drugs that come from doctors. Our position? Nonsense. Herbs also can be dangerous if not used intelligently with knowledge and caution.

According to Winston, it really depends on the herb. He believes, as the Cherokee Indians did, that herbs can be put into one of three categories: foods, medicines, or poisons.

Herbs that can be considered foods have a very mild, nourishing effect on the body and are generally safe for most people to take on a long-term basis. Some herbs that fall into this category are garlic, turmeric, ginger, ginsengs, flaxseed oil, cayenne pepper, and cardamom.

Herbs that are considered medicines are stronger-acting, with a greater potential to adversely affect the body. Like drugs, they are used to treat a specific condition for a given period of time, and they have a definite, pronounced pharmacologic effect. Some herbs that fall into this category are devil's claw, kava-kava, *Tribulus terrestris*, ephedra, and willow bark.

Finally, there are poisons. These have a high potential for toxic effects on the body if not used properly. They should only be utilized by herbal experts, and not for self-treatment. A few examples are poke, aconite, and arnica. (This does not nec-essarily include homeopathic or topical applications of these herbs.)

A lot of prescription drugs were derived from herbs (and some still are). While the specific active ingredients usually are well-known in marketed drugs, less is known about precisely which ingredients are active in herbs. Most herbs contain many organic constituents that might contribute to their effect.

• Another basic thing we'd like to say about herbs: Your body doesn't require them. Your body requires vitamins and minerals in order to function properly. Not so with herbs.

• Despite their long history of use, some herbs have not been studied and tested extensively, unlike prescription drugs. Your doctor doesn't know what to make of them, for the most part, because your doctor was trained in the use of scientifically studied meds.

• Many herbs should also be approached with caution. "People think that just because an herbal product is sold over the counter, it must be safe," says Fort Worth, Texas, sports medicine doctor

DON'T BE A VITAMIN FATHEAD

Some vitamins can be poison. Be careful with three fat-soluble vitamins in particular: A, D, and K. Fat-soluble means that the vitamins are stored and processed in your fatty bodily tissues.

You must have figured out by now how much work you have to do to get rid of fat. Fat-soluble vitamins don't go poof and disappear, either.

Other vitamins are water-soluble and pass out of your body through your urine. Still, megadoses of some water-soluble vitamins can put a strain on your body's filtration system.

Megadoses of vitamins A, D, and K can be especially harmful, particularly over an extended period. E also is a fat-soluble vitamin, but it has much less risk of toxicity.

Your body is particularly susceptible to toxicity from A and D, and vitamin K increases the ability of blood to clot or clump. We all need our blood to clot, but no one needs gummy blood, a possibility from taking too much K.

The National Research Council says that the bare minimum that you should get every day (Daily Values) of these vitamins is 5,000 IU or international units (1,000 micrograms RE) of vitamin A; 400 IU (10 micrograms) of vitamin D; 30 IU (20 milligrams a-TE) of vitamin E; and 80 micrograms of vitamin K.

Alan R. Stockard, D.O. "That's just plain wrong." Some herbs evoke powerful physiological effects, and you can overdose on some herbs or build up levels of toxicity over time. Also, the FDA has no jurisdiction over the quality of herbal products. "That means you cannot be sure of the potency, freshness, or quality of herbs," says Dr. Stockard. Your wisest strategy is to buy from a well-known, well-established manufacturer or herb supplier who uses certified organic herbs.

Also be aware that some herbs interact negatively with prescription medications. Your physician probably has been alerted to the most common herb-drug interactions and is a good source of advice regarding that.

• In the United States, no agency has determined appropriate, effective daily values for herbal substances. Therefore, to determine the right amount for you, you truly *do* need to consult with an herbalist or naturopathic doctor or with a physician or nutritionist who has been trained in herbal medicine, or consult a reliable reference book.

The most common herbs touted for weight trainers fall into the categories of *adaptogenic* and *thermogenic* herbs and compounds, so we will look at those first.

ADAPTOGENS IN ACTION

Herbal *adaptogens* help the body adapt to and resist physical stress, such as that caused by exercise. The most well-known and most-used herbal adaptogens for men are three forms of ginseng.

Two of them are distantly related: American ginseng and Asian ginseng, which is sometimes called Chinese, Korean, or red ginseng. The third ginseng, Siberian ginseng, is not related to the other two.

It appears that Siberian ginseng is probably the best choice for most men who want a pick-me-up for their workouts.

"Siberian ginseng is perfect for the average guy—the 'home' athlete or average health club member," notes Winston, who is a clinical herbalist and president of the Herbal Therapeutics Research Library. "It's also a useful daily tonic for the average overworked American who's in relatively good health and wants to perk up his immune system."

Asian ginseng has a powerful stimulatory effect and is best for the most severely immunologically depleted and deficient people, says Winston. It is appropriate for use in people who have fibromyalgia, chronic fatigue syndrome, and other deficiency syndromes, says Winston. The Asian varieties generally are not recommended for people who are younger than 40, who have high blood pressure, or who have active infections.

American ginseng is milder than its Asian cousins but very similar in effect. It is considered less effective, but it is tonifying to the immune, nervous, and endocrine systems. As with the Asian ginseng, it's used for deficiency syndromes, but it is more appropriate for younger people, from their twenties to forties.

All three forms of ginseng are available in capsule form, as well as in other preparations such as liquids and powders. The amount of ginseng in a single capsule varies widely depending on the product and manufacturer, but 250 milligrams to 520 milligrams per capsule is very common.

For American or Asian ginseng, the recommended dosage is 500 milligrams to 1 gram per day in two divided doses, for up to 3 months at a time.

For Siberian ginseng, a typical capsule dosage is 250 milligrams to 500 milligrams taken one to three times per day.

Winston feels that Siberian ginseng is safe enough to use indefinitely. Wild American ginseng is an endangered species, so he recommends that people buy organically cultivated, woods-grown ginseng instead. You should be able to tell what kind it is from the product's label.

For a 100-count bottle of ginseng capsules, expect to spend between $8 and $20, give or take. The American and Asian ginsengs tend to be at the higher end of the price range, and Siberian ginseng tends toward the lower end.

THERMOGENIC THERAPY

In theory, thermogenic compounds stimulate the metabolism, thereby increasing calorie burn. These compounds are problematic, says Winston.

"Most of the ones that really work are illegal," Winston says, referring to drugs such as amphetamines that are legal only by prescription. "And the ones that work and are legal contain ephedra, which can cause hypertension, cardiovascular problems, and other unpleasant side effects in excess dosage."

Ephedra, also known as ma huang, among other names, is a plant that contains the alkaloid ephedrine, which is a stimulant whose chemical structure is similar to amphetamines. It is synthesized into forms of pseudoephedrine and norephedrine, which are common, effective, and popular ingredients in both prescription and over-the-counter cold and allergy medications. The federal government limits the amount of ephedrine a customer can buy because it can be converted to methamphetamine in underground drug labs.

The effect of ephedrine can be hopped up—and it often is in "fat burner" and "energy" formulas—by combining it with caffeine and aspirin as well as various other herbs, says Winston. While the combinations may heighten the thermogenic effect, they also heighten the danger of adverse side effects. Ephedrine often is used in much higher and more potentially dangerous potencies in thermogenic compounds than it is in herbal cold and allergy remedies.

"People should just steer clear of ephedrine, which is a potent cardiovascular and nervous system stimulator," Dr. Stockard warns.

Anyone who loses weight solely from taking these herbal products will gain back the weight they lost once they stop taking the herbal preparation, says Incledon.

Other herbal compounds being touted as thermogenic do not seem to have much thermogenic effect, says Winston.

"The only non-ephedra thermogenic combos out there that do seem to work contain synephrine, which supposedly has the same positive qualities as ephedra but without the side effects," Winston reports. "But if it really has thermogenic effects similar to ephedra, chances are good that when studied more closely it will turn out to have similar side effects."

Another school of thought, according to Incledon, is that synephrine is just plain useless from a thermogenic standpoint—that it increases bloodflow, so that the person thinks thermogenesis is taking place, but produces no thermogenic effects.

HERBAL POTPOURRI

Here's the scoop on a few other herbs often pitched to weight trainers.

Devil's claw (Harpagophytum procumbens): Some believe that this herb may have an indirect effect on increasing body weight by enhancing appetite.

It is probably better, however, to use devil's claw for its anti-inflammatory properties. It may help reduce muscle stress during workouts, thus reducing muscle pain afterward.

A common dosage is about a gram taken twice daily with water at mealtimes for 9 weeks, then take 2 to 3 weeks off, then begin again. As with all herbs and medications, read and follow warnings and cautions on the labels. Seek medical advice before using devil's claw if you have gastric or duodenal ulcers or gallstones.

Flaxseed oil (Linum usitatissimum): This is one way to add some extra grams of fat to your diet—about 14 per tablespoon—while still getting something healthy out of the deal.

"Flaxseed oil contains both omega-3 and omega-6 fatty acids, which act as anti-inflammatories through the whole body, including the cardiovascular system and connective tissues," Winston explains.

A common dosage is 1 to 2 tablespoons of oil taken in the mornings.

Ginger (Zingiber officinale): Not only is ginger a systemic anti-inflammatory, but it also aids in blood circulation to the muscles and limbs. In addition, it is a digestive aid.

Ginger often comes in capsules with approximately 500 milligrams of powdered root. A typical dosage would be two capsules taken two to four times daily with a glass of water at mealtimes. Use is not advised if you have gallstones.

Kava-kava (Piper methysticum): This won't do anything to enhance your athletic performance, but it can help you relax and perhaps relieve your muscle soreness after a workout, says Winston.

In small, reasonable amounts, Winston feels, kava-kava is quite safe. An effective dosage is 60 to 120 milligrams of kavapyrones (or kavalactones). Check the label to determine how much to take to achieve that. Do not take it daily for more than 3 months without medical advice. Do not mix it with alcohol or barbiturates. And be careful when driving or operating equipment, as this herb is a muscle relaxant.

Tribulus terrestris: Although some sales pitches claim that this herb from Indian Ayurvedic medicine helps to build muscle mass by increasing the body's production of testosterone, these assertions are based on obscure and unsupported case studies rather than diligent research, say Winston and Incledon.

"This is a substance that has been used in India in Ayurvedic medicine as a diuretic and aphrodisiac," Winston notes. "Numerous studies on lab animals have shown that certain chemicals found in this plant have the ability to stimulate sperm production, libido, and fertility. But little or no research has shown that it has these effects on humans." He has serious doubts that it would have any great benefit for increasing muscle mass or stimulating testosterone levels in men. And in any case, *Tribulus terrestris* should only be used under the supervision of a qualified herbal or medical practitioner.

SPICE IT UP

You can find some good ideas in your spice rack too. Here are a couple.

Cayenne pepper (Capsicum annuum; C. frutescens): Capsaicin, the active ingredient in cayenne and other hot peppers, has been touted for its ability to improve blood circulation to muscles and to stimulate the metabolism.

"Regular intake of hot spices can elevate your metabolism," Winston says. "But taking capsaicin supplements or putting a lot of hot sauce on your food is not going to give you significant gains."

A common dose is a 450-milligram capsule taken three times daily at mealtimes. Hot pepper taken on an empty stomach can irritate the gastrointestinal tract.

Turmeric (Curcuma domestica): This spice is a fairly powerful anti-inflammatory agent which can be used for muscle and joint pain and arthritis, according to Winston. Use it to spice up your cooking, or obtain an extract from your local health food store. A typical dose is one or two 400-milligram capsules, three times a day. Follow your product's label directions. Do not use this if you have high stomach acid or ulcers, gallstones, or bile duct obstruction.

The Latest on Creatine, DHEA, Powders, and Potions

The Supplement Game

Some supplements work; most don't. All come with side effects; some are dangerous. Aminos seem to be the safest.

We may not be quick to admit it, but a few of us are looking for a "magic bullet." We dream of a pill or a shake or a machine that will transform us into Hard-Body Man without any serious effort on our parts.

You aren't like that, of course.

But, believe it or not, there are people who down diet soft drinks with their greasy burgers and chow down on chips—ones without fake fat. They buy exercise equipment and videos that promise tight abs in 5 minutes. They buy expensive little bottles of "fat burners" and "energy boosters" and "mega muscle blends."

The fitness industry knows that. Why do you think they stock the shelves with every kind of muscle-building supplement that you can imagine? Some companies promise—or at least strongly imply—that their product is the miracle substance that will forever change how we work out.

It's hype, of course. There is no magic bullet.

Some strength supplements work, but most don't do nearly what they promise, if they do anything at all other than possibly trigger a placebo effect.

Being a Hard-Body Man requires you to put your heart, mind, and body into the Hard-Body Plan. We are not about to tell you that you can buy Hard-Body Man in a Can. It just ain't so.

"There is a cultural bias in the United States in favor of using medications, ergogenic substances, and other physiologic agents to solve most of our problems," notes Gunnar Brolinson, D.O., who practices sports medicine in Toledo, Ohio, "when, in fact, we should be focusing on nutrition and exercise to keep us healthy and fit."

That mouthful is not to say that some of the amino acids, proteins, pro-hormones, and other supplements out there don't have any value. Many actually do something besides make the supplement manufacturer's Mercedes payments.

Doctors wouldn't call them "ergogenic" and "physiologic" if they didn't have measurable effects. *Ergogenic* means performance enhancing. *Physiologic* means that they affect you physically as well as mentally. But just because a manufacturer calls a product physiologic or ergogenic doesn't mean that it is. In fact, most that claim to be physiologic or ergogenic really aren't.

We'll tell you which ones to consider if you have your heart set on a pill, powder, or potion. But keep this in perspective. The real gains come from eating right and working out. Supplements only help you get a leg up or make your workout pay off a little better. And, we should note, even the doctors we consulted who are supplement advocates recommend that you only play with these things under medical supervision.

"Unfortunately, many people figure that if a little bit of a supplement is good, then a lot of it must be better," laments Mark S. Juhn, D.O., a sports medicine expert affiliated with the University of Washington School of Medicine. "And they overestimate the ergogenic benefits of the supplements they take. In combination, those two notions can lead people to overdose on the products."

BRING IN THE AMINOS

Amino acids are the building blocks of proteins. Proteins, in turn, are a critical part of those muscles that you want to develop.

"When I counsel people on fitness and supplements, I always stress the importance of good nutrition," reports Laura Spanbauer, R.D., a registered dietitian and sports nutrition counselor in Albany, New York. "Then I tell them, 'If you still want to try some of the aminos on the market, fine. You might see some benefits.'"

But you should also expect side effects, she warns. Just because it's natural doesn't mean that it won't hurt.

"There are downsides to using aminos, such as bloating and cramping" with some, Spanbauer explains. "That is why I always try to get people to go the route of good nutrition through eating well rather than supplementation. Good nutrition—along with exercise—is what will build endurance and create a better body." Another plus of whole foods: They contain nutrients that haven't even been discovered or studied yet, says Thomas Incledon, R.D., our Hard-Body Plan nutrition advisor. "This is something supplement manufacturers cannot provide because they don't know they exist."

Here's a look at a couple of aminos that actually do something.

CREATINE

Many amino acids are available in supplement form. But a quick trip to any health food store or nutritional outlet will tell you one thing: Right now, creatine is king.

"No other amino acid has been proven to be as useful in building lean muscle mass and improving strength," says Alan R. Stockard, D.O., medical director of sports medicine at the Osteopathic Medical Center of Texas at Fort Worth.

Numerous studies have shown benefits from creatine supplementation in athletes, including:

• An average 6.3 percent increase in fat-free mass compared with 3.1 percent for participants on a placebo, following 12 weeks of heavy resistance training. Also, a 24 percent increase in bench-press performance, compared with 16 percent for the noncreatine group. These results come from a Pennsylvania State University study of 19 athletic men in their midtwenties.

• A 2-kilogram increase in body mass—independent of water retention—after 42 days of strength training and 21 days of detraining. This is according to a study at Université Libre de Bruxelles in Belgium, involving 25 healthy men in their early twenties.

- Gains in fat-free and bone-free mass, in weight lifting ability, and in sprint performance during intense resistance and agility training. These results come from a study of 25 NCAA football players conducted at the University of Memphis.

Creatine also has been shown to help athletes rebound from fatigue more quickly, and it may turn out to have clinical applications in the treatment of heart disease, muscular disease, and Parkinson's disease, says Richard B. Kreider, Ph.D., assistant chair and director of the Exercise and Sports Nutrition Lab at the University of Memphis.

"However, as a physician, it is difficult to wholeheartedly recommend a supplement like this for

HOW TO TAKE CREATINE

Creatine supplementation generally begins with the person taking between 15 and 25 grams of creatine per day for 5 to 7 days, says Richard B. Kreider, Ph.D., assistant chair and director of the Exercise and Sports Nutrition Lab at the University of Memphis. This "loads" the muscles with creatine to maximize the levels of the amino acid. (For your exact loading dose, see "Creatine Loading" on page 322.)

After that, athletic people can maintain the increased levels of creatine in their muscles with a mere 2 to 5 grams of creatine per day. To calculate your precise maintenance dose, divide your body weight in pounds by 2.2 to get its equivalent in kilograms, then multiply that number by 0.03 gram. For example, a guy who weighs 220 pounds, which is equal to 100 kilograms, would take 3 grams a day.

Research data show that dosages up to 15.75 grams per day for 28 days is safe, according to Thomas Incledon, M.S., R.D., designer of the Hard-Body Diet. But people can expect improvements taking as little as 2 to 3 grams per day, he says. To maximize its effects, you should take creatine with carbohydrates—33 to 93 grams of simple sugars. Based on research using rats, some researchers are recommending using a 3-months-on, 1-month-off approach for supplementing with creatine. "Until better data become available, this seems like a prudent recommendation," he says.

Many different creatine preparations are available, from powders to capsules to chewable tablets to—believe it or not—effervescent formulations that bring to mind the old "plop, plop, fizz, fizz" Alka Seltzer commercials.

"The different types are all just bells and whistles," says Alan R. Stockard, D.O., medical director of sports medicine at the Osteopathic Medical Center of Texas at Fort Worth. "There is very little excitement to mixing up a nasty-tasting powder to make a grainy shake. So if people think a fizzy concoction sounds sexier, they will buy that one."

There is really no difference in how the creatine gets into your system. Pills are appealing because all you have to do is swallow. But the creatine won't get into your muscles any better or quicker with one preparation or another, says Incledon. "Effervescent formulas get into the blood faster, but once any creatine is in the blood, it's in the same form so there is no difference in uptake rate by muscle cells."

People seeking creatine supplementation should probably stick to creatine monohydrate, however, which is the most studied and probably most effective form of creatine, says Laura Spanbauer, R.D., a registered dietitian and sports nutrition counselor in Albany, New York.

most people—because when you do, everyone wants to take megadoses of the stuff," Dr. Stockard says. "They think, 'If a little is good, a lot would be better.'"

Short-term side effects of creatine use that have been reported include muscle cramping, muscle tearing, and dehydration. More recent studies show just the opposite effect in some cases.

The debate is about long-term safety. Many health care and fitness professionals fear that use of creatine over many years may have detrimental effects. Creatine is found naturally in the brain as well as the heart, testicles, uterus, and retinas—and creatine research really hasn't addressed what effect supplementation might have on those organs and tissues, says Dr. Juhn. Brain levels of creatine have been shown to increase during supplementation. But whether that could have any long-term detrimental health effect is unknown, and the fact that it is unknown concerns him, Dr. Juhn says.

Such concerns are as overblown as the belief that creatine will turn you into a superman, maintains Dr. Kreider, who has conducted a great deal of research on creatine. He says that several creatine studies have followed participants for 5 years with participants showing no ill effects.

"A lot of the studies out there on commonly used vitamins and minerals don't go out any farther than 5 years," says Dr. Kreider. "Actually, most ergogenic-aid-type studies don't even go past 3 months. For example, the longest carbohydrate supplementation study is 42 days." He maintains that few researchers doubt creatine's safety.

No one should expect massive improvements in exercise gains with the use of creatine.

The average gain in performance in all studies reporting statistically significant results, according to Dr. Kreider, is 10 to 15 percent.

A word to the wise: Taking creatine supplements may suppress your body's own production of creatine. On the bright side, this suppression apparently ceases when you stop taking creatine.

Obtaining "therapeutic" doses of creatine from food is impractical. The average balanced diet offers only 1 gram of creatine per day.

GLUTAMINE

Exercise depletes the body's stores of glutamine. Such depletion may inhibit recovery and reduce gains from exercise. Recent research suggests that taking a glutamine supplement following exercise can help to improve glutamine levels and help replenish muscle glycogen.

But glutamine's coolest potential is as a growth hormone releaser.

Growth hormone supercharges the muscle-building process. And some aminos, taken orally, increase its production and/or its release.

A 1995 study at the Louisiana State University College of Medicine showed that people who received a 2-gram dose of oral glutamine produced growth hormone levels four times that of their normal levels. However, no data measurements of changes in performance or body composition were taken, so we don't know how this affected the people involved, says Incledon. In fact, Incledon says, no study has demonstrated that glutamine supplementation changes body composition or improves performance.

Glutamine is one of the most abundant aminos in the body, notes Ronald Klatz, D.O., president of the American Academy of Anti-Aging Medicine in Chicago. But, he says, your system may not be able to synthesize all the glutamine that it needs when it is under physical stress such as exercise. Dr. Klatz recommends that you take 2 grams per day at bedtime to increase human growth hormone production and release from the anterior pituitary gland.

OTHER GROWTH HORMONE RELEASERS

Several other amino acids appear to stimulate growth hormone secretion, among them arginine, lysine, and ornithine.

Although any one of these aminos can act as growth hormone releasers, you may want to consider "stacking" (combining) lysine with glutamine, arginine, and/or ornithine for the best results, says Dr. Klatz.

He recommends that you have a physician check your blood levels of these aminos to see whether you are low in them. If you are, he suggests boosting them with the following dosages.

• **Arginine:** 2 to 5 grams before exercise and before going to sleep

• **Lysine:** 1-gram doses 1 hour before exercise, and before bedtime

• **Ornithine:** 2 to 5 grams before bedtime

Your metabolism is always changing, so while supplementing, have your blood levels evaluated four times a year to be sure that you are taking the right amounts, Dr. Klatz says.

All three of these amino acids can cause diarrhea when taken in high doses, and arginine can stimulate outbreaks of genital herpes in people who have the virus.

Creatine and other amino acids are not the only powdered wonders on the shelves of your health food store. Sharing space are various protein formulas.

The question is, do you need them to build a hard body? Let's consider a few.

PROTEIN SUPPLEMENTS

Remember that you only need between 1.4 and 1.8 grams of protein per kilogram of body weight per day.

"Beyond that, protein is not substantially beneficial," Dr. Brolinson stresses.

"The excess protein that you consume is excreted through your kidneys or your liver," Dr. Stockard explains. This puts unnecessary stress on your body.

Very few people need supplementation to get the required amount of protein. In fact, most of us eat too much protein.

Athletic people do need slightly more protein than other people, but that's generally made up for by their higher caloric intake.

Although high-protein diets are currently the craze, none of our advisors recommends following them for any sustained period, and some warn that such diets may actually cause kidney damage. With the Hard-Body Plan, you get the protein you need without the risk.

MESSING WITH HORMONES

Hormonal supplementation hit its stride when researchers discovered the myriad health benefits of estrogen replacement therapy for postmenopausal women.

Then, researchers started to explore hormone replacement for middle-age and elderly men, with some promising results.

Now the whippersnappers want to start taking hormones to fend off Mother Nature before she even gets a swing in.

Two hot hormones among fitness-minded men right now are DHEA and androstenedione. We don't recommend either, unless a doctor discovers that you have low levels and need supplementation.

DHEA

Known in clinical and research circles by its tongue-twisting full name of dehydroepiandrosterone, DHEA is a hormonal product that has been touted as a veritable fountain of youth.

Animal studies have shown that DHEA can slow aging, strengthen the immune system, stabilize blood sugar, ward off cancer and heart disease, and burn fat while building muscle mass. Few such studies have been completed using humans. Human studies have shown that it can increase levels of testosterone and other sex steroidal hormones.

"The theory behind DHEA supplementation is to 'supercharge' the hormonal system," Dr. Brolinson says. He is a skeptic.

DHEA is important, and it is sometimes referred to as the mother of all hormones because it is used by the body to create the sex steroids testosterone, estrogen, progesterone, and corticosterone—certainly not "all hormones," but a cool selection.

But even DHEA proponents admit that supplementation may temporarily cripple the body's ability to create DHEA itself.

And side effects of DHEA use can include acne, irritability, irregular heart rhythms, liver problems, enlarged male breasts, accelerated growth of existing tumors, hair loss, and a possible increased risk of prostate cancer.

So, with the questionable benefit-to-risk ratio, is taking DHEA really worth it?

Probably not, says Dr. Brolinson.

ANDROSTENEDIONE

Andro, as its friends call it, is a precursor hormone involved in the production of testosterone. It got a big publicity boost a couple years back when it became public that some heavy hitters in the Major Leagues were using andro supplements.

Andro defenders say that supplementation with just 100 milligrams of the hormone increases testosterone in the body by 300 percent, allowing athletes to train harder and recover more quickly.

Detractors argue that the hormone too closely resembles an anabolic steroid and may pose similar health risks, including liver and heart problems, breast enlargement, personality disorders, and acne.

Furthermore, recent research at Iowa State University's department of health and human performance suggests that andro supplementation doesn't increase serum testosterone levels meaningfully and doesn't increase muscle mass.

"A single dose will elevate testosterone levels briefly," Dr. Brolinson says. "But that increased level drops by half within 90 minutes. It is unlikely that this small, transient increase is of significant benefit to any athlete."

In addition, long-term andro supplementation, like DHEA supplementation, may impair your body's natural ability to produce the hormone, he says. Luckily, however, your body does regain its ability to produce the hormone once supplementation is stopped.

A Vegetarian's Guide to High-Energy Muscle Food
Beef Up without Meat

A WELL-MANAGED VEGETARIAN DIET IS HEALTHY AND RELATIVELY SIMPLE TO FOLLOW. KEEP UP WITH YOUR PROTEIN REQUIREMENTS, YOUR CALORIE INTAKE, AND A FEW IMPORTANT VITAMINS AND MINERALS FOUND MAINLY IN MEAT, AND YOU'LL GET EVERYTHING YOU NEED TO BUILD HARD MUSCLE.

Some real men eat quiche. And they eat nuts, seeds, tofu, tempeh, and dozens of other plant foods. These guys lift weights. They slim down, bulk up, and build rock-hard bodies.

What they don't eat is meat—including fish, in many cases. And some, called vegans, (pronounced VEE-guns) also avoid eggs, dairy, and animal-derived products of any kind. Vegetarian body-builders grow big muscles on broccoli, beans, and other foods that come from the ground.

An example is four-time Mr. Universe Bill Pearl, a longtime vegetarian who gradually gave up meat for health reasons and still kept a hard body.

Throughout this book, we've promoted the benefits of a more plant-based, less meat-centered diet because meat in moderation has a lot of muscle-building benefits for an active guy. But you can go meatless just as well.

Although vegetarians eat better than nonvegetarians on average, don't assume that vegetarian diets are always superior. Unless you replace the nutrients formerly supplied by meat and other animal products, you'll wipe out nutritional balance—and good health. If you throw out the meat, fish, and poultry section of the food pyramid, you've got to replace it with dried beans, nuts, and seeds.

Eating badly, even if your diet sounds healthy, won't power your workouts, speed recovery, or grow muscles. Whether you decide to give up only red meat or to go whole hog and adopt a vegan diet, you need to pay attention to details. It's not hard to learn the details that you need to monitor.

317

"Vegetarian athletes can't just wing it and expect that it will all work out right," says Richard B. Kreider, Ph.D., director of a nutrition laboratory in Memphis.

Vegetarian weight lifters have slightly higher protein requirements than their meat-eating counterparts. But by eating a number of different plant proteins, a vegetarian can get all of his essential amino acids.

Much of the concern about athletes and vegetarian diets centers on—surprise, surprise—protein. Can vegetarian strength trainers get enough protein? The answer is yes, but it takes focused effort.

Vegetarians need to eat slightly more protein than meat eaters do, because plant proteins are slightly more difficult to digest due to the extra fiber in plants.

Some protein seems to get lost in the process, says Virginia Messina, R.D., author of *The Vegetarian Way*.

Weight lifters need somewhere in the range of 1.4 to 1.8 grams of protein per kilogram of body

TYPES OF VEGETARIANS

You go to lunch with this magnificently built woman you met in the history section at the bookstore. Over wine, she describes her passion for early 20th-century labor history, her new Volkswagen Beetle, and *weight lifting*. When the waitress takes the order, your date adds, "Oh . . . and I'm a vegetarian."

"That's cool. That's cool," you say, thinking you'll have the spaghetti and tofu with the organic sauce.

But then she orders the salmon bisque, and you say something like, "Uh . . . isn't fish a meat?"

(For the record, it is a meat, but traditionally some vegetarians have regarded fish differently than they do a steer or sow. Maybe it's because fish swim. But then again, some have regarded fowl differently too. Maybe it's because they fly.)

"Fish is definitely not meat," she retorts.

You would like to disagree, but why have a dietary debate with this brainy beautiful being? You'll lose the argument and, besides, you're hooked. You can already picture her at your place in a T-shirt, eating a bagel-and-yogurt breakfast before you both head off to the gym.

But don't get ahead of yourself. Get your definitions straight first. There are several types of vegetarians. This young lady is a semivegetarian.

Here's a rundown on the latest and most politically correct labels.

- **Semivegetarian:** Usually excludes red meat but may eat poultry, fish, and seafood.

- **Ovo-lactovegetarian:** Eats dairy and eggs but excludes all flesh.

- **Lactovegetarian:** Eats dairy but excludes eggs and all flesh.

- **Ovo-vegetarian:** Eats eggs but excludes dairy and all flesh.

- **Strict vegetarian or vegan:** Eats no animal foods at all.

- **Macrobiotic:** Eats whole cereal grains, vegetables, soups, beans, and sea vegetables.

weight each day. A vegetarian weight lifter needs more, Messina says.

"I would definitely recommend being on the higher end of that range. Two grams per kilogram wouldn't be too much," she says. "If you are eating a high-protein diet, plant protein may be better for you than animal protein because it can lower cholesterol levels and reduce your risk of heart disease."

Protein from vegetables, legumes, and grains differs significantly from animal protein. It has different amino acid content. Meats, eggs, dairy, and all other animal products are called complete proteins because they contain the nine essential amino acids needed by your body. Your liver can manufacture nonessential amino acids as needed, but your body gets the essential amino acids either from food or by breaking down, or "catabolizing," muscle. Catabolizing muscle is not what we want to be doing.

Each of the various plant proteins contains all of the essential amino acids. They may, however, be high in some of the amino acids but low in others. Therefore, a vegetarian must eat a selected variety of plant proteins—basically mixing and matching some essential amino acids here and others there. For example, eating beans and rice turns two incomplete proteins into a complete protein.

If you're a meat eater, the animal has already done this assembly work for you. By eating its flesh, drinking its milk, or eating its eggs, you can take in everything you need in the right proportions.

If you don't eat any animal products, vary the plant proteins you eat at every snack and meal, and emphasize high-quality protein such as soy. Constant variation guarantees that you'll take in adequate amino acids for muscle repair and recovery.

How difficult it is to assemble all the essential amino acids depends on how strict you are in your vegetarianism.

A person who eats some animal products needn't worry about protein. As long as you eat enough calories each day and eat many types of protein-rich plant foods, you should be fine. Vegans, however, have a difficult but not an impossible task.

To shift your diet toward more protein-rich foods, eat more legumes, such as beans, lentils, nuts, tofu, tempeh, and soy nuts, Messina recommends.

Anything with soy is good because soy is nearly as complete a protein as dairy products are. Nuts, legumes, and grains are much less complete.

"Soy is really an amazing, versatile food," Messina says. "You can do a lot with it."

Textured vegetable protein (TVP), made from soy flour, is a favorite among vegetarians. It has the consistency of ground meat and can be used in spaghetti sauces, chili, and sloppy joes. You can even form it into burgers.

Exactly how much of these plant proteins you need to eat really varies with your body weight, but you should shoot for at least six ½-cup servings per day, Messina says.

For many years, vegetarians were told that they needed to pair up certain plant proteins at each meal. This eating strategy, called mutual supplementation, maintained that incomplete proteins had to arrive in the gut at the same time. That's why really strict vegetarians have always been careful about planning their meals, making sure to eat a legume with a grain.

In recent years, there has been much less emphasis on this precision, and for most folks it probably isn't necessary. As long as vegetarians take in adequate calories and eat a wide variety of protein-rich foods over the course of the day, they shouldn't have any problem meeting their amino acid needs.

But during especially intense periods of strength training, vegetarians should stick with the old regimen of always mixing grains and legumes, Dr. Kreider recommends. Also, he says, and as we earlier advised, vegetarians should eat some protein at every meal and snack, instead of bunching the protein into just one or two meals.

"You want to keep the reservoir of amino acids in your body full in order to maximize repair and recovery," he says. "If you don't get enough protein—and enough overall calories—your body will start catabolizing muscle. You want to prevent that breakdown."

Vegetarian athletes who don't pay attention to their protein intake have longer recovery times between workouts and are more prone to plateaus, meaning that they work out regularly but see no results, Dr. Kreider says.

Taking in enough calories can be a problem for active guys who eat few or no animal products. Strict vegetarians should eat high-calorie plant foods and consider meal replacement drinks and smoothies.

One way to take some of the guesswork out of vegetarian eating is to consume a high-carbohydrate/high-protein replacement meal a couple of times a day, Dr. Kreider says.

If you eat dairy products, whey protein powder works well. Soy protein is almost as effective. You can make your own smoothie by blending juice, ice, and fruit with yogurt or soy powder or tofu, says Enette Larson, R.D., Ph.D., a sports nutritionist and consultant to the athletic teams at the University of Alabama at Birmingham.

"The commercial meal replacement can get expensive to drink every day," she says. "It's really easy to make your own—and you can make them good-tasting too."

Not only are meal replacements good sources of carbs and proteins but they also contain an ample supply of calories.

Vegetarian athletes sometimes rob themselves of needed calories by focusing on their carbohydrate intake and eating only bulky and low-calorie food, says Dr. Larson.

"You have to eat more calorie-dense foods which include fats," she says. "It's okay to eat a certain quantity of fat, especially when you have really high-calorie needs like most athletes."

Fill your calorie and fat needs with cheese, eggs, and dairy products. You can also add fats strictly from plant sources, with olive and canola oil, avocados, and soy milk, tofu, soybeans, and other soy products. Nuts and seeds also contain good amounts of fatty acids, antioxidants, and fiber. Your best bets are almonds, peanuts, and sunflower seeds, and peanut and almond butter, says Messina.

"I'm really big on nuts and seeds. They contain all kinds of good stuff in addition to fat. I think every vegetarian should have a couple of tablespoons every day," Messina says.

Carbohydrates, not surprisingly, are rarely a problem for vegetarians—except for maybe having too much, Dr. Larson says. Fruits and vegetables; legumes; and rice, pasta, bread, and other types of grains—the staples of a veggie diet—supply all the carbohydrate muscle fuel a Hard-Body guy needs.

Vitamins and minerals that are supplied in small amounts—or not at all—in a vegetarian diet can be obtained through a daily multivitamin/mineral supplement.

Vegetarians usually take in enough vitamins and minerals, the occasional exceptions being iron, calcium, vitamin B$_{12}$, and zinc. Whether you should be concerned about a deficiency really depends on the type of vegetarianism you practice. And most of the time, you can avoid any problem by eating a certain way or taking a common daily vitamin/mineral supplement, says Dr. Larson.

If you drink milk and eat yogurt or other dairy products, don't worry about calcium. If not, you need to load up on collard greens, kale, and other dark leafy vegetables, as well as tofu and calcium-fortified orange juice, says Messina. That may give you enough calcium, since a man's calcium needs are 1,000 milligrams a day.

Vegetarians may, however, experience iron deficiency because of problems with iron absorption. Meats and fish contain heme iron, the easily absorbed form of iron. Whole grains, legumes, vegetables, dried fruits, and nuts contain nonheme iron, says Dr. Larson. One of the things that will make nonheme more absorbable is vitamin C (ascorbic acid).

You should eat vitamin C–rich food at every meal. Have fruits, especially citrus, and vegetables such as peppers, broccoli, and cauliflower, says Dr. Larson. Tomatoes, which contain both iron and vitamin C, do both jobs at once. Even using cast-iron cookware can improve iron absorption.

In addition to supplying easily absorbable iron, meat satisfies most guys' zinc requirements, and there is some evidence that vegetarians may be zinc-deficient. Ironically, a meatless diet that includes whole grains, nuts, pumpkin seeds, legumes, and wheat germ is rich with zinc. But chemicals called phytates in some grains and legumes seem to block zinc absorption. And most vegetarians eat loads of legumes and grains.

Don't take megadoses of zinc supplements, though, Messina says. "All you really need is a daily vitamin/mineral supplement that contains the DV for zinc." The recommended Daily Value for men is 15 milligrams.

BECOMING VEGETARIAN

So you wanna veg out? You'll have to break a few habits, like hitting the drive-thru for a burger on the way home from work or having beer and steaks with your buddies on football Sundays. But you can do it.

The best advice is to ease into a vegetarian diet. Changing from a flesh eater to a plant muncher isn't something you do overnight, says Susan Kleiner, R.D., Ph.D., a sports nutritionist in Mercer Island, Washington. Here's what Dr. Kleiner suggests:

- Start off by eating several vegetarian meals each week.

- Don't stop all meats immediately. Start with red meat and then, if you want, cut back on pork, chicken, and fish.

- Gradually introduce more high-fiber vegetarian foods. Fiber bulks up your stool and slows digestion. But too much fiber too soon may give you a pain in the gut and embarrassing flatulence.

- Try many types of vegetarian fare. Don't settle on eating just a few foods. You'll soon grow bored.

- Experiment with recipes in vegetarian cookbooks. Don't just eat boiled or fried zucchini; make a zucchini calzone or casserole. Forget the bland. Spice it up.

A daily vitamin supplement will also take care of any deficiencies of vitamin B_{12}, an especially important vitamin for the manufacture of red blood cells and nerves. You only get B_{12} from animal products. If you're a vegan, you definitely need to supplement B_{12} or eat some type of food fortified with B vitamins; you should be able to find a B-vitamin-enriched cereal, says Messina.

The recommended Daily Value isn't much: just 6 micrograms per day.

A vegetarian bodybuilder who eats no meat or fish cannot internally manufacture all the creatine he requires for muscle building. Consider using a synthetic creatine supplement.

Low amounts of creatine probably don't concern most vegetarians, but you're a weight lifter, and you need a generous amount of creatine in your muscles. Creatine is a natural substance that aids muscle contractions and forms a short-term energy source.

Creatine comes primarily from meats and fish. There are only trace amounts in vegetables and a few other plant foods. Cranberries, for example, have just 0.01 gram per pound, while salmon has 2 grams per pound and herring has 4.5 grams per pound.

Your body manufactures some creatine internally by assembling three amino acids. A Hard-Body Man who's a vegetarian is missing the additional creatine from meats, though, and he'll need to supplement, says Dr. Kreider.

CREATINE LOADING

As you creatively imagine how you'll look as a muscular creature—a true Hard-Body creation!—don't forget one of the details: creatine. Depending on how deep you are into your veggie lifestyle, you may not have enough creatine in your body to support serious weight lifting, says Richard B. Kreider, Ph.D., an exercise nutrition expert and coauthor of *Creatine: The Power Supplement*.

"If you don't eat meat but eat fish regularly, you probably won't have any problem," Dr. Kreider says. "Otherwise you should be supplementing with synthetic creatine."

Initially, Dr. Kreider recommends taking 0.3 gram of creatine per kilogram of body weight each day for about 5 days. This relatively high dosage loads the muscles, Dr. Kreider says. To figure your need for this 5-day period, divide your weight in pounds by 2.2 to give you kilograms, then multiply that number by 0.3. If you're 175 pounds, here's your math:

$$175 \text{ pounds} \div 2.2 \text{ pounds per kilogram} = 79.5 \text{ kilograms}$$

$$79.5 \text{ kilograms} \times 0.3 \text{ gram of creatine per kilogram of body weight} = \text{about 24 grams of creatine}$$

Thomas Incledon, M.S., R.D., points out that 5 grams equals 1 level teaspoon—an easy way to measure.

"With vegetarians, you need to supersaturate the muscle and get the levels up," Dr. Kreider says. "After that, reduce to about 2 grams per day."

To calculate your precise maintenance dose, divide your body weight in pounds by 2.2 to get its equivalent in kilograms, then multiply that number by 0.03 gram. For example, a guy who weighs 220 pounds, which is equal to 100 kilograms, would take 3 grams a day.

And since you've probably been deficient in creatine for a long time, you might want to load up at first, though it isn't necessary, says Hard-Body Diet designer Thomas Incledon, M.S., R.D. He says that if you take a 5-gram dose daily, you'll reach full-load levels in 30 days. Or you can do more intense loading and reach full load in 5 days. After 5 days of loading, it is important to reduce your intake to a maintenance dose. (See "Creatine Loading.")

Now you know that a range of different eating styles can take you to a hard body, just as different paths leading up a mountain can bring you to its summit. A vegetarian deep ecologist can get there with food he likes, as can a meat-eating lumberjack and all the varied types and styles of men in between.

You don't need to cram into a one-size-fits-all fad diet or torture yourself with huge amounts of any one type of food. Your body just needs a variety of wholesome foods and drinks, spaced throughout your waking hours.

The Hard-Body Plan does that. Vegetarians need to adapt it only slightly, as we've indicated, and, of course, to their personal needs.

Vegetarian or not, you will adapt this plan to your own goals and starting weight, and to your own tastes and lifestyle. In the next chapter, called Personalizing the Plan, we'll tell you exactly how to mold this plan so it fits you perfectly as you accomplish your Hard-Body goals.

INDIVIDUAL PRECISION
PERSONALIZING THE PLAN

Like comedy teams throughout history, David Spade and the late Chris Farley of *Saturday Night Live* fame operated on the "heavy + skinny = wacky fun" formula. The lumbering Farley would stumble around, crushing furniture under his bulk, and the bony Spade would offer flinty, biting insults.

Whether you have the heft of one or the wiriness of the other (or, more likely, a weight and build somewhere in between), you'll approach the Hard-Body Plan in the same way that they approached punch lines: uniquely and with variations that likely will work only for you.

You will need and want to customize the Hard-Body Plan to your specific weight and goals.

To illustrate concepts throughout the book, we've used a 5-foot-10, 175-pound reference man who wants to bulk up a little. But we know that a one-size-fits-all approach won't fit every reader any more than one pair of pants would. That's why we offer two sets of nutritional stats here: one for the thin guy whose Hard Body will require more bulk, and another for a guy who'll need to trim away flab to find his Hard Body.

You already have a pretty good idea of which guy you are. If you have any uncertainty, a body fat measurement can point you in the right direction, says Thomas Incledon, M.S., R.D., designer of the Hard-Body Diet. You should be able to get your body composition checked at a health club—preferably, he says, by someone with an advanced degree in exercise science or exercise physiology, or by a registered dietitian. (Many noncredentialed strength trainers know how to wield the calipers and can make the calculations just fine, but credentials assure you that they've been properly taught the procedure.)

The tester will probably measure skin folds at several sites around your body to determine how much fat you're carrying. An ideal body fat range to shoot for would be about 12 to 18 percent, says Incledon. Under 8 percent is getting too trim for best health, and you may need to add a bit of padding. Over 25 percent means that you probably need to trim some calories and slim your waistline.

Pick your scenario. Are you Weight-Loss Man or Weight-Gain Man? (If you aren't concerned about losing fat and just want to put on muscle, you're a weight-gain man. We know some of them, and we know a lot more weight-loss men. No shame in being either. This program is all about improvement no matter where you start.) Choose your nutrition stats (see page 326) and familiarize yourself with them. You'll notice that the protein amounts are the same for both kinds of guys. Weight-loss guys will be cutting calories by eating fewer grams of carbohydrates and fat.

This plan isn't one-size-fits-all, and it's not just two-sizes-fit-all, either. If you're a jackhammer operator or other type who puts plenty of sweat into your occupation, you're going to burn a lot more energy before you even put in your workout than a sedentary guy who works behind a desk does. Therefore, you'll need to take in more calories than the chart recommends.

So, as you progress through the plan, keep an eye on your weight. If you're dropping more than 2 pounds a week, you need to bump up your caloric intake a notch. You're going too fast. Try adding 300 to 500 calories to your daily total to slow down the rate of weight loss. Similarly, if you're gaining more than 2 pounds a week, you need to cut back and slow down. Cut 300 to 500 calories from your daily total. Why? Because it's really hard to gain that much muscle that quickly, so in all likelihood you're packing on fat as well, Incledon explains.

Remember, you'll just be in the weight room a few hours a week, but food is *everywhere.*

The endless stream of decisions that you make in front of the refrigerator and at restaurants, quick-stops, vending machines, and grocery stores will play a big role in how far your gym work will take you.

In part 4, we'll lead you through menus at the places where you'll be making those decisions—from Burger King to the salad bar to your own kitchen—and we'll train your eye to judge the nutritional value of the foods that you encounter.

Find where you fit on the weight-loss or weight-gain "Daily Quotas" chart we provide on page 326. Write down the numbers from that line on the back of a business card or on an index card that you can slip into your wallet for frequent reference. Write down your daily quotas for calories, carbohydrates, protein, and fat.

Then, do a little math. Divide each of those numbers by six and write down those results. Those numbers are your target at each meal or snacktime. (Technically, on workout days, you eat seven times, because your workout snack is divided into a preworkout snack and a postworkout snack. The combined total calories, though, equal one regular snack.)

You'll need to have these numbers in hand when you look through the menus that follow. Compare your quotas with the numbers listed for each meal. If you're working on weight loss, you may need to have smaller portion sizes than the ones listed in the menus. If you're bulking up, you might spoon yourself bigger portions. Only you will know, and you will know based on your own numbers. Carry this book with you for a few days for reference as you encounter real-world foods. You'll quickly get a handle on portion sizes and food types.

As you work through the Hard-Body Plan, your weight will change. When it changes, your numbers will change. You'll need to come back to the chart and calculate new numbers.

We suggest that you check your weight, on the same scale, and recalculate your portions at least every 2 weeks. This is scientific, Hard-Body eating. And, believe it, you aren't going to starve!

There's a world of food out there and a right way to eat it. Get ready to dig in.

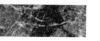

DAILY QUOTAS

Body Weight (lb)	For Weight-Loss Man				For Weight-Gain Man			
	Calories	Protein (g)	Fat (g)	Carbs (g)	Calories	Protein (g)	Fat (g)	Carbs (g)
170	2,135	139	47	288	3,235	139	72	508
175	2,213	143	49	299	3,313	143	74	519
180	2,290	147	51	311	3,390	147	75	531
185	2,368	151	53	322	3,468	151	77	542
190	2,445	155	54	334	3,545	155	79	554
195	2,523	159	56	345	3,623	159	81	565
200	2,600	163	58	357	3,700	163	82	577
205	2,678	168	60	368	3,778	168	84	588
210	2,755	172	61	379	3,855	172	86	599
215	2,833	176	63	391	3,933	176	87	611
220	2,910	180	65	402	4,010	180	89	622
225	2,988	184	66	414	4,088	184	91	634
230	3,065	188	68	425	4,165	188	93	645
235	3,143	192	70	436	4,243	192	94	656
240	3,220	196	72	448	4,320	196	96	668
245	3,298	200	73	459	4,398	200	98	679
250	3,375	204	75	471	4,475	204	99	691
255	3,453	208	77	482	4,553	208	101	702
260	3,530	212	78	494	4,630	212	103	714
265	3,608	217	80	505	4,708	217	105	725
270	3,685	221	82	516	4,785	221	106	736
275	3,763	225	84	528	4,863	225	108	748
280	3,840	229	85	539	4,940	229	110	759
285	3,918	233	87	551	5,018	233	112	771
290	3,995	237	89	562	5,095	237	113	782
295	4,073	241	91	573	5,173	241	115	793
300	4,150	245	92	585	5,250	245	117	805

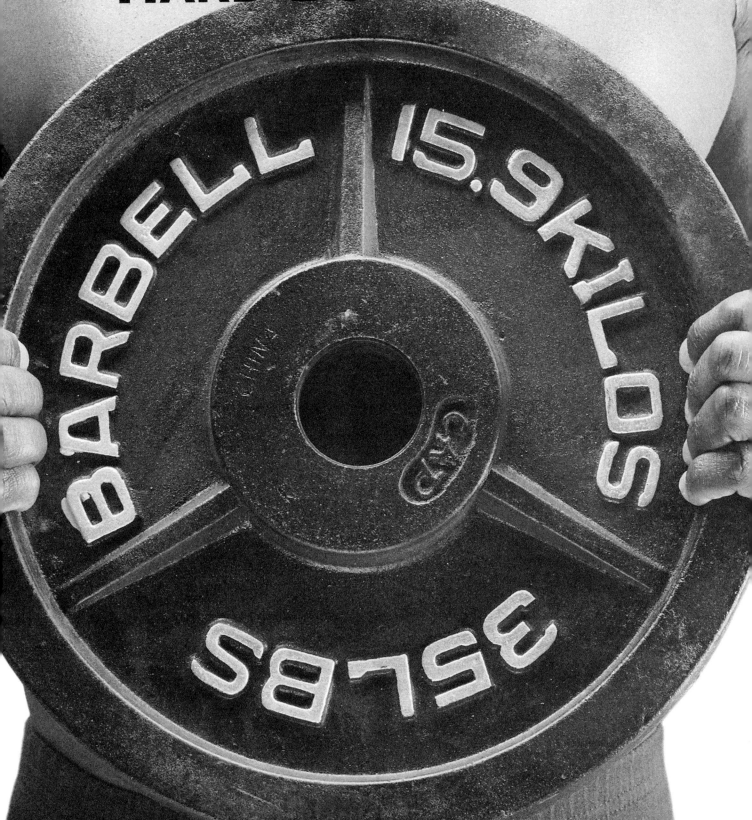

PART 4

THE
HARD-BODY DIET

16 PERFECT MORNING FEASTS

BREAKFAST

When your alarm clock jangles, do you smack the snooze button until the final instant that you have to haul your sorry carcass out of bed, jump into your clothes, and race to work?

Bad idea. While you sleep, your blood sugar levels nosedive. If you don't replenish them by breaking your fast (*breakfast*, pretty clever, huh?), chances are that the day's demands will break you. You won't have enough energy to even compete in the rat race, much less win it.

A good, nutritional breakfast is essential to the Hard-Body Plan. And it's strategic. Because you burn food more efficiently in the morning, you'll start the day with foods that are most quickly converted into energy: carbohydrates and proteins. If you consistently eat a Hard-Body breakfast of cereals, fruits, and fat-free milk instead of a Homer Simpson breakfast of doughnuts, bacon, and half-and-half, you'll look less and less like the Pillsbury Doughboy and more like the stud muffin that nature intended you to be.

Remember, these breakfasts are for our 175-pound, 5-foot-10-inch reference man. You will need to adjust portions up or down a bit relative to your own weight and goals as you determined in Personalizing the Plan on page 324. Also if you can't find some of these items in your area, feel free to make healthy substitutions.

FOR THE WEIGHT-LOSS MAN

Scrambled-Egg Sandwich/Cook and eat it in a flash

- 1   large whole egg
- 3   large egg whites
- 2   slices whole-wheat bread
- 1   tomato, sliced
- ½   cup orange juice

Scramble the whole egg and egg whites in a bowl. Fry them in a pan spritzed with vegetable oil spray, dump them onto the bread, and garnish with sliced tomato. Coat the bread with spicy mustard if you like. If you're wide awake or ambitious, or if you just want to impress yourself, add green peppers, onions, or other vegetables to the eggs. If you're in a hurry, munch on some of the tomato slices while cooking the eggs, toss a couple of slices on the sandwich, wrap the works in a napkin, and eat it while you drive. Gulp down a glass of orange juice on your way out the door.

Totals: 355 calories, 46 g carbohydrates, 24.1 g protein, 8.4 g fat

	Whole Egg	Egg Whites	Whole-Wheat Bread	Tomato	OJ
Calories	75	46	146	31	57
Carbohydrates (g)	0.6	1	25.8	5.7	12.9
Protein (g)	6.3	10.5	5.4	1	0.9
Fat (g)	5.3	0	2.4	0.4	0.3

Boiled-Egg Sandwich/Just the thing for a hard-boiled guy

- 3   whole eggs, boiled
- 2   slices wheat bread
- ¾   cup orange juice
- ½   cup fat-free milk

Hate to cook in the A.M.? Boil eggs the night before while you watch *The Late Show*, then stick 'em in the fridge. At rise and shine, peel and slice the eggs. (Save all the whites, and toss two of the yolks.) Sip the OJ while you're working with the eggs. Put the eggs on the bread and wash 'em down with the milk.

Totals: 369 calories, 52 g carbohydrates, 23 g protein, 7.6 g fat

	Whole Egg	Egg Whites	Wheat Bread	OJ	Milk
Calories	75	29	134	84	47
Carbohydrates (g)	0.6	0.3	24.8	20.3	6
Protein (g)	6.3	7	4.4	0.8	4.5
Fat (g)	5.3	0	2	0	0.3

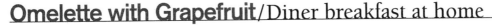

Omelette with Grapefruit/Diner breakfast at home

- 1 large whole egg
- 3 large egg whites
- 1 slice rye bread
- 1 grapefruit
- 1 cup regular or decaf coffee
- 1 teaspoon sugar
- ½ cup fat-free milk

Cook the eggs in a nonstick pan coated with vegetable oil spray, fold 'em over, cook some more, and *voilà!*— you have a really boring omelette. To make it more conversational, add some peppers and mushrooms. Have the bread and fruit on the side, and pour yourself some joe. If you hate grapefruit, substitute an orange.

Totals: 361 calories, 49.2 g carbohydrates, 25 g protein, 6.8 g fat

	Whole Egg	Egg Whites	Rye Bread	Grapefruit	Coffee	Sugar	Milk
Calories	75	46	68	103	5	17	47
Carbohydrates (g)	0.6	1	12.7	23.8	0.9	4.2	6
Protein (g)	6.3	10.5	2.3	1.2	0.2	0	4.5
Fat (g)	5.3	0	0.9	0.3	0	0	0.3

Bagel Breakfast to Go/Throw it together and eat it in the car

- ½ cinnamon-raisin bagel
- 1 tablespoon smooth, no-salt-added peanut butter
- 1 small banana
- 1½ cups fat-free milk

Spread peanut butter on the bagel. Stick it in an empty margarine tub or other container so it won't end up face-down on your car seat. (If you use reduced-fat peanut butter, you can have 2 tablespoons, big guy.) Stash the banana in your briefcase, or put some slices atop the peanut butter and inhale the rest. Fill a water bottle or car mug with fat-free milk to wash the peanut butter down your throat in time for the morning meeting.

Totals: 382 calories, 52 g carbohydrates, 19.8 g protein, 9.8 g fat

	Bagel	Peanut Butter	Banana	Milk
Calories	36	102	103	141
Carbohydrates (g)	7.2	3.1	23.7	18
Protein (g)	1.3	4	1	13.5
Fat (g)	0.2	8.2	0.5	0.9

Waffles with Frozen Fruit/My cherry amour

- 1½ whole-grain frozen waffles
- ½ cup frozen cherries
- 2 cups fat-free milk

This dessertlike breakfast is great for guys who hate real cooking. Just microwave the waffles and cherries for a minute, then wash 'em down with fat-free milk.

Totals: 376 calories, 56.7 g carbohydrates, 22.1 g protein, 5.8 g fat

	Waffles	Cherries	Milk
Calories	129	59	188
Carbohydrates (g)	20.2	12.5	24
Protein (g)	3.1	1	18
Fat (g)	4.1	0.5	1.2

Yogurt That Packs a Crunch/Mix it up, eat it on the go

- 1 cup low-calorie, fat-free yogurt
- 1 ounce low-fat granola
- 1 teaspoon flaxseed oil (Yes, some oil is good for you!)
- 1 ounce toasted plain wheat germ

Choose any flavor of yogurt you want, as long as it has 90 to 100 calories per cup. Dump it into a plastic container, mix in the goodies, and spoon it down as you speed along the freeway.

Totals: 365 calories, 49.7 g carbohydrates, 20.7 g protein, 9.2 g fat

	Yogurt	Granola	Flaxseed Oil	Wheat Germ
Calories	92	114	42	117
Carbohydrates (g)	13	22.6	0	14.1
Protein (g)	10	2.4	0	8.3
Fat (g)	0	1.5	4.7	3

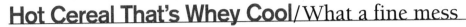

Hot Cereal That's Whey Cool/What a fine mess

- 6 ounces Maypo (or other whole-grain cereal)
- ½ cup fat-free milk
- 1 teaspoon flaxseed oil
- 1 ounce seedless raisins
- 1 scoop powdered whey protein, such as Designer Protein Chocolate Whey

Mix the Maypo with unsalted water and nuke it. Then mix the milk, flaxseed oil, raisins, and powdered protein into the cereal. The result: a great hot breakfast and only one lousy bowl to wash.

Totals: 395 calories, 53.5 g carbohydrates, 27 g protein, 7.8 g fat

	Maypo	Milk	Flaxseed Oil	Raisins	Whey Protein
Calories	122	47	42	95	89
Carbohydrates (g)	22.6	6	0	22.4	2.5
Protein (g)	4.1	4.5	0	0.9	17.5
Fat (g)	1.7	0.3	4.7	0.1	1

Hot Cereal with Vanilla Whey/More than plain vanilla

- 6 ounces Quaker Creamy Wheat Enriched Farina
- ½ cup fat-free milk
- 1 teaspoon flaxseed oil
- 1 cup unsweetened frozen blackberries
- 1 scoop whey protein, such as Designer Protein French Vanilla Whey

Not a chocolate lover? Try this vanilla variation. Mix farina and unsalted water, and nuke 'em in a bowl. Mix the milk, flaxseed oil, frozen blackberries, and vanilla whey into the cereal.

Totals: 364 calories, 50.9 g carbohydrates, 24.9 g protein, 6.5 g fat

	Farina	Milk	Flaxseed Oil	Blackberries	Whey Protein
Calories	88	47	42	108	79
Carbohydrates (g)	19.2	6	0	23.7	2
Protein (g)	2.6	4.5	0	1.8	16
Fat (g)	0.1	0.3	4.7	0.6	0.8

Hot Cereal That's Peachy Keen/Is Georgia on your mind?

- **4   ounces Wheatena**
- **1   cup fat-free milk**
- **1   teaspoon flaxseed oil**
- **1   ounce whole grain amaranth**
- **1   medium-size fresh peach**

Mix Wheatena and unsalted water, then microwave. Add milk, flaxseed oil, amaranth, and the peach minus the pit. (We like crunchy, but not that crunchy.) If you prefer, have the peach on the side.

Totals: 358 calories, 55.1 g carbohydrates, 16.1 g protein, 7.8 g fat

	Wheatena	Milk	Flaxseed Oil	Amaranth	Peach
Calories	68	93	42	108	47
Carbohydrates (g)	13.4	12	0	18.8	10.9
Protein (g)	2.3	9	0	4.1	0.7
Fat (g)	0.6	0.5	4.7	1.9	0.1

Bacon and Cold Cereal/The bacon diet? You bet!

- **6   slices light, lean Canadian-style bacon**
- **2   ounces plain shredded wheat**
- **½   cup fat-free milk**

Cook the bacon in a pan. Serve it alongside the cereal and milk. Lean meats are okay once in a while, but don't overdo it. Most bacon is so high in sodium and chemicals that it's a wonder it doesn't glow in the dark.

Totals: 321 calories, 52 g carbohydrates, 28.5 g protein, 3.3 g fat

	Canadian-Style Bacon	Shredded Wheat	Milk
Calories	66	208	47
Carbohydrates (g)	0	46	6
Protein (g)	18	6	4.5
Fat (g)	3	0	0.3

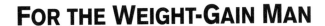

FOR THE WEIGHT-GAIN MAN

Turkey Sausage with Cereal/Gobble this quick and tasty meal

- 2 ounces cooked Louis Rich Turkey Smoked Sausage
- ¾ cup Kellogg's Complete Oat Bran Flakes
- 1 cup fat-free milk
- 1 teaspoon flaxseed oil
- 2 sliced small bananas

Cook the sausage in a pan. Serve alongside the cereal, which gets topped with the milk and oil. If you'd rather not go bananas this morning, substitute 12 ounces of OJ.

Totals: 550 calories, 84.8 g carbohydrates, 23 g protein, 12.8 g fat

	Sausage	Bran Flakes	Milk	Flaxseed Oil	Banana
Calories	90	119	93	42	206
Carbohydrates (g)	2.2	23.2	12	0	47.4
Protein (g)	8.1	3.9	9	0	2
Fat (g)	5.4	1.2	0.5	4.7	1

Carrot Muffins and Fruit/It doesn't get much easier than this

- 2 low-fat carrot muffins, about 1½ ounces each (or any other muffin with 3 grams of fat or less)
- 2 teaspoons soft margarine
- 1 cup fat-free milk
- 1 small orange

If you really hate cleaning up after yourself, this ready-made, grab-and-go breakfast will only dirty a knife and a glass. One knife, one glass? Hell, toss 'em in the trash. Who's gonna miss 'em . . .

Totals: 545 calories, 90.3 g carbohydrates, 24.4 g protein, 9 g fat

	Muffins	Margarine	Milk	Orange
Calories	313	67	93	72
Carbohydrates (g)	62	0	12	16.3
Protein (g)	14	0	9	4
Fat (g)	1	7.4	0.5	1

Grits 'n' Raspberries/You'll wanna tag "Bob" onto the end of your first name

- 2   packets Quaker Plain Instant Corn Grits
- 4   ounces fresh raspberries
- 1   scoop Designer Protein French Vanilla Whey
- 1   teaspoon flaxseed oil
- 1   cup vanilla soy milk

Microwave or cook the grits and mix in the raspberries, whey, and flaxseed oil. If you're lactose intolerant or just plain tired of moo juice, the vanilla soy milk will hit the spot.

Totals: 523 calories, 80 g carbohydrates, 29 g protein, 9.6 g fat

	Grits	Raspberries	Whey Protein	Flaxseed Oil	Soy Milk
Calories	188	63	79	42	151
Carbohydrates (g)	41.2	13.1	2	0	23.7
Protein (g)	4.4	1	16	0	7.6
Fat (g)	0.6	0.7	0.8	4.7	2.8

Strawberry Shake with Milk/Berry, berry cool

- 2   cups fat-free milk
- 16   ounces frozen unsweetened strawberries
- 2   teaspoons flaxseed oil
- 1   ounce toasted plain wheat germ

Pour the milk in the blender, then toss in the rest of the goodies. The frozen strawberries will make the shake so thick that you'll need a spoon.

Totals: 568 calories, 79.5 g carbohydrates, 28.3 g protein, 14.2 g fat

	Milk	Strawberries	Flaxseed Oil	Wheat Germ
Calories	188	179	84	117
Carbohydrates (g)	24	41.4	0	14.1
Protein (g)	18	2	0	8.3
Fat (g)	1.2	0.6	9.4	3

Blue-Plate Breakfast: Diner Pancakes and Eggs/Go ahead, order the pancakes

- 3 blueberry pancakes, approximately 1.3 ounces each
- 2 tablespoons reduced-calorie syrup
- 2 teaspoons soft margarine
- • 3-egg omelette
- • black coffee

Diners are pure Americana. You can find them just about everywhere. And you can eat hearty without bumping up your pants size.

Totals: 680 calories, 72 g carbohydrates, 24.9 g protein, 32.4 g fat

	Pancakes	Syrup	Margarine	Omelette
Calories	220	121	67	272
Carbohydrates (g)	40	30.2	0	1.8
Protein (g)	6	0	0	18.9
Fat (g)	4	0	7.4	21

Eating Healthy at McDonald's/Make it a McMuffin

- 1 McDonald's Egg McMuffin
- 3 containers orange juice

As guilty pleasures go, the Egg McMuffin isn't the worst offender. Burger King's breakfast biscuit sandwiches contain considerably more fat. Just make sure that the McMuffin is only an occasional indulgence.

Totals: 541 calories, 87 g carbohydrates, 20 g protein, 12.5 g fat

	Egg McMuffin	OJ
Calories	284	257
Carbohydrates (g)	27	60
Protein (g)	17	3
Fat (g)	12	0.5

16 OUTSTANDING SANDWICHES, SALADS, AND SOUPS
LUNCH

Even if you don't work in a factory, you can almost hear the sound of the noon whistle reverberating in the pit of your stomach.

And although half the day is already gone, there are still battles to be fought, fires to be put out, deadlines to be met. To meet the challenges that lie ahead, you can't go back to the front lines on an empty stomach or, worse, a stomach filled with junk food. These Hard-Body lunch suggestions will give you the energy to hop the hump.

Remember: These lunches are for our 175-pound, 5-foot-10 reference man. You will need to adjust portions up or down a bit relative to your own weight and goals as you determined in Personalizing the Plan on page 324. Also, if you can't find these items in your area, feel free to make healthy substitutions.

FOR THE WEIGHT-LOSS MAN

Tuna-Salad Sandwich/Tastes like chicken (of the sea)

- 1   oat bran bagel
- 2½ ounces white, water-packed tuna, drained solids
- 1   teaspoon mayo
- 4   leaves romaine lettuce
- 1   medium apple

Mix the tuna with mayo, spread it on the bagel, and garnish it with lettuce. If you're not a bagel boy, substitute any whole-grain bread. Munch the apple for dessert.

Totals: 398 calories, 59.9 g carbohydrates, 25.4 g protein, 7.3 g fat

	Bagel	Tuna	Mayo	Lettuce	Apple
Calories	181	86	34	7	90
Carbohydrates (g)	37.8	0	0.1	1	21
Protein (g)	7.6	16.7	0.1	0.7	0.3
Fat (g)	0.9	2.1	3.7	0.1	0.5

Fortified Beef-Vegetable Soup/For the ground-round hound

- 1   cup beef-vegetable soup
- 2   ounces extra-lean ground beef, cooked well-done and drained
- 1   medium whole-wheat dinner roll

Start with basic beef-vegetable soup and add the cooked hamburger, and you have something that'll stick to your ribs. Sop up the leftover juice with the dinner roll.

Totals: 390 calories, 41.7 g carbohydrates, 28.8 g protein, 12.2 g fat

	Soup	Ground Beef	Roll
Calories	144	145	101
Carbohydrates (g)	23.3	0	18.4
Protein (g)	9.5	16.2	3.1
Fat (g)	1.5	9	1.7

Beyond Chicken-Noodle Soup/Everyone likes this except the chicken

- 1 cup chicken-noodle soup
- 1 ounce cooked chicken breast
- ½ piece Sahara oat bran pita
- 1 small pear
- 1 slice American cheese

Start with basic chicken-noodle soup, add cooked chicken breast, and you have a soup that's not a grueling chore to eat. The pita, pear, and cheese side dishes give the meal additional heft.

Totals: 363 calories, 46 g carbohydrates, 22.1 g protein, 10.1 g fat

	Soup	Chicken	Pita	Pear	Cheese
Calories	75	44	74	91	79
Carbohydrates (g)	9.4	0	15.3	21	0.3
Protein (g)	5.7	8.8	2.4	0.5	4.7
Fat (g)	1.6	1.0	0.3	0.6	6.6

Ready-Made Chicken-Salad Sandwich/Buy it, refrigerate it, bring it to work

- 1 Mrs. Winners Chicken Salad sandwich
- 1 tomato, sliced
- 1 cup fat-free milk

Open the ready-to-eat sandwich and spruce it up with tomato slices. Wash it down with the milk.

Totals: 350 calories, 50.7 g carbohydrates, 20 g protein, 6.9 g fat

	Sandwich	Tomato	Milk
Calories	226	31	93
Carbohydrates (g)	33	5.7	12
Protein (g)	10	1	9
Fat (g)	6	0.4	0.5

Arby's Chef Salad/Just be sure to bring your own fruit

- 1 Arby's chef salad
- ½ cup fat-free milk
- 1 whole-wheat pita
- 1 small orange

If you've gotta eat on the run, this fast-food platter will hold you until your midafternoon snack. Just remember, it's BYOO (bring your own orange).

Totals: 410 calories, 50.7 g carbohydrates, 27.1 g protein, 10.6 g fat

	Salad	Milk	Pita	Orange
Calories	212	47	79	72
Carbohydrates (g)	13	6	15.4	16.3
Protein (g)	18.5	4.5	2.7	1.4
Fat (g)	9.5	0.3	0.7	0.1

Homemade Chicken Salad/Pretend you're Mr. Gourmet

- 2 ounces grilled chicken breast
- 1 cup romaine lettuce
- 1 tomato
- 1 small green pepper
- 1 medium carrot
- 3 tablespoons Hidden Valley Italian dressing, 94% fat-free
- 1 tablespoon Progresso grated Parmesan cheese

This lunch gives you not only an excuse to fire up your grill but also an opportunity to brag to your coworkers about your advanced cooking skills. Grill the chicken breast in the evening, make it into a salad with the other ingredients, and store it in the fridge till morning. If you want, make a really big batch without the dressing, then take the recommended amount to work each day. (Just don't forget to take the dressing.)

Totals: 268 calories, 26.5 g carbohydrates, 22.8 g protein, 7.7 g fat

	Chicken	Lettuce	Tomato	Pepper	Carrot	Dressing	Cheese
Calories	89	10	31	23	28	57	30
Carbohydrates (g)	0	1.3	5.7	4.8	6.2	7.5	1
Protein (g)	17.6	0.9	1	0.7	0.6	0	2
Fat (g)	2	0.1	0.4	0.1	0.1	3	2

Homemade Ham Salad/A lean meal that won't make you porky

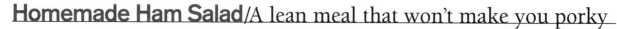

- 1 **cup romaine lettuce**
- 1 **tomato**
- 1 **small green pepper**
- 1 **medium carrot**
- 2 **tablespoons Marzetti's Caesar light dressing**
- 3 **ounces Boar's Head Boiled Deluxe Ham**
- 1 **medium pear**

Here's another salad option that mixes lean meat with lots of vegetables. If you want to, you can liven it up as you did the homemade chicken salad by adding cheese. Have the pear for an appetizer while you make the salad.

Totals: 369 calories, 46.6 g carbohydrates, 19.8 g protein, 11.4 g fat

	Lettuce	Tomato	Pepper	Carrot	Dressing	Ham	Pear
Calories	10	31	23	28	69	99	109
Carbohydrates (g)	1.3	5.7	4.8	6.2	0.5	3	25.1
Protein (g)	0.9	1	0.7	0.6	1	15	0.6
Fat (g)	0.1	0.4	0.1	0.1	7	3	0.7

Homemade Tuna Salad/Conduct a little fishy business at your desk

- 1 **cup romaine lettuce**
- 1 **tomato**
- 1 **small green pepper**
- 1 **medium carrot**
- 3 **ounces white, water-packed tuna, drained solids**
- 1 **tablespoon light Italian salad dressing**
- 1 **large orange**

Tuna is an all-purpose fish, and here it's the basis for a super salad. Just mix all the ingredients together except the orange, which you'll eat for dessert. For variety, fortify the salad with onions, red peppers, celery, squash, or any dark leafy vegetable. You can steam the squash if you wish to, or just chop it raw into the mix.

Totals: 321 calories, 40.6 g carbohydrates, 25 g protein, 6.4 g fat

	Lettuce	Tomato	Pepper	Carrot	Tuna	Dressing	Orange
Calories	10	31	23	28	103	31	95
Carbohydrates (g)	1.3	5.7	4.8	6.2	0	1	21.6
Protein (g)	0.9	1	0.7	0.6	20.1	0	1.7
Fat (g)	0.1	0.4	0.1	0.1	2.5	3	0.2

FOR THE WEIGHT-GAIN MAN

Cold Pasta with Tuna/Eat it like a salad

- 1   cup elbow macaroni, cooked
- 2   ounces light, water-packed tuna, drained solids
- 2   tablespoons Spectrum Lite Canola Mayo
- 1   cup romaine lettuce
- 1   small green pepper
- 1   tomato
- 1   medium carrot
- 2   small oranges

Attention, pasta lovers: Just boil up some macaroni, add everything but the oranges, and stick it in the refrigerator. Looks like salad, tastes like salad.

Totals: 564 calories, 94.6 g carbohydrates, 26.5 g protein, 8.7 g fat

	Macaroni	Tuna	Mayo	Lettuce	Pepper	Tomato	Carrot	Oranges
Calories	194	62	62	10	23	31	28	154
Carbohydrates (g)	39.7	0	2	1.3	4.8	5.7	6.2	34.9
Protein (g)	6.7	14.5	0	0.9	0.7	1	0.6	2.1
Fat (g)	0.9	0.5	6	0.1	0.1	0.4	0.1	0.6

Pizza with Side Salad/Kick back with a couple of slices

- 2   slices pepperoni pizza
- 1   cup romaine lettuce
- 1   tomato
- 1   small green pepper
- 1   medium carrot
- 1   tablespoon Hidden Valley Italian dressing, 94% fat-free
- 1   cup fat-free milk

As long as you can hold yourself to two slices, you can indulge your pizza passion without looking like a pizza pork. With this lunch, you even get a practically fat-free salad with Italian dressing.

Totals: 570 calories, 72.3 g carbohydrates, 32.4 g protein, 16.2 g fat

	Pizza	Lettuce	Tomato	Pepper	Carrot	Dressing	Milk
Calories	366	10	31	23	28	19	93
Carbohydrates (g)	39.8	1.3	5.7	4.8	6.2	2.5	12
Protein (g)	20.2	0.9	1	0.7	0.6	0	9
Fat (g)	14	0.1	0.4	0.1	0.1	1	0.5

DIY Pizza Treat/All you need is heat

- 1 Lender's 2-ounce bagel
- 1 teaspoon Blue Bonnet soft margarine
- 2 tablespoons Ragu Old World Style Smooth Pasta Sauce
- 2 ounces Dorman's reduced-fat, low-sodium cheese
- 2 tomato slices
- ¼ small green pepper
- 2 large oranges

If you can't head out for pizza but still have a hankering for one, prepare this pizzalike treat—you can even do it at work. Just spread a little margarine on a bagel, spread on the pasta sauce, cover it with cheese and tomato and pepper slices, and stick it in the microwave or toaster oven for 1 minute or less.

Totals: 560 calories, 80.4 g carbohydrates, 28.3 g protein, 13.9 g fat

	Bagel	Margarine	Sauce	Cheese	Tomato	Pepper	Oranges
Calories	153	33	21	152	5	6	190
Carbohydrates (g)	30	0	3.1	2	0.9	1.2	43.2
Protein (g)	6	0	0.5	18	0.2	0.2	3.4
Fat (g)	1	3.7	0.7	8	0.1	0	0.4

Subway's Cheesesteak Sandwich/Hop aboard and fight the fat

- 1 Subway 6-inch steak and cheese hot sub on whole-wheat bread
- 1 cup romaine lettuce
- 1 medium carrot
- 1 small green pepper
- 1 tomato
- 1 tablespoon Kraft Reduced-Calorie Creamy Italian
- 1 large orange

As fast foods go, Subway's 6-inch sandwiches are definitely on the lean side. If you know that you're going to be on the road during your lunch hour, pack a salad made from the lettuce, tomato, pepper, and carrot, with dressing on the side and an orange, and order Subway's sinful-sounding but low-fat 6-inch cheesesteak hot sub.

Totals: 579 calories, 81.6 g carbohydrates, 33.9 g protein, 12.9 g fat

	Sandwich	Lettuce	Carrot	Pepper	Tomato	Dressing	Orange
Calories	370	10	28	23	31	22	95
Carbohydrates (g)	41	1.3	6.2	4.8	5.7	1	21.6
Protein (g)	29	0.9	0.6	0.7	1	0	1.7
Fat (g)	10	0.1	0.1	0.1	0.4	2	0.2

Arby's Roast Chicken Sandwich/Low-cal, but not featherweight

- 1   **Arby's Deluxe Light Roast Chicken Sandwich**
- 1   **Arby's Old Fashioned Noodle Soup**
- ½   **small serving french fries**
- 1   **small orange**

While other customers are loading up on fat-filled entrées, you can munch your way through a sandwich, soup, and half an order of fries. Bring an orange from home for dessert.

Totals: 585 calories, 79 g carbohydrates, 32.5 g protein, 15.5 g fat

	Sandwich	Soup	French Fries	Orange
Calories	291	99	123	72
Carbohydrates (g)	33	14.8	14.9	16.3
Protein (g)	24	6	1.1	1.4
Fat (g)	7	1.8	6.6	0.1

Burger King's Broiled Chicken Sandwich/
Get a Whopperless whopper lunch

- 1   **Burger King Broiler chicken sandwich without mayo**
- 1   **Burger King garden salad without dressing**
- 1   **Burger King Italian Dressing, reduced-calorie**
- 6   **ounces orange juice**
- 1   **large apple**

While other customers are clogging their arteries with double-beef Whoppers with cheese, you can enjoy a chicken sandwich and a garden salad. Bring an apple from home for dessert.

Totals: 544 calories, 69.1 g carbohydrates, 28.9 g protein, 16.8 g fat

	Sandwich	Salad	Dressing	OJ	Apple
Calories	202	101	17	86	138
Carbohydrates (g)	7	8	3	18.8	32.3
Protein (g)	21	6	0	1.5	0.4
Fat (g)	10	5	0.5	0.5	0.8

Wendy's Spicy Chicken Sandwich/Little fat, lotsa food

- 1 **Wendy's Spicy Chicken Fillet**
- 12 **ounces cola**

If you don't want to follow Dave's path to the heart surgeon, skip the burgers. Go for the spicy chicken sandwich, and wash it down with a cola.

Totals: 573 calories, 81.5 g carbohydrates, 28 g protein, 15 g fat

	Sandwich	Cola
Calories	419	154
Carbohydrates (g)	43	38.5
Protein (g)	28	0
Fat (g)	15	0

Pizza Hut's Veggie Lovers Pizza/Thin 'n' crispy 'n' unfattening

- 2 **medium-size slices Pizza Hut Thin 'n' Crispy Veggie Lovers Pizza**
- 12 **ounces cola**

Just a whiff of Pizza Hut should be enough to make you shout "Danger, danger! Warning, warning!" Still, there's one item on the menu that's calorically safe: the Thin 'n' Crispy Veggie Lovers Pizza. The catch: You can only eat two slices, so you'll either have to share the others or bring them home to Rover.

Totals: 546 calories, 78.5 g carbohydrates, 22 g protein, 16 g fat

	Pizza	Cola
Calories	392	154
Carbohydrates (g)	40	38.5
Protein (g)	22	0
Fat (g)	16	0

18 PERFECT PLATES OF FOOD
DINNER

Remember that voracious man-eating plant in *Little Shop of Horrors* who couldn't stop shouting "Feed me! Feed me! Feed me!"? Ever felt like that when dinnertime rolled around?

You won't on the Hard-Body Plan. Sure, you'll be looking forward to some fantastic food, but you won't be crying for it—as long as you stick with the meal-timing program. Don't skip. Don't do this "eating fashionably late" thing—unless you're wanting some unfashionable fat hanging around your belly and butt. The later in the day you cram down the calories, the more likely it is that your body will store them as fat.

Hard-Body dinners aren't the kind of stomach-stuffers that leave you praying to the Alka-Seltzer gods for a good burp. Stick with the plan and you'll find little or no appetite for dinner-time pigouts. And you'll enjoy dinners that contain satisfying, man-sized portions of the foods you love to eat.

Remember: These dinners are for our 175-pound, 5-foot-10-inch reference man. You will need to adjust portions up or down a bit relative to your own weight and goals as you determined in Personalizing the Plan on page 324. Also, if you can't find some of these items in your area, feel free to make healthy substitutions.

FOR THE WEIGHT-LOSS MAN

Meat and Potatoes—and Dessert/You can cook it while you watch the news

- 3   ounces boneless chicken breast, broiled, grilled, or roasted
- ½   cup frozen mixed vegetables, boiled and drained, no salt
- 1   baked potato, no salt
- 1   teaspoon unsalted butter
- ½   cup strawberries

Cook the chicken breast by the low-fat method of your choice. If a baked spud sounds too boring, substitute a sweet potato or wild rice.

Totals: 399 calories, 50.6 g carbohydrates, 32.5 g protein, 7.4 g fat

	Chicken	Vegetables	Potato	Butter	Strawberries
Calories	133	59	148	35	24
Carbohydrates (g)	0	11.9	33.6	0	5.1
Protein (g)	26.4	2.6	3.1	0	0.4
Fat (g)	3	0.1	0.2	3.8	0.3

Whitefish with Brown Rice/Have a deep-sea adventure

- 1½ cups tossed salad without dressing
- 2   ounces light salad dressing
- ¾   cup cooked brown rice
- 3½ ounces grilled whitefish fillet

Pick up a pretossed salad at the supermarket and top it with your favorite low-cal dressing. Boil the rice, grill the fish, and you've got a feast fit for Ernest Hemingway (in his younger, thinner days, of course).

Totals: 442 calories, 52.6 g carbohydrates, 30.8 g protein, 12.2 g fat

	Salad	Dressing	Rice	Fish
Calories	38	79	161	164
Carbohydrates (g)	6.7	12.3	33.6	0
Protein (g)	2.6	0.1	3.8	24.3
Fat (g)	0.1	3.3	1.3	7.5

Salmon with Wild Rice/Jammin' with salmon

- 3 ounces cooked salmon fillet
- 1 cup wild rice, cooked
- 1 cup squash or zucchini, boiled and drained, no salt

What guy hasn't thrilled to the sight of a bear scooping a big, fat salmon out of a raging river? While you bake, broil, or grill the fish, pretend you're the bear that caught it—just as strong, but not nearly as fat.

Totals: 354 calories, 42.1 g carbohydrates, 29.3 g protein, 7.6 g fat

	Salmon	Rice	Squash
Calories	149	171	34
Carbohydrates (g)	0	35	7.1
Protein (g)	21.6	6.5	1.2
Fat (g)	6.9	0.6	0.1

Filet Mignon/Sweet meat with a sweet spud

- 1 large baked sweet potato, no salt
- 2½ ounces grilled or broiled filet mignon
- 1 cup frozen chopped broccoli, boiled and drained, no salt
- ¼ lemon

While the potato is baking (keep the skin on when you eat it), grill or broil the filet mignon, and boil the broccoli. Squeeze the lemon over the cooked broccoli, and there you have it: a healthy version of a meal that's toppled many a titan.

Totals: 417 calories, 54 g carbohydrates, 30.4 g protein, 8.8 g fat

	Sweet Potato	Steak	Broccoli	Lemon Juice
Calories	189	162	64	2
Carbohydrates (g)	43.7	0	9.8	0.5
Protein (g)	3.1	21.6	5.7	0
Fat (g)	0.2	8.4	0.2	0

Pork Chop with Mashed Potatoes/A low-calorie pigfest

- 3 ounces cooked boneless pork chop
- 1 cup mashed potatoes, made with about 1 ounce fat-free milk and no butter
- ⅔ cup Green Giant Select Harvest Fresh green beans with almonds, no butter

Grill, broil, or bake the pork chop. Make the mashed potatoes and boil the green beans. You've got the makings of a Midwestern favorite.

Totals: 396 calories, 41.9 g carbohydrates, 25.1 g protein, 14.2 g fat

	Pork Chop	Mashed Potatoes	Green Beans
Calories	166	175	55
Carbohydrates (g)	0	36.9	5
Protein (g)	19	4.1	2
Fat (g)	10	1.2	3

Hamburger Helper Beef Teriyaki/A little touch of the Orient

- ⅔ cup Hamburger Helper beef teriyaki
- 1 ounce cooked lean ground beef
- 1 cup romaine lettuce
- 1 tomato
- 1 small green pepper
- 1 medium carrot
- 1 tablespoon Hidden Valley Italian salad dressing, 94% fat-free
- ½ cup fat-free milk

Take our word for it: Hamburger Helper really helps. Just cook the beef teriyaki per the instructions on the box, mix up a big, bountiful salad, and, bam, you're riding on the Orient Express.

Totals: 396 calories, 51.8 g carbohydrates, 21 g protein, 11.3 g fat

	H. Helper	Beef	Lettuce	Tomato	Pepper	Carrot	Dressing	Milk
Calories	126	112	10	31	23	28	19	47
Carbohydrates (g)	25.3	0	1.3	5.7	4.8	6.2	2.5	6
Protein (g)	3.3	10	0.9	1	0.7	0.6	0	4.5
Fat (g)	1.3	8	0.1	0.4	0.1	0.1	1	0.3

Grilled Chicken Salad/More than just wabbit food

- **2 ounces grilled boneless chicken breast**
- **1 cup romaine lettuce**
- **1 tomato**
- **1 small green pepper**
- **1 medium carrot**
- **3 tablespoons Wish-Bone Fat-Free Italian! salad dressing**
- **1 tablespoon grated Parmesan cheese**
- **1 cup fat-free milk**

Between the chicken, the Parmesan cheese, and the Italian dressing, this is a grilled chicken salad worth putting on the witness stand. If you want, add more veggies than the recipe calls for—lots more, if you like.

Totals: 319 calories, 34 g carbohydrates, 31.8 g protein, 5.5 g fat

	Chicken	Lettuce	Tomato	Pepper	Carrot	Dressing	Cheese	Milk
Calories	89	10	31	23	28	15	30	93
Carbohydrates (g)	0	1.3	5.7	4.8	6.2	3	1	12
Protein (g)	17.6	0.9	1	0.7	0.6	0	2	9
Fat (g)	2	0.1	0.4	0.1	0.1	0.3	2	0.5

Quick Vegetable Salad/It's cold and bold

- **1 cup romaine lettuce**
- **1 tomato**
- **1 small green pepper**
- **1 medium carrot**
- **¼ cup Green Giant Niblets corn (No Salt or Sugar Added)**
- **¼ cup canned kidney beans**
- **1 ounce Kraft natural, mild, shredded Light Naturals Cheddar cheese**
- **2 tablespoons Wish-Bone Fat-Free Italian! salad dressing**
- **½ cup fat-free milk**

On those nights when you'd rather starve than cook, this cold salad made from refrigerated and canned ingredients can be a lifesaver.

Totals: 331 calories, 45 g carbohydrates, 21.7 g protein, 6.5 g fat

	Lettuce	Tomato	Pepper	Carrot	Corn	Beans	Cheese	Dressing	Milk
Calories	10	31	23	28	47	54	81	10	47
Carbohydrates (g)	1.3	5.7	4.8	6.2	9	10	0	2	6
Protein (g)	0.9	1	0.7	0.6	1.5	3.5	9	0	4.5
Fat (g)	0.1	0.4	0.1	0.1	0.5	0	5	0	0.3

The You-Can Tuna Salad/But you can't tune a fish

- 1   apology
- 1   cup romaine lettuce
- 1   tomato
- 1   small green pepper
- 1   medium carrot
- 3   ounces white, water-packed tuna, drained solids
- 1   tablespoon light Italian salad dressing
- ½   cup fat-free milk
- 1   large orange

Whip up this salad in less time than it takes to remember an old StarKist commercial. Eat the orange for dessert. Remember, you can add a little bit o' Charlie the Tuna to any salad to bring up the protein.

Totals: 347 calories, 47.6 g carbohydrates, 29.5 g protein, 3.7 g fat

	Lettuce	Tomato	Pepper	Carrot	Tuna	Dressing	Milk	Orange
Calories	10	31	23	28	103	10	47	95
Carbohydrates (g)	1.3	5.7	4.8	6.2	0	2	6	21.6
Protein (g)	0.9	1	0.7	0.6	20.1	0	4.5	1.7
Fat (g)	0.1	0.4	0.1	0.1	2.5	0	0.3	0.2

Spaghetti with Side Salad/Mama Mia, it's almost Italian

- 2   ounces extra-lean pan-fried (medium) ground beef, drained
- ¼   cup Ragu Old World Style Smooth Pasta Sauce, Traditional
- 1   cup enriched spaghetti, cooked without added salt
- 1   cup romaine lettuce
- ¼   small green pepper
- ¼   tomato
- ½   medium carrot

Just add some cooked ground beef to the Ragu, dump it on boiled spaghetti, and whip up a salad, and you have a dinner you can't refuse.

Totals: 412 calories, 52.8 g carbohydrates, 23.4 g protein, 11.8 g fat

	Beef	Sauce	Spaghetti	Lettuce	Pepper	Tomato	Carrot
Calories	140	40	194	10	6	8	14
Carbohydrates (g)	0	6.1	39.7	1.3	1.2	1.4	3.1
Protein (g)	14.1	0.9	6.7	0.9	0.2	0.3	0.3
Fat (g)	9.3	1.3	0.9	0.1	0	0.1	0.1

FOR THE WEIGHT-GAIN MAN

Spaghetti with White Clam Sauce/Clam it and slam it

- 1 **cup enriched spaghetti, cooked without added salt**
- ½ **cup canned Progresso White Clam Sauce**
- 2 **ounces light, water-packed tuna, drained solids**
- 1 **cup frozen chopped broccoli, boiled without salt**
- 1 **cup romaine lettuce**
- 1 **tomato**
- 1 **small green pepper**
- 2 **medium carrots**
- 1 **tablespoon Hidden Valley Italian salad dressing, 94% fat-free**

Boil the spaghetti, mix it with the clam sauce, tuna, and broccoli, and you've got a pasta dish that'll rip you out of your shell. Round it out with a salad.

Totals: 571 calories, 77.2 g carbohydrates, 39.7 g protein, 11.4 g fat

	Spaghetti	Sauce	Tuna	Broccoli	Lettuce	Tomato	Pepper	Carrots	Dressing
Calories	194	112	62	64	10	31	23	56	19
Carbohydrates (g)	39.7	1	0	9.8	1.3	5.7	4.8	12.4	2.5
Protein (g)	6.7	9	14.5	5.7	0.9	1	0.7	1.2	0
Fat (g)	0.9	8	0.5	0.2	0.1	0.4	0.1	0.2	1

Chili with Beans and Cheese/Socially acceptable, politically correct

- 1 **cup chili with beans, canned entrée**
- 1 **ounce reduced-fat Cheddar or Colby cheese**
- ¾ **cup cooked brown rice**
- 1 **large apple**
- **Beano drops**

Heat the chili and top with cheese, or eat the cheese separately. Toss down the rice and apple. Use the Beano on the chili and no one will ever have to know what you had for dinner.

Totals: 576 calories, 99.5 g carbohydrates, 29.1 g protein, 6.9 g fat

	Chili	Cheese	Rice	Apple
Calories	229	48	161	138
Carbohydrates (g)	33.1	0.5	33.6	32.3
Protein (g)	18	6.9	3.8	0.4
Fat (g)	2.8	2	1.3	0.8

Turkey Breast with Ham and Swiss/A gobbler in a blanket

- 3 ounces broiled boneless, skinless turkey breast
- 1 slice Jones Dairy Farm 97% fat-free, hickory smoked Lean Choice Ham
- 1 ounce sliced, nonprocessed, reduced-fat Swiss cheese
- 1 cup romaine lettuce
- 1 tomato
- 1 small green pepper
- 1 medium carrot
- 3 ounces fresh mushrooms

- 2 tablespoons light Italian salad dressing
- 1 potato, baked without salt
- 1 teaspoon Blue Bonnet soft margarine

If you'd rather not see another turkey breast, try this. Bake a potato. Broil a turkey breast. Stay tuned. When the turkey's almost done, top it off with the ham and Swiss cheese. Finish broiling. The salad and baked potato give this meal some heft.

Totals: 519 calories, 58.6 g carbohydrates, 47.2 g protein, 10.4 g fat

	Turkey	Ham	Cheese	Lettuce	Tomato	Pepper
Calories	108	25	76	10	31	23
Carbohydrates (g)	0	0	1	1.3	5.7	4.8
Protein (g)	25.6	4.5	9	0.9	1	0.7
Fat (g)	0.6	0.8	4	0.1	0.4	0.1

	Carrot	Mushrooms	Dressing	Potato	Margarine
Calories	28	27	20	148	33
Carbohydrates (g)	6.2	4	4	33.6	0
Protein (g)	0.6	1.8	0	3.1	0
Fat (g)	0.1	0.4	0	0.2	3.7

Burger King's Cheeseburger/
Have it your way, as long as that doesn't involve fries

- 1 Burger King Cheeseburger
- 6 ounces orange juice

If you're hungry for Burger King, this dinner won't force you to surrender your Hard Body.

Totals: 461 calories, 46.8 g carbohydrates, 24.5 g protein, 19.5 g fat

	Cheeseburger	OJ
Calories	375	86
Carbohydrates (g)	28	18.8
Protein (g)	23	1.5
Fat (g)	19	0.5

Burger and French Fries/Simple, basic, classic

- 3   ounces extra-lean, pan-fried (medium) ground beef patty, drained
- 1   hamburger roll
- 20 strips frozen french-fried potatoes
- 1   cup California blend mixed vegetables (cauliflower, broccoli, zucchini, carrot), no salt
- 2   inner leaves romaine lettuce
- 1   tomato slice

Can you say "all-American"? Pan-fry the burger, bake the fries, boil the veggies, plop the lettuce and tomato on the burger, and you're John Wayne.

Totals: 569 calories, 59.5 g carbohydrates, 30.5 g protein, 23.2 g fat

	Beef	Roll	Fries	Vegetables	Lettuce	Tomato
Calories	211	115	208	26	4	5
Carbohydrates (g)	0	21.2	31.6	5.3	0.5	0.9
Protein (g)	21.2	4.3	3.2	1.3	0.3	0.2
Fat (g)	14	1.5	7.6	0	0	0.1

McDonald's Quarter Pounder/A lean alternative to the Big Mac

- 1   McDonald's Quarter Pounder
- 1   Side Garden Salad
- ½   packet low-fat salad dressing
- 1   container orange juice

If you're cruising for burgers, you could do worse than choose McDonald's Quarter Pounder with side salad and OJ. How much worse? Look at the Big Mac.

Totals: 577 calories, 71.3 g carbohydrates, 26.5 g protein, 25.8 g fat

	Quarter Pounder	Salad	Dressing	OJ
Calories	429	27	35	86
Carbohydrates (g)	37	4	11.5	18.8
Protein (g)	23	2	0	1.5
Fat (g)	21	0.3	4	0.5

Arby's Turkey Sandwich/Gobble and gulp

- 1   **Arby's Light Roast Turkey Deluxe sandwich**
- ½   **small serving french fries**
- 1   **Arby's Side Salad**
- 1   **Arby's Reduced Calorie Italian salad dressing**

If you're stuck in Strip Mall City at dinnertime, check out Arby's Light Roast Turkey Deluxe Sandwich. You'll even have room left over for a salad and a half-order of fries. Of course, they don't make half-orders of fries. You've got to toss out half. You're on the honor system here. (Secret: Toss half of them in the trash before you sit down.)

Totals: 440 calories, 55.4 g carbohydrates, 23.1 g protein, 14 g fat

	Sandwich	French Fries	Salad	Dressing
Calories	266	123	27	24
Carbohydrates (g)	33	14.9	4	3.5
Protein (g)	20	1.1	2	0
Fat (g)	6	6.6	0.3	1.1

Denny's Ham Sandwich/For all the nighthawks at the diner

- 1   **Denny's Ham Sandwich made with 2 slices of ham, special-ordered on 2 slices of whole-wheat bread with 1 teaspoon of yellow mustard instead of mayo**
- 4   **ounces mashed potatoes, no gravy or butter**
- 16 **ounces soda**

Denny's will serve this sammich whenever you want it, in an environment that's pure plastic, Formica, and uniformed-waitress Americana. Leave a bigger-than-usual tip if she wears rhinestone glasses or calls you "Hon."

Totals: 608 calories, 81 g carbohydrates, 35 g protein, 16 g fat

	Ham	Whole-Wheat Bread	Mustard	Mashed Potatoes	Soda
Calories	246	111	3	72	176
Carbohydrates (g)	2	19.8	0.2	15	44
Protein (g)	28	4.8	0.2	2	0
Fat (g)	14	1.4	0.2	0.4	0

48 GREAT GUY CHOW CHOICES
SNACKS

In the bad old days, the food police routinely handed out citations for eating between meals. They viewed snacking as the dietary equivalent of cheating on your wife, an immoral act that would inevitably lead you into Pavarotti's Inferno.

Strict fidelity to the three squares. That was their credo.

Not anymore. Although they still frown on cheese curls, bear claws, and other vending-machine atrocities, they now say that low-fat noshing throughout the day is a great way to keep yourself on the straight and narrow.

Snacks are an essential element in the Hard-Body Plan. They top off your tank so it keeps repairing and building muscle.

MORNING SNACKS

In this section we've included 10 morning snacks for the weight-loss man and 8 morning snacks for the weight-gain man. Since these munchies include the meats, cheeses, and fruits that taste especially good in the A.M., they'll keep you satisfied during the long, dry stretch between breakfast and lunch.

Remember, these snacks are for our 175-pound, 5-foot-10 reference man. You will need to adjust portions up or down a bit relative to your own weight and goals as you determined in Personalizing the Plan on page 324. Also, if you can't find these items in your store, feel free to make healthy substitutions.

MORNING SNACKS FOR THE WEIGHT-LOSS MAN

Oatmeal with Blueberries/Feel your oats and eat 'em

- ¾ cup quick or instant oatmeal
- 1 cup fat-free milk
- 1 ounce toasted, plain wheat germ
- 3 ounces frozen, unsweetened blueberries

Nuke the oatmeal in unsalted water and mix in the milk, wheat germ, and blueberries. If you splatter some on your tie, don't worry. Your coworkers will just think it's abstract art.

Totals: 368 calories, 55.5 g carbohydrates, 22.3 g protein, 5.8 g fat

	Oats	Milk	Wheat Germ	Blueberries
Calories	110	93	117	48
Carbohydrates (g)	19	12	14.1	10.4
Protein (g)	4.6	9	8.3	0.4
Fat (g)	1.8	0.5	3	0.5

Fruit and Cheese Platter/A finger-food feast

- 1 medium apple
- 5 1" reduced-fat Cheddar cheese cubes
- 30 seedless grapes

Go ahead, munch 'em at your desk. No one will notice if you close your eyes and pretend that your main squeeze is dropping 'em into your mouth.

Totals: 353 calories, 49.3 g carbohydrates, 22.4 g protein, 7.5 g fat

	Apple	Cheese	Grapes
Calories	90	145	118
Carbohydrates (g)	21	1.7	26.6
Protein (g)	0.3	21.1	1.0
Fat (g)	0.5	6.1	0.9

Tuna on Rye/For the wry guy

- 2   slices rye bread
- 3   ounces water-packed tuna, drained
- 1   teaspoon Kraft Light mayo
- 1   celery stalk
- 2   leaves romaine lettuce
- 12 ounces no-salt-added V-8 juice

Unless you're the sort of badass who raids other people's refrigerated food, you'll have to bring this one from home. Feel free to pile on extra tomatoes, onions, and other low-fat vegetables.

Totals: 366 calories, 49.2 g carbohydrates, 28.1 g protein, 6.3 g fat

	Rye Bread	Tuna	Mayo	Celery	Lettuce	V-8 Juice
Calories	164	103	16	7	4	72
Carbohydrates (g)	30.9	0	0.3	1.5	0.5	16
Protein (g)	5.4	20.1	0	0.3	0.3	2
Fat (g)	2.1	2.5	1.7	0	0	0

Turkey on Pumpernickel/A pumped-up morning snack

- 2   slices Arnold pumpernickel bread
- 3   ounces (3 slices) Louis Rich smoked, 98% fat-free turkey breast
- 1   ounce (1 slice) Hickory Farms Light Choice Low Sodium provolone
- 1   teaspoon Kraft Light mayo
- 2   leaves romaine lettuce
- 2   plums

Between the heavy bread, the cheese, and the turkey, this sandwich may exceed your calorie quota. Just make the next meal or snack a little lighter.

Totals: 435 calories, 50.9 g carbohydrates, 25.7 g protein, 14.3 g fat

	Pumpernickel	Turkey	Provolone	Mayo	Lettuce	Plums
Calories	155	87	93	16	4	80
Carbohydrates (g)	29.4	3	0.5	0.3	0.5	17.2
Protein (g)	5.4	12	7	0	0.3	1
Fat (g)	1.8	3	7	1.7	0	0.8

Ham on Rye/Ham it up at the office

- 2   slices rye bread
- 3   ounces (3 slices) extra-lean ham (approximately 5% fat)
- 2   teaspoons Grey Poupon mustard
- 12 ounces no-salt-added V-8 juice

Fix it at home, eat it at your desk, and wash it down with the V-8. If some smart aleck asks "Do you have any Grey Poupon?" answer "Yes" and smear some on his suit.

Totals: 351 calories, 49.7 g carbohydrates, 23.9 g protein, 6.3 g fat

	Rye Bread	Ham	Grey Poupon	V-8 Juice
Calories	164	107	8	72
Carbohydrates (g)	30.9	0.8	2	16
Protein (g)	5.4	16.5	0	2
Fat (g)	2.1	4.2	0	0

Chicken Breast on Rye/Are we feeling peckish yet?

- 2   slices rye bread
- 3   ounces (3 slices) Louis Rich boneless, oven-roasted chicken breast, 96% fat-free
- 2   leaves romaine lettuce
- 2   teaspoons Grey Poupon mustard
- 12 ounces no-salt-added V-8 juice

Fix it at home, eat it in the break room, make your coworkers jealous. If you're getting sick of rye, remember that this and the other sandwiches can be made from any whole-grain bread containing comparable calories.

Totals: 347 calories, 52.4 g carbohydrates, 22.7 g protein, 5.1 g fat

	Rye Bread	Chicken	Lettuce	Grey Poupon	V-8 Juice
Calories	164	99	4	8	72
Carbohydrates (g)	30.9	3	0.5	2	16
Protein (g)	5.4	15	0.3	0	2
Fat (g)	2.1	3	0	0	0

Hard-Boiled Egg Sandwich/For the hard-boiled man

- 2 slices rye bread
- 1 large hard-boiled egg
- 2 large hard-boiled egg whites
- 2 leaves romaine lettuce
- 1 teaspoon Kraft Light mayo
- 12 ounces no-salt-added V-8 juice

Nothing hits the spot in the morning like eggs, even if they're cold. Boil the eggs ahead of time and make the sandwich whenever you feel like it.

Totals: 362 calories, 49 g carbohydrates, 21 g protein, 9.1 g fat

	Rye Bread	Egg	Egg Whites	Lettuce	Mayo	V-8 Juice
Calories	164	75	31	4	16	72
Carbohydrates (g)	30.9	0.6	0.7	0.5	0.3	16
Protein (g)	5.4	6.3	7	0.3	0	2
Fat (g)	2.1	5.3	0	0	1.7	0

Roast Beast on Rye/Beef up with beef

- 2 slices rye bread
- 2 ounces (2 slices) Boar's Head roast beef
- 2 leaves romaine lettuce
- 1 teaspoon Kraft Light mayo
- 12 ounces no-salt-added V-8 juice

Slap it together at home, gnaw on it next to the water cooler, casually flex your pecs in view of desirable coworkers.

Totals: 338 calories, 49.7 g carbohydrates, 21.7 g protein, 5.8 g fat

	Rye Bread	Roast Beef	Lettuce	Mayo	V-8 Juice
Calories	164	82	4	16	72
Carbohydrates (g)	30.9	2	0.5	0.3	16
Protein (g)	5.4	14	0.3	0	2
Fat (g)	2.1	2	0	1.7	0

PB&J Sandwich/AT&T (always tasty and tremendous)

- 2 slices wheat bread
- 2 tablespoons Jif Reduced Fat Peanut Butter, creamy-style
- 1 tablespoon Polaner Apricot All Fruit Spreadable Fruit
- ½ cup fat-free milk

You can't improve on a classic, so we won't even try. This snack includes ample amounts of spread, plus a little milk to wash down the peanut butter that's stuck in your throat.

Totals: 391 calories, 48.8 g carbohydrates, 20.9 g protein, 12.3 g fat

	Wheat Bread	Peanut Butter	Fruit Spread	Milk
Calories	134	162	48	47
Carbohydrates (g)	24.8	6	12	6
Protein (g)	4.4	12	0	4.5
Fat (g)	2	10	0	0.3

Strawberry Shake/Whey in, way out

- 1 scoop Designer Protein Strawberry Whey
- 1 teaspoon flaxseed oil
- ½ cup fat-free milk
- 1 cup red grape juice

Mix the ingredients in a blender and serve in a malt glass. Feel free to experiment with other whey products, juices, or fruits as long as you stay within the protein, fat, carbohydrate, and calorie totals.

Totals: 330 calories, 46.1 g carbohydrates, 22.9 g protein, 5.7 g fat

	Whey Protein	Flaxseed Oil	Milk	Grape Juice
Calories	82	42	47	159
Carbohydrates (g)	2.3	0	6	37.8
Protein (g)	17	0	4.5	1.4
Fat (g)	0.5	4.7	0.3	0.2

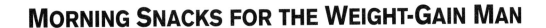

MORNING SNACKS FOR THE WEIGHT-GAIN MAN

Chocolate-Banana Shake/Enough to feed a banana republic

- 1 scoop Designer Protein Chocolate Whey
- ½ cup fat-free milk
- 2 extra-large bananas
- 2 tablespoons flaxseed meal

Blenderize the ingredients into a serious shake, and eat it with a long spoon. Note that this recipe uses flaxseed meal instead of flaxseed oil. The meal is a great source of fiber.

Totals: 537 calories, 83.7 g carbohydrates, 28.2 g protein, 9.7 g fat

	Whey Protein	Milk	Bananas	Flaxseed Meal
Calories	89	47	310	91
Carbohydrates (g)	2.5	6	71.2	4
Protein (g)	17.5	4.5	3.2	3
Fat (g)	1	0.3	1.4	7

Apples and Peanuts/A pair to draw to

- 2 medium apples
- 1 ounce peanuts, dry-roasted, without salt
- 2 cups fat-free milk

Apples and peanuts make a crunchy combination that won't stick to the roof of your mouth like a caramel apple.

Totals: 545 calories, 72.2 g carbohydrates, 25.4 g protein, 16.2 g fat

	Apples	Peanuts	Milk
Calories	179	178	188
Carbohydrates (g)	42	6.2	24
Protein (g)	0.6	6.8	18
Fat (g)	1	14	1.2

Bagels and Margarine/The best kind of chew

- **2 Lender's 2-ounce bagels**
- **4 teaspoons Blue Bonnet soft margarine**
- **1 cup fat-free milk**

So what if you don't get to smother them with lox and cream cheese? Toasted bagels taste good even when they're just smeared with margarine. Plus, they give your jaw muscles a great workout. Chomp away, and wash 'em down with fat-free milk.

Totals: 532 calories, 72 g carbohydrates, 21 g protein, 17.3 g fat

	Bagels	Margarine	Milk
Calories	306	133	93
Carbohydrates (g)	60	0	12
Protein (g)	12	0	9
Fat (g)	2	14.8	0.5

Chocolate Pudding with Banana/Satisfies your midmorning sweet tooth

- **1 cup Jell-O Chocolate Flavor Instant Pudding, sugar-free, fat-free**
- **1 scoop Designer Protein Chocolate Whey**
- **¼ cup flaxseed meal**
- **1 large banana**
- **1 cup grapes**

Make the pudding with fat-free milk and mix in the whey. When you're ready to scarf it down, add banana slices and you've got a chocolatey treat that's a helluva lot better for you than a bag of M&M's. If you want, try vanilla pudding with vanilla whey. The grapes? Pelt anyone with them who tries to scarf your snack.

Totals: 554 calories, 78.5 g carbohydrates, 24.7 g protein, 15.7 g fat

	Pudding	Whey Protein	Flaxseed Meal	Banana	Grapes
Calories	128	45	182	139	60
Carbohydrates (g)	24	1.3	8	31.9	13.3
Protein (g)	8	8.8	6	1.4	0.5
Fat (g)	0	0.5	14	0.7	0.5

Jell-O and Yogurt with Raspberries/
A whey-out midmorning dessert

- **2 cups sugar-free Jell-O Brand Raspberry Flavor Gelatin prepared as directed**
- **10 ounces plain, fat-free yogurt**
- **1 cup fresh raspberries**
- **2 tablespoons flaxseed meal**
- **1½ ounces raisins**

If you're not into the powdered protein thing, prepare the Jell-O and add the rest of the goodies for a tasty treat.

Totals: 474 calories, 73.6 g carbohydrates, 25.8 g protein, 8.4 g fat

	Jell-O	Yogurt	Raspberries	Flaxseed Meal	Raisins
Calories	16	157	68	91	142
Carbohydrates (g)	0	21.8	14.2	4	33.6
Protein (g)	4	16.3	1.1	3	1.4
Fat (g)	0	0.5	0.7	7	0.2

Ready-to-Eat Apple-Bran Muffins/Hey, it's a bran-new day

- **2 Total Health apple-bran muffins**
- **2 teaspoons Blue Bonnet soft margarine**
- **2 cups fat-free milk**

If you want simple, this is simple. Just smear on margarine, munch away, and try not to spill too many crumbs onto your lap. Wash down with fat-free milk.

Totals: 568 calories, 86 g carbohydrates, 32 g protein, 9.6 g fat

	Muffins	Margarine	Milk
Calories	313	67	188
Carbohydrates (g)	62	0	24
Protein (g)	14	0	18
Fat (g)	1	7.4	1.2

Crackers with Cheese and Tomatoes/Nuke 'em and nosh 'em

- **18 Triscuit crackers, low-salt (½-ounce serving)**
- **2 ounces shredded, fat-free cheese (your choice)**
- **4 cherry tomatoes**

Place the crackers on a plate, load on the cheese and tomatoes, and microwave for however long it takes to melt the fat-free cheese. A minute oughta do it.

Totals: 469 calories, 65.2 g carbohydrates, 24.6 g protein, 12.2 g fat

	Tricuits	Cheese	Tomatoes
Calories	372	80	17
Carbohydrates (g)	60	2	3.2
Protein (g)	6	18	0.6
Fat (g)	12	0	0.2

Strawberry and Blueberry Smoothie/A purple eater, people

- **7 ounces fresh strawberries**
- **7 ounces fresh blueberries**
- **1 scoop Designer Protein Strawberry Whey**
- **½ cup fat-free milk**
- **1 tablespoon flaxseed oil**
- **6 ounces red grape juice**

Blenderize the listed ingredients. Pretend that the finished product is puree of Barney the purple dinosaur.

Totals: 527 calories, 67.4 g carbohydrates, 25.2 g protein, 17.1 g fat

	Strawberries	Blueberries	Whey Protein	Milk	Flaxseed Oil	Grape Juice
Calories	67	85	82	47	126	120
Carbohydrates (g)	13.9	16.8	2.3	6	0	28.4
Protein (g)	1.2	1.4	17	4.5	0	1.1
Fat (g)	0.7	1.4	0.5	0.3	14	0.2

AFTERNOON SNACKS

By midafternoon, your batteries are probably running so low that they couldn't light a nightlight. Quick—before you start to flicker, grab a snack.

To give you extra voltage, here are some no-fuss snacks that'll fill you up without blowing your diet. These creamy shakes and crunchy treats are sure to hit the spot during slump times when your stomach is growling like a Rottweiler and you're on the verge of nodding off at your desk.

Remember: These snacks are for our 175-pound, 5-foot-10 reference man. You will need to adjust portions up or down a bit relative to your own weight and goals as you determined in Personalizing the Plan on page 324. Also, if you can't find some of the ingredients listed, feel free to make healthy substitutions.

AFTERNOON SNACKS FOR THE WEIGHT-LOSS MAN

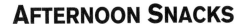Cottage Cheese with Fruit/Munch it at your desk

- ½ ounce Planters dry-roasted sunflower seeds
- 4 ounces fat-free cottage cheese
- 1¼ cups canned peaches (light syrup pack with solids and liquids)

Spoon out a mound of cottage cheese and garnish it with a mixture of peaches and sunflower seeds. If you want, substitute other fruits for the peaches or replace the cottage cheese with yogurt.

Totals: 367 calories, 50.8 g carbohydrates, 23.9 g protein, 7.6 g fat

	Seeds	Cottage Cheese	Peaches
Calories	87	91	189
Carbohydrates (g)	3	2.1	45.7
Protein (g)	3	19.5	1.4
Fat (g)	7	0.5	0.1

Peanut Butter 'n' Celery/Munch and crunch

- 2 teaspoons reduced-fat peanut butter, smooth-style, without salt
- 2 celery stalks
- 8 ounces fat-free yogurt
- ½ ounce toasted plain wheat germ
- 1 ounce raisins

This one's not just healthy—it might also bring back snacktime memories from grade school (too bad there's no recess anymore). Spread peanut butter on celery stalks and eat them with a cup of mixed-up yogurt, wheat germ, and raisins.

Totals: 361 calories, 51.9 g carbohydrates, 21.3 g protein, 7.6 g fat

	Peanut Butter	Celery	Yogurt	Wheat Germ	Raisins
Calories	68	15	125	58	95
Carbohydrates (g)	2.1	3	17.4	7	22.4
Protein (g)	2.7	0.6	13	4.1	0.9
Fat (g)	5.4	0.2	0.4	1.5	0.1

Tuna Sandwich with Mayo/Tastes like chicken of the sea

- 3 ounces white, water-packed tuna, drained solids
- 1 teaspoon Kraft Light mayo
- 1 celery stalk, 7½" long
- 2 inner leaves romaine lettuce
- 2 slices seven-grain Hearty Slice bread
- 1 small orange

Mix the tuna and mayo and spread it on one slice of bread. Sprinkle chopped celery and lettuce on the other slice. Wrap it in a paper towel and eat it at the kitchen counter. Chase with an orange.

Totals: 385 calories, 54.6 g carbohydrates, 27.1 g protein, 6.4 g fat

	Tuna	Mayo	Celery	Lettuce	Bread	Orange
Calories	103	16	8	4	182	72
Carbohydrates (g)	0	0.3	1.5	0.5	36	16.3
Protein (g)	20.1	0	0.3	0.3	5	1.4
Fat (g)	2.5	1.7	0.1	0	2	0.1

Turkey and Cheese Sandwich/Gobble it at your desk

- 3 ounces Louis Rich Smoked Turkey Breast, 98% fat-free
- 1 teaspoon Kraft Light mayo
- 2 slices cracked-wheat bread
- 2 inner leaves romaine lettuce
- 1 ounce (1 slice) fat-free cheese
- 1 small banana

Spread mayo on a slice of bread; load on the turkey, lettuce, and cheese; and send it down the chute. Eat the banana for dessert.

Totals: 380 calories, 53.3 g carbohydrates, 25.7 g protein, 7.2 g fat

	Turkey	Mayo	Bread	Lettuce	Cheese	Banana
Calories	87	16	134	4	36	103
Carbohydrates (g)	3	0.3	24.8	0.5	1	23.7
Protein (g)	12	0	4.4	0.3	8	1
Fat (g)	3	1.7	2	0	0	0.5

Ham 'n' Cheese Sandwich/A healthy pig-out

- 2 slices cracked-wheat bread
- 2 ounces extra-lean sliced ham (approximately 5% fat)
- 1 ounce (1 slice) fat-free cheese
- 2 inner leaves romaine lettuce
- 1 teaspoon Kraft Light mayo
- 1 small banana

Assemble the bread, ham, cheese, lettuce, and mayo. You know the rest of the story. You want something really different? Slice the banana and put it on the sandwich, too.

Totals: 364 calories, 50.9 g carbohydrates, 24.7 g protein, 7 g fat

	Bread	Ham	Cheese	Lettuce	Mayo	Banana
Calories	134	71	36	4	16	103
Carbohydrates (g)	24.8	0.6	1	0.5	0.3	23.7
Protein (g)	4.4	11	8	0.3	0	1
Fat (g)	2	2.8	0	0	1.7	0.5

Oven-Roasted Chicken Sandwich/It's finger-lickin' good

- **2**   **slices cracked-wheat bread**
- **3**   **ounces Louis Rich boneless, deluxe, oven-roasted chicken breast, 96% fat-free**
- **1**   **ounce (1 slice) fat-free cheese**
- **2**   **inner leaves romaine lettuce**
- **1**   **teaspoon Kraft Light mayo**
- **1**   **small banana**

Following the customary rules, stack your bread, chicken, cheese, lettuce, and mayo; deal yourself a sandwich; and raise the bid by one banana.

Totals: 392 calories, 53.3 g carbohydrates, 28.7 g protein, 7.2 g fat

	Bread	Chicken	Cheese	Lettuce	Mayo	Banana
Calories	134	99	36	4	16	103
Carbohydrates (g)	24.8	3	1	0.5	0.3	23.7
Protein (g)	4.4	15	8	0.3	0	1
Fat (g)	2	3	0	0	1.7	0.5

Egg and Cheese Sandwich/A Grade-A energy booster

- **2**   **slices cracked-wheat bread**
- **1**   **large whole hard-boiled egg, sliced**
- **1**   **large hard-boiled egg white, sliced**
- **2**   **inner leaves romaine lettuce**
- **1**   **teaspoon Kraft Light mayo**
- **1**   **ounce (1 slice) fat-free cheese**
- **1**   **small banana**

Make the sandwich with eggs, lettuce, mayo, and cheese. Just for a change of pace, eat the banana first.

Totals: 383 calories, 51.2 g carbohydrates, 23.5 g protein, 9.5 g fat

	Bread	Egg	Egg White	Lettuce	Mayo	Cheese	Banana
Calories	134	75	15	4	16	36	103
Carbohydrates (g)	24.8	0.6	0.3	0.5	0.3	1	23.7
Protein (g)	4.4	6.3	3.5	0.3	0	8	1
Fat (g)	2	5.3	0	0	1.7	0	0.5

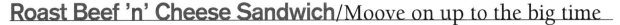

Roast Beef 'n' Cheese Sandwich/Moove on up to the big time

- 2 slices cracked-wheat bread
- 2 ounces Boar's Head Roast Beef
- 2 inner leaves romaine lettuce
- 1 teaspoon Kraft Light mayo
- 1 ounce (1 slice) fat-free cheese
- 1 large orange

Beef up your afternoon snack with a sandwich made from roast beef, lettuce, mayo, and cheese. Orange you glad we didn't say to chase it with a banana?

Totals: 367 calories, 50.2 g carbohydrates, 28.4 g protein, 5.9 g fat

	Bread	Roast Beef	Lettuce	Mayo	Cheese	Orange
Calories	134	82	4	16	36	95
Carbohydrates (g)	24.8	2	0.5	0.3	1	21.6
Protein (g)	4.4	14	0.3	0	8	1.7
Fat (g)	2	2	0	1.7	0	0.2

Peanut Butter and Jelly Bagel/PB&J is A-okay

- 1 oat bran bagel
- 2 tablespoons Jif Reduced Fat Peanut Butter, creamy-style
- 2 teaspoons Polaner All Fruit Spreadable Fruit, black cherry flavor

Spread peanut butter and fruit spread on a bagel. Shave off a few calories by using a smaller bagel or a slice of whole-grain bread.

Totals: 375 calories, 51.8 g carbohydrates, 19.6 g protein, 10.9 g fat

	Bagel	Peanut Butter	Fruit Spread
Calories	181	162	32
Carbohydrates (g)	37.8	6	8
Protein (g)	7.6	12	0
Fat (g)	0.9	10	0

Strawberry Short Shake/It's berry, berry good

- 1 scoop Designer Protein Strawberry Whey
- 1 cup fat-free milk
- 1 cup red grape juice

Blenderize the whey, fat-free milk, and grape juice into a heady froth.

Totals: 334 calories, 52.1 g carbohydrates, 27.4 g protein, 1.2 g fat

	Whey Protein	Milk	Grape Juice
Calories	82	93	159
Carbohydrates (g)	2.3	12	37.8
Protein (g)	17	9	1.4
Fat (g)	0.5	0.5	0.2

AFTERNOON SNACKS FOR THE WEIGHT-GAIN MAN

Chocolate-Banana Shake/A P.M. picker-upper

- 1 scoop Designer Protein Chocolate Whey
- 2 cups fat-free milk
- 2 large bananas

Can you say "blenderize"?

Totals: 556 calories, 90.3 g carbohydrates, 38.3 g protein, 3.6 g fat

	Whey Protein	Milk	Bananas
Calories	89	188	279
Carbohydrates (g)	2.5	24	63.8
Protein (g)	17.5	18	2.8
Fat (g)	1	1.2	1.4

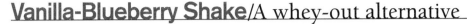

Vanilla-Blueberry Shake/A whey-out alternative

- 10 ounces Healthy Choice Vanilla old-fashioned Dairy Dessert
- 2 cups fat-free milk
- 6 ounces blueberries, fresh or frozen, unsweetened

Blenderize the dairy dessert, fat-free milk, and blueberries. Save the leftovers for videotaping so you can tell your friends that it's a blue movie.

Totals: 556 calories, 91 g carbohydrates, 29.2 g protein, 7.4 g fat

	Dairy Dessert	Milk	Blueberries
Calories	295	188	73
Carbohydrates (g)	52.6	24	14.4
Protein (g)	10	18	1.2
Fat (g)	5	1.2	1.2

Cheese and Veggie Salad/Chop it up, chow it down

- 3 ounces reduced-fat Cheddar cheese
- 2 tablespoons Kraft Reduced-Calorie Creamy Italian salad dressing
- 2 medium carrots
- 1½ small green peppers
- 1 cup romaine lettuce
- 1 tomato
- 2 cups orange juice

Chop the lettuce and veggies and toss them to make a salad. Sprinkle on the grated cheese and dressing. Wash it down with OJ.

Totals: 551 calories, 80.2 g carbohydrates, 28.9 g protein, 12.2 g fat

	Cheese	Dressing	Carrots	Peppers	Lettuce	Tomato	OJ
Calories	147	44	56	34	10	31	229
Carbohydrates (g)	1.6	2	12.4	7.2	1.3	5.7	50
Protein (g)	20.7	0.1	1.2	1	0.9	1	4
Fat (g)	6	4	0.2	0.1	0.1	0.4	1.4

Blueberry-Bran Muffins/Tastes great, keeps you regular

- 2 **Muffin-A-Day Total Health Muffins, blueberry bran**
- 2 **teaspoons Blue Bonnet soft margarine**
- 2 **cups fat-free milk**

Spread the muffins with margarine, open your mouth, and bombs away. Wash 'em down with fat-free milk.

Totals: 568 calories, 86 g carbohydrates, 32 g protein, 9.6 g fat

	Muffins	Margarine	Milk
Calories	313	67	188
Carbohydrates (g)	62	0	24
Protein (g)	14	0	18
Fat (g)	1	7.4	1.2

Chips, Chips, and More Chips/Satisfy your crunch tooth

- 3 **ounces baked potato chips**
- 1 **small orange**
- 1 **cup fat-free milk**
- ½ **cup fat-free yogurt**

Nosh the chips at your computer, and get extra pleasure revenge by pretending that they're Pentium III's. Then satisfy your sweet tooth by mixing orange slices in the yogurt and washing it all down with the milk.

Totals: 559 calories, 106.7 g carbohydrates, 23.4 g protein, 3.8 g fat

	Chips	Orange	Milk	Yogurt
Calories	327	72	93	67
Carbohydrates (g)	69	16.3	12	9.4
Protein (g)	6	1.4	9	7
Fat (g)	3	0.1	0.5	0.2

EVENING SNACKS

Evening snacks are the downfall of many a would-be Hard-Body Man. You've finished your evening chores, showered and shaved, and put on your flannel pajamas. All you want to do is relax in front of the tube for an hour so you can catch David Letterman's Top 10 list.

But as soon as you sit down, your stomach is growling like a drill sergeant, demanding that you march straight to the refrigerator for leftover pizza, Jell-O, or the fixings for a 1,000-calorie Dagwood sandwich.

A stomach full of food can lull you to sleep. Carbohydrates such as rice, potatoes, and bread are rich in tryptophan, an amino acid that transports the brain to the Land of Nod. When your body is on autopilot, though, high-calorie noshes are more likely to be stored as fat. So here are some carbohydrate-rich, low-calorie snacks that'll satisfy your munchies and help you catch your Zzzz's without wrecking your ripples.

Remember, these snacks are for our 175-pound, 5-foot-10 reference man. You will need to adjust portions up or down a bit relative to your own weight and goals as you determined in Personalizing the Plan on page 324. And as usual, you can substitute healthy alternatives if necessary.

EVENING SNACKS FOR THE WEIGHT-LOSS MAN

Rice 'n' Beans/A Third World classic

- ½ cup long-grain brown rice, cooked without salt and butter
- 1 cup Progresso Black Beans, canned
- 1 teaspoon Fleischmann's soft margarine

Half the world subsists on this stuff, so be grateful that you can have it as a snack. Boil and simmer the rice, bring on the beans, and top it off with a teaspoon of margarine. If you're desperate for more flavor, add a dash of Tabasco.

Totals: 343 calories, 57 g carbohydrates, 16 g protein, 5.7 g fat

	Rice	Beans	Margarine
Calories	100	210	33
Carbohydrates (g)	23	34	0
Protein (g)	2	14	0
Fat (g)	0	2	3.7

Ice Cream 'n' Cantaloupe/Scoop it 'n' scarf it

- 4   ounces cantaloupe
- 1   cup fat-free milk
- ¾   cup vanilla ice cream

Blend it. Sounds more sinful than it is. Just make sure that you exercise strict portion control.

Totals: 348 calories, 56 g carbohydrates, 14.5 g protein, 6.8 g fat

	Cantaloupe	Milk	Ice Cream
Calories	45	93	210
Carbohydrates (g)	9.5	12	34.5
Protein (g)	1	9	4.5
Fat (g)	0.3	0.5	6

Tuna Sandwich and Stuff/Some nighttime fishy business

- 3   ounces white, water-packed tuna, drained solids
- 2   teaspoons Kraft Light mayo
- 2   leaves romaine lettuce
- 2   slices wheat bread
- 1   medium apple
- 1   celery stalk

Place the tuna on one slice of bread and the mayo and lettuce on the other, and slap 'em together. Save the apple and celery for a crunchy dessert.

Totals: 373 calories, 48.5 g carbohydrates, 25.4 g protein, 8.4 g fat

	Tuna	Mayo	Lettuce	Bread	Apple	Celery
Calories	103	33	4	135	90	8
Carbohydrates (g)	0	0.7	0.5	24.8	21	1.5
Protein (g)	20.1	0	0.3	4.4	0.3	0.3
Fat (g)	2.5	3.3	0	2	0.5	0.1

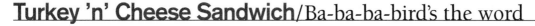

Turkey 'n' Cheese Sandwich/Ba-ba-ba-bird's the word

- **2 slices Pepperidge Farm seven-grain Hearty Slice bread**
- **3 ounces Louis Rich smoked turkey breast, 98% fat-free**
- **2 leaves romaine lettuce**
- **1 teaspoon Kraft Light mayo**
- **1 ounce (1 slice) fat-free cheese**
- **12 seedless grapes**

Place the turkey on one slice of bread, and the mayo, lettuce, and cheese on the other slice. Get your main squeeze to drop the grapes into your mouth.

Totals: 372 calories, 51.5 g carbohydrates, 25.7 g protein, 7.1 g fat

	Bread	Turkey	Lettuce	Mayo	Cheese	Grapes
Calories	182	87	4	16	36	47
Carbohydrates (g)	36	3	0.5	0.3	1	10.7
Protein (g)	5	12	0.3	0	8	0.4
Fat (g)	2	3	0	1.7	0	0.4

Ham 'n' Cheese Sandwich/Pork it in your mouth

- **2 slices Pepperidge Farm seven-grain Hearty Slice bread**
- **2 ounces extra-lean sliced ham (approximately 5% fat)**
- **1 ounce (1 slice) fat-free cheese**
- **2 leaves romaine lettuce**
- **1 teaspoon Kraft Light Mayo**
- **12 seedless grapes**

Place the ham on one slice of bread and the lettuce, mayo, and cheese on the other slice. If you have any grapes left over, see if you can get Rover to eat one. (Most dogs just gum 'em.)

Totals: 356 calories, 49.1 g carbohydrates, 24.7 g protein, 6.9 g fat

	Bread	Ham	Cheese	Lettuce	Mayo	Grapes
Calories	182	71	36	4	16	47
Carbohydrates (g)	36	0.6	1	0.5	0.3	10.7
Protein (g)	5	11	8	0.3	0	0.4
Fat (g)	2	2.8	0	0	1.7	0.4

Chicken 'n' Cheese Sandwich/It'd better taste like chicken

- 2 slices Pepperidge Farm seven-grain Hearty Slice bread
- 3 ounces Louis Rich Chicken Breast, boneless, deluxe, oven-roasted, and 96% fat-free
- 1 ounce (1 slice) fat-free cheese
- 2 leaves romaine lettuce
- 1 teaspoon Kraft Light mayo
- 12 seedless grapes

Place the chicken on one slice of bread and the mayo, lettuce, and cheese on the other slice. Manually combine. For fun, try balancing as many grapes as you can on a table knife.

Totals: 384 calories, 51.5 g carbohydrates, 28.7 g protein, 7.1 g fat

	Bread	Chicken	Cheese	Lettuce	Mayo	Grapes
Calories	182	99	36	4	16	47
Carbohydrates (g)	36	3	1	0.5	0.3	10.7
Protein (g)	5	15	8	0.3	0	0.4
Fat (g)	2	3	0	0	1.7	0.4

Boiled-Egg and Cheese Sandwich/Tell 'em Humpty sent ya

- 2 slices Pepperidge Farm seven-grain Hearty Slice bread
- 1 large egg, hard-boiled
- 1 large egg white, hard-boiled
- 2 leaves romaine lettuce
- 1 teaspoon Kraft Light mayo
- 1 ounce (1 slice) fat-free cheese
- 10 seedless grapes

Slice the eggs and put 'em on one piece of bread. Load the mayo, lettuce, and cheese on the other piece. Now eat the grapes. Save the sandwich for dessert.

Totals: 368 calories, 47.6 g carbohydrates, 23.4 g protein, 9.3 g fat

	Bread	Whole Egg	Egg White	Lettuce	Mayo	Cheese	Grapes
Calories	182	75	15	4	16	36	40
Carbohydrates (g)	36	0.6	0.3	0.5	0.3	1	8.9
Protein (g)	5	6.3	3.5	0.3	0	8	0.3
Fat (g)	2	5.3	0	0	1.7	0	0.3

Roast Beef 'n' Cheese Sandwich/Beefalicious and buffalicious

- 2 slices Pepperidge Farm seven-grain Hearty Slice bread
- 2 ounces Boar's Head Roast Beef, top round, oven-roasted
- 2 leaves romaine lettuce
- 1 teaspoon Kraft Light mayo
- 1 ounce (1 slice) fat-free cheese
- 10 seedless grapes

Place the roast beef on one slice of bread. Load the rest of the goods (minus the grapes) on the other slice. Assemble the sandwich. If you're watching late-night sports, especially football, let loose with a good, satisfying "moo."

Totals: 360 calories, 48.7 g carbohydrates, 27.6 g protein, 6 g fat

	Bread	Roast Beef	Lettuce	Mayo	Cheese	Grapes
Calories	182	82	4	16	36	40
Carbohydrates (g)	36	2	0.5	0.3	1	8.9
Protein (g)	5	14	0.3	0	8	0.3
Fat (g)	2	2	0	1.7	0	0.3

PB&J Sandwich/AT&T (always tempting and tasty)

- 2 slices Pepperidge Farm seven-grain Hearty Slice bread
- 2 tablespoons Jif Reduced Fat Peanut Butter, creamy-style
- 2 teaspoons Smuckers Simply 100% Fruit, blueberry
- ½ cup fat-free milk

Smear the peanut butter on one slice of bread and the fruit spread on the other slice. Clamp together, chase with milk, and think about the little red-haired girl you liked in grade school.

Totals: 423 calories, 56 g carbohydrates, 21.5 g protein, 12.3 g fat

	Bread	Peanut Butter	Fruit Spread	Milk
Calories	182	162	32	47
Carbohydrates (g)	36	6	8	6
Protein (g)	5	12	0	4.5
Fat (g)	2	10	0	0.3

Ice Cream Crunch/An any-night sundae

- ½ cup fat-free ice cream
- 1 ounce toasted, plain wheat germ
- ½ ounce sunflower seed kernels, dry-roasted, with salt added
- 1 cup fat-free milk

Dish the ice cream and sprinkle on the wheat germ and sunflower seeds. To quench your post-sundae thirst, gulp a cup of fat-free milk.

Totals: 402 calories, 52.5 g carbohydrates, 23 g protein, 10.6 g fat

	Ice Cream	Wheat Germ	Sunflower Seeds	Milk
Calories	104	117	88	93
Carbohydrates (g)	23	14.1	3.4	12
Protein (g)	3	8.3	2.7	9
Fat (g)	0	3	7.1	0.5

EVENING SNACKS FOR THE WEIGHT-GAIN MAN

Ice Cream 'n' Almonds/Go all the whey

- 1½ cups Sealtest fat-free ice cream
- 1 ounce Flanigan Farms Almonds, dry-roasted, unsalted, chopped
- ½ scoop Designer Protein Vanilla Whey

Dish the ice cream and top with the rest of the goodies. Laugh all the "whey" to the bathroom scale.

Totals: 559 calories, 79 g carbohydrates, 23 g protein, 16.6 g fat

	Ice Cream	Almonds	Whey Protein
Calories	333	185	41
Carbohydrates (g)	72	6	1
Protein (g	9	6	8
Fat (g)	1	15.2	0.4

Cookies 'n' Milk/It's legal

- 10 **Health Valley Delight Apricot Cookies**
- 1 **cup fat-free milk**
- 2 **tablespoons flaxseed meal**
- ½ **scoop Designer Protein Chocolate Whey**

Dole out the cookies from the bag, mix the flaxseed meal and chocolate whey into the milk, and you've got a healthy version of a favorite bedtime snack.

Totals: 504 calories, 77.3 g carbohydrates, 27.4 g protein, 9 g fat

	Cookies	Milk	Flaxseed Meal	Whey Protein
Calories	275	93	91	45
Carbohydrates (g)	60	12	4	1.3
Protein (g)	6.6	9	3	8.8
Fat (g)	1	0.5	7	0.5

Chocolate Chip Cookies 'n' Milk/An irresistible combination

- 5 **Chocolate Chips Deluxe reduced-fat cookies**
- 2 **cups fat-free milk**

Chomp, slurp, and pity the poor peons who think that they can't have any.

Totals: 563 calories, 79 g carbohydrates, 23 g protein, 16.2 g fat

	Milk	Cookies
Calories	188	375
Carbohydrates (g)	24	55
Protein (g)	18	5
Fat (g)	1.2	15

Oatmeal Cookies and Cottage Cheese/Another combo

- **7 Weight Watchers Oatmeal Cookies with raisins**
- **6 ounces 1% cottage cheese**
- **¾ ounce unsalted, roasted, shelled sunflower seeds**

Eat the cookies separately. Eat the cottage cheese and sunflower seeds separately, or mix them if you want.

Totals: 577 calories, 79.7 g carbohydrates, 28.6 g protein, 15.9 g fat

	Cookies	Cottage Cheese	Sunflower Seeds
Calories	326	118	133
Carbohydrates (g)	70	4.6	5.1
Protein (g)	3.5	21	4.1
Fat (g)	3.5	1.7	10.7

Milk 'n' Chocolate Cake/Happy birthday to you

- **2 cups fat-free milk**
- **5 ounces Weight Watchers Chocolate cake (approximately 1 package)**

Even if it's not your birthday, you can indulge in this guilty pleasure with no morning-after regrets.

Totals: 566 calories, 86 g carbohydrates, 28 g protein, 11.2 g fat

	Milk	Cake
Calories	188	378
Carbohydrates (g)	24	62
Protein (g)	18	10
Fat (g)	1.2	10

100-PLUS BEERS, DESSERTS, AND OTHER RECKLESS PLEASURES
SPLURGES

The Hard-Body Plan draws together all kinds of foods that guys like: turkey sandwiches, pastas with tangy sauces, seafood, scrambled eggs, and the occasional sweet.

What it *doesn't* recommend are the treats that figure more heavily into the Homer Simpson Body Plan, namely . . . mmmm, beer and desserts and desserts and beer.

If you're the sort who can make the investment of time and effort to get into great shape, your willpower will probably help you resist most of the belly-softening foods and drinks that come your way, most of the time.

But sometimes you just *have to* share a few tall, cold ones with your buddies, or dig a spoon into a tasty chocolate or creamy one with your lady friend.

Keeping those special occasions in mind, here is a listing of nutritional information for some of the beers and desserts that you might encounter. If you can't find them on the shelves, feel free to choose a healthy substitution.

BEERS

We can't offer the nutritional breakdown on every single one of the gazillion big-brewery domestics, microbrews, and imports that you can find throughout this fine country and the world. But we can offer nutritional data on some of the brands that you're likely to encounter (see next page).

If you have a particular microbrew fave, ask the brewery for the nutritional breakdown so you can determine how tipping a few tall ones will affect your Hard-Body strategy.

BEERS				
	Calories	Protein (g)	Carbs (g)	Alcohol (g)
Anheuser Marzen	168	2.3	15.2	14
Beck's	148	1.7	10	14.5
Budweiser	144	1.2	11.3	13.4
Bud Light	110	1.1	6.9	11.1
Busch	144	1.2	11.9	13.1
Carlsberg	149	1.2	11.9	13.8
Carlsberg Light	110	1.1	6.5	11.4
Coors	137	0.6	11.6	12.6
Coors Dry	119	0.4	6	13.3
Coors Extra Gold	151	1.3	12.5	13.7
Coors Light	103	0.7	4.7	11.6
Dribeck's	94	1	7	8.9
Keystone	121	0.6	6.8	13.1
Keystone Dry	121	0.6	6.4	13.3
Keystone Light	100	0.6	4.4	11.4
Killian's	161	1	15	13.9
Knickerbocker	140	0.9	12.3	12.5
Lowenbrau Dark Special	158	1.4	14.3	13.6
Meister Brau	141	1	12.8	12.3
Meister Brau Light	98	0.8	3.5	11.5
Michelob	156	1.5	13.6	13.7
Michelob Dry	133	1.3	7.8	13.8
Michelob Light	134	1.2	11.9	11.7
Miller Genuine Draft	147	1	13.1	12.9
Miller Genuine Draft Lite	110	0.8	7	11.5
Miller High Life	147	1	13.1	12.9
Milwaukee's Best	133	0.9	11.4	12
Milwaukee's Best Light	98	0.8	3.5	11.5
Natural Light	110	1.1	6.6	11.3
Prior Double Dark	171	1.4	15.4	14.8
Rheingold	148	1	12.9	13.2
Rheingold Light	96	0.7	2.8	11.7
Rolling Rock Premium	145	0.4	10	14.8
Rolling Rock Light	104	0.4	8	10.1
Schmidt's	148	1	12.9	13.2
Schmidt's Light	96	0.7	2.8	11.7

NOTE: 12-oz serving and 0 g fat

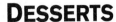

DESSERTS

Special occasions are special occasions and are celebrated in special ways. As long as you regard desserts as special-occasion treats and go lightly on the portions, you can enjoy yourself—and the sinful, sumptuous flavors and textures—without blowing your Hard-Body work.

We'll give you nutritional breakdowns on some typical desserts so that you can understand the potential damage. Take a look, then go ahead and have a good time.

ICE CREAM AND FROZEN YOGURT

	Calories	Protein (g)	Carbs (g)	Fat (g)
Regular Ice Cream				
Häagen Dazs Butter Pecan	352	5	29	24
Häagen Dazs Chocolate	269	5	24	17
Häagen Dazs Chocolate Chocolate Chip	312	5	28	20
Häagen Dazs Coffee	265	5	23	17
Häagen Dazs Vanilla	265	5	23	17
Fat-Free Ice Cream				
Sealtest Black Cherry "Free"	100	2	25	0
Sealtest Chocolate "Free"	100	3	23	0
Sealtest Peach "Free"	100	2	23	0
Sealtest Strawberry "Free"	100	2	23	0
Sealtest Vanilla "Free"	100	3	24	0
Sealtest Vanilla-Chocolate-Strawberry "Free"	100	3	23	0
Sealtest Vanilla-Fudge Royale "Free"	100	3	24	0
Sealtest Vanilla-Strawberry Royale "Free"	100	3	25	0
Frozen Yogurt				
Ben & Jerry's Cherry Garcia Low Fat	167	4	31	3
Ben & Jerry's Chocolate Fudge Brownie Low Fat	200	6	35	4
Breyers All Natural Chocolate	117	3	24	1
Breyers All Natural Strawberry	109	3	22	1
Breyers All Natural Vanilla	113	3	23	1
Sealtest Black Cherry "Free"	104	2	24	0
Sealtest Chocolate "Free"	108	3	24	0
Sealtest Peach "Free"	100	2	23	0
Sealtest Red Raspberry "Free"	100	2	23	0
Sealtest Strawberry "Free"	96	2	22	0
Yoplait Vanilla, Light	105.5	3	20	1.5

NOTE: ½-cup serving

CAKES, PIES, AND PUDDINGS

	Size	Calories (g)	Protein (g)	Carbs (g)	Fat
Cakes	3.6 oz				
Angel food, store-bought		262	5.9	57.8	0.8
Cheesecake, store-bought		327	5.5	25.5	22.5
Chocolate with chocolate frosting, store-bought		382.4	4.1	54.6	16.4
Fruitcake, store-bought		340	2.9	61.6	9.1
Pineapple upside-down, homemade		325	3.5	50.5	12.1
Pound, butter, store-bought		396	5.5	48.8	19.9
Sponge, store-bought		290	5.4	61.1	2.7
Yellow with chocolate frosting, store-bought		393	3.8	55.4	17.4
Yellow with vanilla frosting, store-bought		380	3.5	58.8	14.5
Packaged Snack Cakes					
Creme-filled, chocolate with frosting	1 cupcake	193	1.7	30.2	7.3
Creme-filled, sponge	1 cake	158	1.3	27.2	4.8
Cupcake, low-fat chocolate, with frosting	1 cupcake	137	1.8	28.9	1.6
Pies	⅛ of a 9-in. pie				
Apple, store-bought		243	1.9	34	11
Banana cream, no-bake, homemade from mix		256	3.4	31.6	12.9
Blueberry, store-bought		237	1.8	34.9	10
Boston cream, store-bought		258	2.4	42.9	8.5
Cherry, store-bought		266	2	39.8	11
Chocolate creme, store-bought		319	2.6	33.6	19.4
Chocolate mousse, no-bake, homemade from mix		271	3.5	29.6	15.4
Coconut creme, store-bought		307	2.1	37.2	16.6
Lemon meringue, store-bought		273	1.5	47.2	8.7
Pecan, store-bought		411	4	57.2	18.5
Pumpkin, store-bought		210	3.9	27.3	9.5
Ready-to-Eat Puddings	4 oz				
Banana		144	2.7	24	4
Chocolate		150	3.1	25.8	4.5
Lemon		142	0.1	28.4	3.4
Rice		185	2.3	25	8.4
Tapioca		135	2.3	22	4.2
Vanilla		147	2.6	24.7	4.1

Pastries, Toaster Pastries, and Marshmallow Treats

	Size	Calories	Protein (g)	Carbs (g)	Fat (g)
Pastries					
Cream puffs, shell with custard filling, homemade	1 cream puff	335	8.7	29.8	20.2
Danish (apple, cinnamon, raisin, or strawberry)	3 oz	539	7.7	67.9	26.3
Eclairs, custard-filled with chocolate glaze, homemade	1 3½-in. by 2-in.	295	7.2	27.1	17.6
Toaster Pastries					
Kellogg's Low Fat Pop-Tarts, Cherry	1 pastry	194	2.3	39.8	2.9
Kellogg's Pop-Tarts, Blueberry	1 pastry	214	2.4	35.6	6.9
Kellogg's Pop-Tarts, Brown Sugar Cinnamon	1 pastry	222	2.7	32.2	9.2
Kellogg's Pop-Tarts, Frosted Blueberry	1 pastry	206	2.4	37.3	5.2
Kellogg's Pop-Tarts, Frosted Brown Sugar Cinnamon	1 pastry	213	2.5	34.2	7.4
Kellogg's Pop-Tarts, Frosted Cherry	1 pastry	206	2.2	37.4	5.3
Kellogg's Pop-Tarts, Frosted Chocolate Fudge	1 pastry	204	2.7	37.3	4.8
Marshmallow Treats					
Kellogg's Rice Krispies Treat	3.6 oz	90	1	18	2

ROAD EATS
EATING WELL ON THE RUN

In Jack Kerouac's classic novel *On the Road*, the characters subsisted on standard diner fare: chicken-fried steak, mashed potatoes with gravy, and lemon meringue pie.

But that was the 1950s, when the rules of the road were simple: Load up your stomach with enough high-calorie grub to hold you until the next truck stop. That's why so many aging truckers look at least as jowly and bulky, to put it politely, as that bulldog hood ornament on one make of big rigs.

For Hard-Body Man, today's rules of the road are a little more complicated. If you'd rather resemble the sleek greyhound painted on the sides of buses, you have to eat smart. Here are some meal suggestions for when you're forced to patronize places where the air is so heavy with cooking grease that you feel fatter just inhaling it. If you can't find these items, feel free to substitute similar foods.

THE RULES OF THE ROAD

1. Get the doggie bag/box with your order. That way, you can keep the extra portions out of harm's way while you eat, and save them for another meal.

2. Skip sugary sodas that add unnecessary calories. Instead, slake your thirst with no-cal sodas, black coffee, tea, or just plain water.

3. Send your stomach some fiber. When you're really ravenous, drinking a sugar-free psyllium fiber supplement such as Metamucil or Equate before you eat can take the edge off your appetite. It might even improve your cholesterol profile. Be sure to follow the directions on the label. If you aren't that extreme, munch on an apple or a pear instead.

4. Bank your calories. If you know that you're going out for dinner, eat a little less breakfast, lunch, and snacks so you stay within your calorie limit for the day.

5. Go for the salad. Stick with tossed salads containing 1 to 1½ cups of vegetables and 2 tablespoons of low-calorie dressing. Always order salad dressings on the side (likewise potato toppings).

Since most of these meals exceed your calorie totals, it's best to minimize the number of meals that you eat out. But if you can't, at least stick to the following generic meal plan:

• 3 ounces of lean broiled or roasted beef, fish, or chicken

• a salad with low-calorie dressing and no cheese

• 1 cup of steamed vegetables

• 1 small plain baked potato or ½ cup rice

Check out these menus and restaurants will never intimidate you again. You can eat ethnic, you can eat truck-driver-fare, but wherever you eat you'll do it with class and Hard-Body smarts.

Seafood Dinner No. 1/Eat lobster, live to tail about it

- 1 salad with low-cal dressing
- ½ cup steamed vegetables, no butter
- 4 ounces steamed or broiled lobster tail, no butter
- ½ cup rice pilaf

Believe it or not, this meal is only about 60 calories more than your normal meals. Just remember to dribble the lobster with lemon instead of butter, order low-cal salad dressing, and ask that your vegetables be steamed.

Totals: 393 calories, 59.8 g carbohydrates, 32.8 g protein, 4.3 g fat

	Salad	Vegetables	Lobster Tail	Rice Pilaf
Calories	37	36	102	218
Carbohydrates (g)	6.7	7	1.1	45
Protein (g)	1.6	2	23.2	6
Fat (g)	2.1	0.2	0.5	1.5

Seafood Dinner No. 2/Flounder for success

- 1 salad with low-cal dressing
- 1 flounder stuffed with 3 ounces breading
- ½ cup steamed vegetables, no butter

You gotta love a fish that looks like a pancake with eyes, and this dinner allows you to love it without leaving it.

Totals: 419 calories, 34.7 g carbohydrates, 28.6 g protein, 20.3 g fat

	Salad	Flounder	Vegetables
Calories	37	346	36
Carbohydrates (g)	6.7	21	7
Protein (g)	1.6	25	2
Fat (g)	2.1	18	0.2

Chinese Food/Stir-fry won't fry your diet

- 1   3-ounce egg roll
- 1   cup wonton soup
- 1   cup stir-fry chicken and vegetables (no rice)
- 1   salad with low-cal dressing

Sorry, no fried wonton or fortune cookies. But it's enough Chinese to make you feel like you've had Chinese.

Totals: 486 calories, 48.4 g carbohydrates, 46.7 g protein, 11.4 g fat

	Egg Roll	Soup	Stir-Fry	Salad
Calories	156	108	185	37
Carbohydrates (g)	24	10	7.7	6.7
Protein (g)	6	8	31.1	1.6
Fat (g)	4	2	3.3	2.1

Mexican Food No. 1/Go south of the border without "going south"

- 1   6½-ounce bean and cheese burrito
- 1   salad with low-cal dressing

Yes, you can indulge your passion for Mexican food. Just remember, one burrito is a whole meal.

Totals: 423 calories, 61.7 g carbohydrates, 16.7 g protein, 13.8 g fat

	Burrito	Salad
Calories	386	37
Carbohydrates (g)	55	6.7
Protein (g)	15.1	1.6
Fat (g)	11.7	2.1

Mexican Food No. 2/Fajita your face

- 1   7-ounce chicken fajita
- 1   salad with low-cal dressing

Tempted to eat a fajita? If you stick with the chicken variety, you don't have to chicken out.

Totals: 364 calories, 42.7 g carbohydrates, 22.6 g protein, 13.1 g fat

	Fajita	Salad
Calories	327	37
Carbohydrates (g)	36	6.7
Protein (g)	21	1.6
Fat (g)	11	2.1

Fast Food/Hot diggity dawg

- 1   hot dog with chili
- 1   salad with low-cal dressing

If you have no alternative but the local Wiener World, you can still have your dog and eat it too.

Totals: 337 calories, 38 g carbohydrates, 15.1 g protein, 15.5 g fat

	Hot Dog	Salad
Calories	300	37
Carbohydrates (g)	31.3	6.7
Protein (g)	13.5	1.6
Fat (g)	13.4	2.1

Out with the Guys/Nosh on some nachos

- **6 to 8**   **nachos with cheese and jalapeño peppers**
- **2**   **light beers**

An occasional night of nachos and beer is okay, but it'll eat up your entire calorie quota for dinner and your evening snack. It's also filled with empty calories. To paraphrase Woody Allen, though, as empty-calorie experiences go, it's one of the best.

Totals: 835 calories, 73.5 g carbohydrates, 18.8 g protein, 34.1 g fat

	Nachos	Beers
Calories	615	220
Carbohydrates (g)	60.1	13.4
Protein (g)	16.8	2
Fat (g)	34.1	0

American Style/Spring for a spud

- **1**   **baked potato with 2 tablespoons of cheese sauce, broccoli, and roughly 1 level teaspoon of bacon bits**
- **1**   **salad with low-cal dressing**

An occasional spud won't preclude you from achieving stud-muffinhood.

Totals: 540 calories, 53.2 g carbohydrates, 16.2 g protein, 30.8 g fat

	Potato	Salad
Calories	503	37
Carbohydrates (g)	46.5	6.7
Protein (g)	14.6	1.6
Fat (g)	28.7	2.1

Fried Chicken Dinner/Fry me a river

- 1   piece white-meat fried chicken
- 1   salad with low-cal dressing

Take it from us: One piece of fried chicken is company, but two will crowd your arteries.

Totals: 524 calories, 26.3 g carbohydrates, 37.3 g protein, 31.6 g fat

	Chicken	Salad
Calories	487	37
Carbohydrates (g)	19.6	6.7
Protein (g)	35.7	1.6
Fat (g)	29.5	2.1

Steakhouse Dinner/Steak your claim to good eating

- 1   salad with low-cal dressing
- 1   6-ounce filet mignon
- 1   baked sweet potato, cinnamon only, no butter

If the filet mignon weighs 12 ounces, cut it in half and stash one half in a doggie bag/box. If the potato is extra large, do the same. If you save some for the microwave, you'll get to do the steak-and-potato thing two nights in a row.

Totals: 507 calories, 34.4 g carbohydrates, 52.1 g protein, 19.5 g fat

	Salad	Steak	Sweet Potato
Calories	37	350	120
Carbohydrates (g)	6.7	0	27.7
Protein (g)	1.6	48.5	2
Fat (g)	2.1	17.3	0.1

Italian Dinner/Please pasta spaghetti

- 1   **salad with low-cal dressing**
- 1   **cup spaghetti with meat sauce**
- 1   **piece garlic bread**

Mama Mia, you get garlic bread with this dinner, and it won't stink up your calorie count.

Totals: 360 calories, 52.1 g carbohydrates, 15 g protein, 11.8 g fat

	Salad	Spaghetti	Bread
Calories	37	221	102
Carbohydrates (g)	6.7	33	12.4
Protein (g)	1.6	11	2.4
Fat (g)	2.1	5	4.7

Quick Dinner-on-the-Go/A wrap that's music to your mouth

- 1   **tortilla or pita-type steak wrap**
- •   **Unsweetened iced tea or sparkling water**

Tune in an oldies station and get your kicks on Route 66 while gnawing on this Southwest-inspired hybrid.

Totals: 517 calories, 52 g carbohydrates, 21 g protein, 25 g fat

	Wrap	Tea or Water
Calories	517	0
Carbohydrates (g)	52	0
Protein (g)	21	0
Fat (g)	25	0

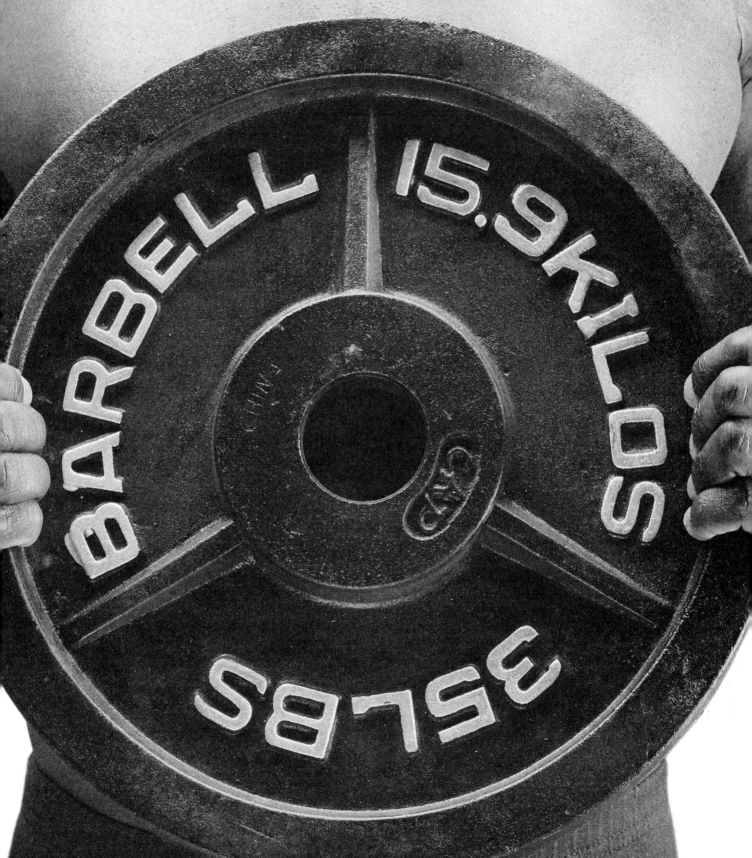

How to Create the Ultimate Workout Space
The Perfect Home Gym

We're going to assume that you have the space, the desire, and the money to set up your very own home gym. What are the essentials and what are some fun extras you might want to have? It's only limited by space, desire, and money. Here are our suggestions.

- A few full-length mirrors on walls
- Boom box
- Your six favorite enlivening, make-you-wanna-boogie CDs
- Fan
- Fridge with a case of sports drinks or juice drinks
- Hooks for three towels—one to wipe your sweat off you, one to wipe your sweat off your equipment, and one for a buddy
- Chair for rest breaks
- Padded carpeting on floor, or rubber gym flooring. You will break tile and scar wood and most other surfaces, not to mention make terrific noise if anyone's ceiling is also your floor.
- Noticeably absent: beepers and phones. None. Not one.
- Wall clock with a second hand to time your workouts
- TV and VCR
- Jump rope
- Exercise bike (Schwinn Air-Dyne style)
- Stairmaster
- Concept II rowing machine
- Treadmill. Skip this unless you're willing to pay $1,000 or more for one that meets these criteria: It should have a 2.5 horsepower continuous-duty motor and a welded frame; it should be at least 18 inches wide on the running surface and at least 50 inches long; and it should be capable of being raised and lowered while you're running on it, so you can adjust terrain while working out.
- Swiss ball
- Pullup bar
- Dip bar
- Plate tree and dumbbell rack
- Light (as opposed to dark) posters on the walls to brighten up the place if it's a basement. Good visuals. Whatever motivates you. Our publisher likes posters of jazz greats. Some of us prefer posters of Pamela Anderson. Wives probably appreciate jazz greats—or buff football players. Put up what moves *you* without your having to move *out*.
- Full-spectrum lights or halogen lighting if it's a dark room, such as a basement, to give it a lively, summery feel
- Blackboard or whiteboard on which you have your workouts charted for each day
- Air filter
- Water cooler
- Scale
- Extra sweats and T-shirts to layer on if you start to chill
- Measuring tape . . . to chart those gains
- Legal pad or clipboard, and hook to hang it on
- Corner sauna and portable hot tub
- Shower
- More towels for use after a shower

WEIGHT TRAINING EQUIPMENT

- One bar (either a standard 6-foot or Olympic-style 7-foot-long weight bar)

- One set of weights: four 5-pounds, four 10s, two 25s, two 35s, and two 45s to start. You'll add more later.

- One easy-curl bar (20 to 25 pounds)

- Two collars. Newer collars that use spring tension to anchor the weights (instead of bolts screwed down against the bar) are easier to use, more reliable, and more expensive. Still, a good set should run less than $50.

- Six pairs of dumbbells. Get 10-, 15-, 20-, 25-, 30-, and 35-pound sets.

- Good-quality bench that can incline and decline. Make sure that the supports are at least 36 inches wide for stability. Cheap ones are too narrow and flimsy.

- Set of squat racks

- Smith machine

- Hyperextension machine

- Incline board (to stand on for calf raises)

NOTE: These recommendations were reviewed by exercise physiologist Peter Lemon, Ph.D.

THE RIGHT CLOTHES FOR WORKING OUT
THE HARD-BODY CLOSET

How much workout clothing do you need? Here's a beautifully stocked closet to use as your guide, courtesy of the style and fitness gurus at *Men's Health* magazine. Understand that to do this to the hilt will mean spending between $500 and $1,000.

Our assumptions:

- You do indoor workouts three times per week.

- You do outdoor aerobic activities (running, biking, softball, leaf raking, whatever) three times a week.

- You wash your clothes once a week.

- You use each article of clothing just one time before washing it. You can wear your shorts for a couple of days if you want. Most guys do. Always wear fresh underwear, T-shirts, and socks.

TOWELS

- Six oversize cotton bath towels. Splurge on this one; great towels aren't much more costly than cheap ones and are a great luxury after a shower. Wash after each use.

- Four cotton hand towels. Keep one with you while weight training to wipe your brow and clean up the sweat you leave on the gear. Wash after each use.

PANTS

- Two pairs of running shorts made of high-tech, lightweight, wicking fabric with a built-in (underwear) liner

- Three pairs of all-cotton sweat shorts

- Two pairs of all-cotton sweatpants

- One pair of North Face cross-training pants made of a vapor-wick, stretch jersey, poly-Lycra blend

- Two pairs of swim trunks (come summer or vacation, you'll need them)

- Two pairs of running tights (if you live in a cold-winter region)

UNDERWEAR

- Six pairs of all-cotton boxers or briefs (comfortable ones you can move in)

- Two pairs of Champion biking shorts (These not only wick away sweat on hot days but are also amazingly comfortable. If you're modest, wear sweat shorts over them.)

SHOES

- One pair of running shoes

- One pair of cross-trainers (for your indoor workouts)

- One pair of walking/hiking shoes

- Specialty shoes, based on your preferred activities (baseball cleats, biking shoes . . .)

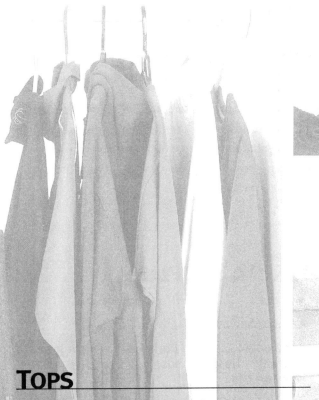

TOPS

- Six short-sleeve T-shirts made of cotton or synthetic wicking material (or mix 'em up)
- Two long-sleeve cotton henley shirts
- Two all-cotton sweatshirts, one of them hooded
- One long-sleeve shirt made of wicking, warmth-holding material
- One long-sleeve, unlined shell windbreaker/rain jacket

SOCKS

- Six pairs of full-calf, all-cotton white socks
- Three pairs of low-cut, all-cotton white socks
- Two pairs of polypropylene socks (for hiking and winter activities)
- Two pairs of wool outdoor socks (these go over the polypropylene socks)

OTHER

- Baseball cap
- Weight lifting gloves
- Sports gloves (baseball, golf, biking—whatever your sport)
- Two pairs of sunglasses
- Key holder (for running or biking; the around-the-neck type is most convenient)
- Canvas bag or backpack (useful for stuffing dirty clothes in)
- Exercise bag (collapsible but strong, with pockets for carrying gear to and from the gym)
- Prepacked toiletry bag (have it always ready for trips to the gym or for business or pleasure travel)

WHAT EVERY GUY SHOULD STOCK
THE PERFECT PANTRY

What should a man interested in eating well keep in stock in his kitchen cabinets? Here's a very full list. Remember the obvious rule of space management: Keep the stuff you use a lot (cereals, cooking oils, boxes of pasta) close by, at a convenient height. Put the occasional-usage stuff low, high, or in the basement.

And, of course, you will need to adjust the quantities that are suggested to your own rate of consumption and needs.

BASIC COOKING SUPPLIES

- Oils. You need two: vegetable (preferably canola) and olive.

- Vinegars. Again, two versions: red wine and apple cider.

- Herbs: oregano, basil, thyme, Italian seasoning, parsley, rosemary

- Spices: chili powder, cinnamon, cumin, garlic powder, and some shakers of special blends, such as the McCormick Spice Blends

- Sugar

- Flour or flour mix, such as Bisquick

- Salt

- Pepper

- Soy sauce

- Chicken broth (stock both small and large cans)

- Pasta. Have both strand types (for instance, linguine or spaghetti) and shape types (such as fusilli or wagon wheels).

- Wild rice (2 pounds uncooked or a large box of instant)

- Ramen noodles, six bags

DRINK SUPPLIES

- Cocoa

- Lemonade powder

- Tea bags: assorted herbal; jasmine or green (great antioxidant booster); English Breakfast or Earl Grey

PREPARED FOODS

- Spaghetti sauces, low-fat

- Prepared soups, six cans. Keep a selection, such as minestrone, lentil, and low-fat clam chowder.

- Side dishes, four or five boxes. Get starches such as rice pilaf, black beans and rice, low-fat macaroni and cheese, and couscous blends.

READY-TO-EAT ITEMS

- Cereals, three boxes. Keep a mix, such as fruit or nut brans, flake cereals, wheat germ, and low-fat granolas.

- Oatmeal, either in packets or in a canister or box. (The canister type offers more healthy fiber.)

- Cereal bars (good for breakfasts or snacks)

- Raisins

- Crackers, two types. Try sesame rounds and wheat.

- Microwave popcorn. Buy it by the case, in reduced-fat or fat-free versions.

- Tortilla chips, baked

- Nuts. Get chopped unsalted nuts and sunflower seeds—they're great for adding to salads and very healthy.

CANNED GOODS (TWO OF EACH)

- Pineapple chunks in juice or light syrup

- Pears

- Water chestnuts

- Bamboo shoots

- Beans. Always keep a variety, such as black beans, chili beans, chickpeas, baked beans, and low-fat refried beans.

- Whole tomatoes

- Tomato sauce

- Tomato paste

INTERMEDIATE-LEVEL COOKING SUPPLIES

- Nuts, three 1-pound bags (peanuts, walnuts, cashews, pistachios)

- Favorite specialty items. We recommend hearts of palm, artichoke hearts, roasted peppers, and capers.

- Sesame oil

- Rice wine vinegar

- Chocolate Chambord sauce or any premade dessert sauce. Spoon on ice cream, brownies, or even just bananas.

- Tofu. Buy brands that come in a tightly sealed box; these store at room temperature for up to a year.

IF YOU HAVE A BREAD MACHINE OR BAKE

- Baking powder

- Wheat flour

- Bread flour

- Baking soda

- Cornstarch

- Honey

- Yeast

REFRIGERATOR BACKUPS

- Jar of salsa

- Ketchup

- Mustard

- Fruit spreads

- Peanut butter (reduced fat)

FRESH FOODS

- Onions, 2 pounds

- Potatoes, four loose russets or reds and/or sweet potatoes

- Garlic, one large head

- Bananas, small bunch

- Tropical fruit, such as a pineapple, mango, kiwi, or papaya. They're hell to peel but heaven to eat.

OTHER BACKUP ITEMS

- Whey protein powder (for those rush days)

- Psyllium fiber, such as Metamucil

The advice here was reviewed by Thomas Incledon, M.S., R.D.

WHAT HARD-BODY MAN KEEPS ON ICE
THE SMART REFRIGERATOR

You can't eat well if the only green stuff in your refrigerator is mold. Here's how Mr. Perfect would stock his icebox if he wanted to eat healthy and well—and impress visiting photographers, mothers, women, and small children. You may need to adjust the specific amounts of food items listed below according to your needs.

The assumptions:

- You eat most breakfasts and dinners at home, but just a few lunches.
- You shop once a week, so you keep meats and produce for the coming week and not much more.
- You're stocking this just for yourself, plus enough for a few dinner guests through the week.

DRINKS

- Fat-free milk, 1 gallon
- Orange juice, ½ gallon
- Other fruit juices such as grape juice, or sports drinks
- Vegetable juice, such as V-8
- Six-pack of beer
- Large pitcher of filtered water

CONDIMENTS (FOR THE DOOR)

- Ketchup
- Barbecue sauce
- Hot sauces, two types: Tabasco and one crazy-named scorcher
- Salsa
- Mustard, three types: golden, brown, and something fancy, such as honey
- Mayonnaise, low-fat (not fat-free)
- Two salad dressings: Italian and blue cheese (low-fat, not fat-free)
- Crushed garlic in a jar
- Maple syrup (reduced-calorie syrup)

THE ADVENTURE SHELF IN THE DOOR (FOR COOKS ONLY)

- Chinese condiments: chili garlic paste, black bean sauce, hoisin sauce, oyster sauce, plum sauce
- Italian condiments: sun-dried tomatoes in oil, cured olives, stuffed green olives, capers
- Latin condiments: marinated jalapeño peppers; salsa; flour tortillas
- Lemon juice
- Lime juice
- Mysterious food jars given to you as holiday presents

OTHER DOOR STUFF

- Butter or soft margarine
- Cheddar cheese, reduced-fat
- Grated Parmesan cheese
- Flax oil (a.k.a. flaxseed oil)

SHELF STUFF

- Plain yogurt, low-fat, 1 quart
- Fruit spreads, two flavors
- Eggs, one dozen
- Sour cream, low-fat, 1 pint
- Applesauce
- Plastic containers (leftovers)
- Pudding cups
- Peanut butter (reduced-fat)
- Chocolate syrup

MEAT DRAWER

Keep chicken breast and ground beef in the refrigerator for 2 days of meals; freeze the leftovers.

- Turkey bacon, 1 pound
- Boneless, skinless chicken breasts
- Ground beef, extra-lean
- Cooked shrimp, small tub
- Sliced lean ham or turkey, ½ pound
- Cheese slices, reduced-fat, ¼ pound
- Cheese block, reduced-fat, ¼ pound

FRUIT DRAWER

Start each week with 15 to 20 servings of fresh fruit on hand.

- Apples, half-dozen
- Oranges, half-dozen
- Summer fruit or berries as available
- Melon: a cantaloupe or one-quarter watermelon

VEGETABLE DRAWER

Stock enough vegetables for a salad and a cooked vegetable for each of the week's home-cooked dinners.

- Lettuces: one head iceberg, one head leaf lettuce such as romaine or premixed greens
- Cucumbers, two
- Tomatoes, three
- Green onions, one bunch
- Celery
- Carrots
- Green pepper
- Four cooking vegetables, such as zucchini, broccoli, eggplant, green beans, Chinese cabbage
- Fresh ginger, small hunk

FREEZER

- Meats for four meals: unbreaded fish fillets, extra-lean steaks, chicken breasts, extra-lean sausage
- Prepared foods for one or two dinners: veggie burgers, 1-pound bag of dumplings (wontons, ravioli, pierogies . . .), low-fat frozen dinners
- Vegetables in 1-pound bags or boxes. Try different types of mixed vegetables, plus chopped broccoli and spinach.
- Coffee. This stores best when frozen.
- Berries. Keep blueberries, strawberries, and other more exotic berries if you like, for fruit shakes or topping for ice cream, pancakes, and more.
- Soft pretzels, one box
- Bagels, half-dozen. The small Lender's variety are fine.
- Whole-wheat bread, one loaf
- Low-fat vanilla ice cream or yogurt
- Whole-grain waffles, low-fat, one box

The advice here was reviewed by Thomas Incledon, M.S., R.D.

For First-Aid and Do-It-Yourself Doctoring
The Protective Medicine Cabinet

You aren't supposed to hurt yourself, muscle man. You aren't supposed to get sick, bruised, sore, strained, sprained, or scratched. But you're a man, and this is the real world and you're supposed to "Be Prepared." Remember? Stock these essentials and extras, and you'll be ready for minor mishaps.

The Usual Stuff

- Instant ice packs
- Elastic wrap in 3-, 4-, and 6-inch widths (all the same length)
- Rubbing alcohol
- Aspirin or ibuprofen for relieving pain and reducing inflammation
- Adhesive tape and gauze
- Antibacterial cream for dressing wounds
- Variety pack of flesh-colored adhesive bandages, such as Band-Aids
- Cotton balls or pads
- Cotton swabs
- List of emergency phone numbers, including your doctor and the ambulance service
- Photo of Meg Ryan smiling to remind you that no matter how bad you hurt, there *are* things worth living for

Tubes and Bottles

- Cortizone brand cream for itches, or calamine lotion
- Antiseptic such as Betadine
- Hydrogen peroxide
- Antifungal cream or liquid
- Sunscreen with at least SPF 15
- Lip balm with at least SPF 8
- Arnica cream or gel for muscle pain or inflammation
- Insect repellent

THE PROTECTIVE MEDICINE CABINET   405

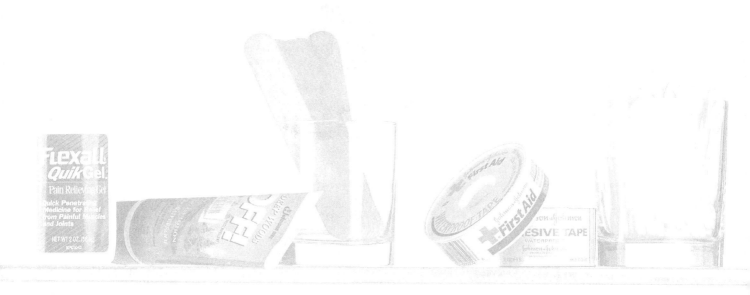

BASIC EQUIPMENT

- Blunt-ended scissors
- Thermometer
- Tweezers
- Tongue depressors for splinting fingers and toes (and depressing tongues)

EXTRAS

- Massager (ones with the motor in the head give the most satisfying vibration)
- Back roller

All products listed and pictured here are approved by James Garrick, M.D., director of the Center for Sports Medicine at Saint Francis Memorial Hospital in San Francisco.

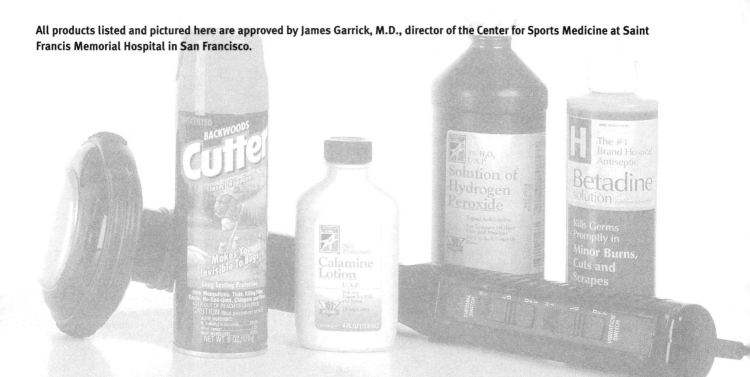

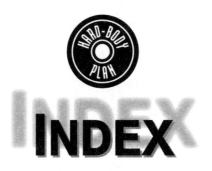

INDEX